Moses
The First Author of Health

by Jay Nelson, OD

SDL Press
110 Executive Center
Hilton Head, South Carolina
29928

SDL Press
110 Executive Center
Hilton Head, South Carolina
29928
fax 1-973-423-1362
1-800-468-2646
1-800-878-2646
ISBN 0 – 9656589 –2 – 9

------------------------------------ **acknowledgements** ------------------------------------

The author is indebted to many people for the publication of this book, including: Rev. Bob Miles; Tracy Knight, OD; Don Seavy, PhD; Dave Gamble, PhD; Cindy O'Brien; Sam Windsor; Dave Lewis; Don Patten; Ron Lowrie; Paul Genung, DDS; & Brent Emery for editing–proof-reading–consultations: Andrew Gause; Donna Pontrelli; & Gina Pontrelli for graphics: Marty Love; & Diane Woods for prayer: Singh Dhillion, PhD; John Weckel, PhD; Richard Nelson, PhD; & Harold Barnett for consultations: Jana Walsh; Victor Esposito; Audrey Williams; Chris Stapleton; & Heather Russell for illustrations: John Stockton; Michael Cunliffe; Jeff Nelson; & Margot Nelson for computers: all faculty/staff at Pacific University, Seattle University, Olympic College and East Bremerton School District for my education: and all the librarians and staff at Kitsap Co. Library for research assistance and reference material.

If I have seen farther, it is only because I have had the shoulders of giants upon which to stand. Dr. Chuck Missler, Dr. J. Vernon McGee and Rev. Chuck Smith teach the Scriptures on radio and tape. William Ludlam, OD, taught vision therapies and eye exercises for patients with special vision needs. Donald Seavy, PhD teaches his biology students more than can ever be expressed in mere words. Bernard Jensen, DC, taught principles of healthy living and proper nutrition. Dr. Ludlam and Dr. Jensen also related how their therapies brought patients results. Thank you all.

Dr. Seavy taught me how to reason as a scientist.

Dr. Ludlam taught his Optometry students:

"If what is taught in a classroom doesn't work in the clinic, then the teaching from books may need to be amended."

Dr. Jensen taught me how to think as a nutritionist; plus, when to search for experts who were willing teachers.
Dr. Ludlam and Dr. Jensen taught me the adaptive nature of the body and the sequential aspect of health problems.

The author helps Dr. Seavy with his sand dollar research. – (right)

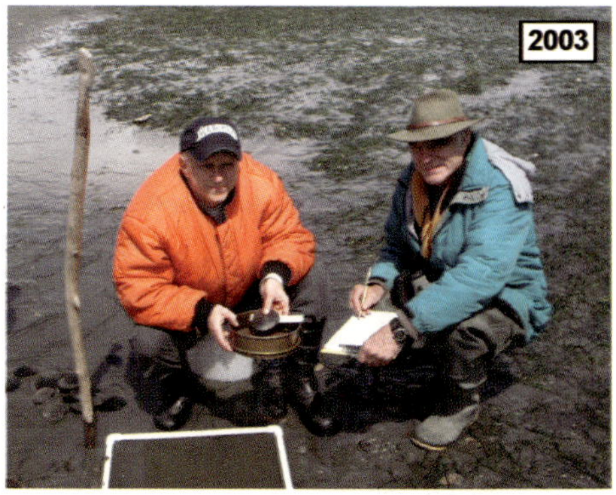

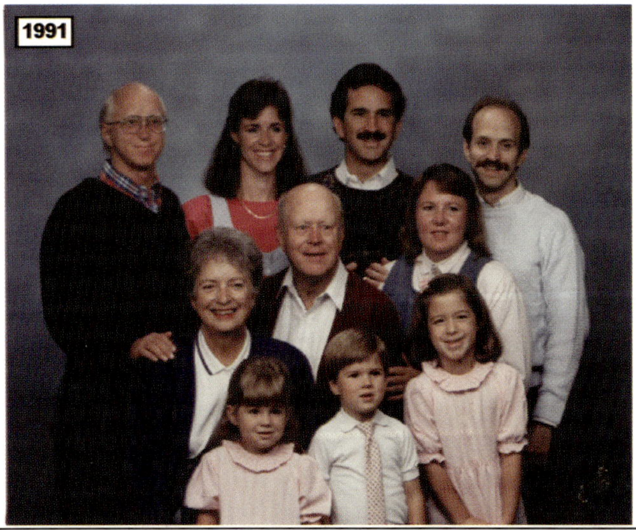

Jay – Margo – Jeff – Jim // Betty – Jorgen – Patti // Lisa – Tyler – Laura

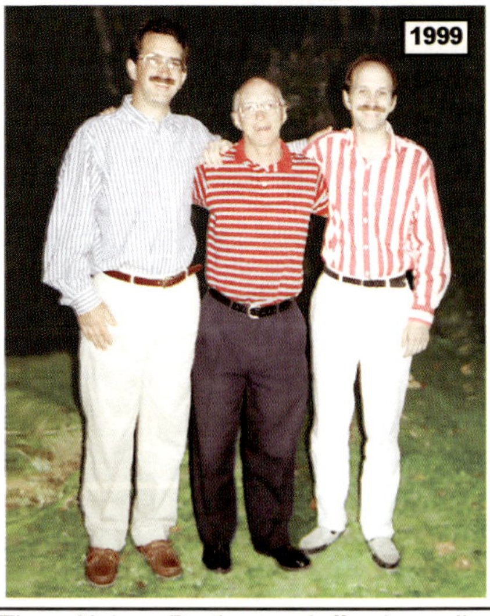

Three Nelson Brothers – Jeff – Jay – Jim

Four Vessels – diagramed

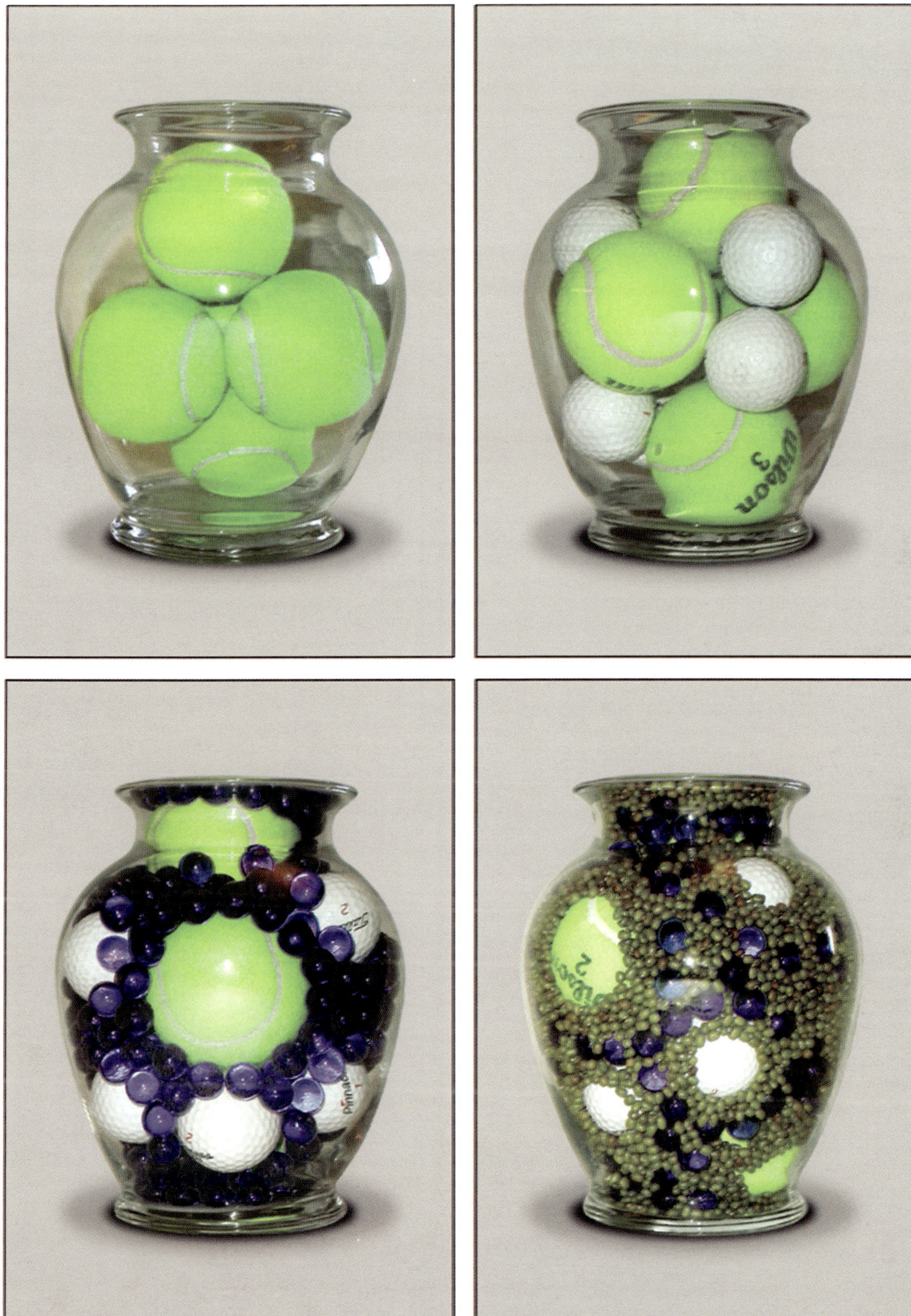

∗ A full vessel allows people to overcome obstacles. Obstacles destroy people with an empty vessel.

(see Ch 2 – pg 39)

This book is dedicated to the memory of:

Sherrill (Polum) McCleary
Linda Higgins
Mary Gates
Janice Kirk
Robin (Ragsdale) Cameron

Bill Riddell
David Kay
Bernard Jensen
Bill Ludlam
Jeffrey Arthur Nelson

My brother, Jeff

I asked my parents for a brother, and
I prayed to God for a brother, and
God blessed me with two brothers.
A brother initially is someone for play,
for fun and for games.
A brother becomes someone
to trust and love.
A brother becomes someone who is
always there for you.
A brother is someone to walk beside
and someone to work beside
and someone to worship beside.
A brother is someone who supports you
when you need it the most.
A brother is someone to learn from and
with whom to share lessons learned.
A brother is someone to confide in and
with whom to share a laugh or a smile.
A brother is someone to give to and then
receive back more than you gave.
A brother becomes your best friend.
A brother is your own flesh and blood.
A brother is a part of who you are.
To lose a brother is to lose a part of self.
My brother, Jeff, is now home with the LORD
in his new room in a heavenly mansion.
My life on Earth will forever be
impoverished without my brother, Jeff.
I have shed my tears.
I have said my good-bye.
But I will never forget my brother, Jeff.

by brother, Jay Nelson
Jeffrey Arthur Nelson – (10-07-1955 to 08-14-2001)

Hugs ...
The Perfect Cure

No movable parts
No periodic checkups
No batteries to wear out
Low energy consumption
No harmful side-effects
No monthly payments
High energy yield
Reduces stress
Inflation proof
Non-polluting
Theft proof
Non-taxable
100% Natural
Fully returnable
Never out-of-style
Approved for all ages
Try it ... hugs are healthy!

Anonymous

Jeff believed in the health value of Hugs.
'Hug everyone you love every day.'
This admonition was read at Jeff's memorial service and is included on Jeff's gravestone.

In Proverbs, Solomon discusses the Spirit of the LORD, who may stick closer than a brother.
JPS Pr 18:24(b) But there is a friend that sticketh closer than a brother.

In the past, I have relied on my brother, Jeff, for wise counsel in everything that I have done. Thank the LORD I still have my brother, Jim, from whom to seek wise counsel. But now, more than ever, I need the Spirit of the LORD to be my best friend, who may become even closer than a brother.

∗ Everyone needs the friendship of a brother, as well as One who may be even closer than a brother.

Persistence

"Nothing in the world can take the place of persistence.
Talent will not; nothing is more common than unsuccessful men with talent.
Genius will not; unrewarded genius is almost a proverb.
Education will not; the world is full of educated derelicts.
Persistence and determination are alone omnipotent."

Calvin Coolidge

30th President of the United States

The quote on 'Persistence' by President Coolidge is not directly related to Moses or the ***Torah***, but it has everything to do with the author's determination to ask questions and to seek answers. (My brother, Jeff, gave me this quote, which is the best description of me that I have ever read.)

Perspective

Torah teacher Chuck Missler, PhD stated;
"Perspective is the most important insight"
– with Persistence any data required to substantiate the proper Perspective can always be obtained.

Geologist Stephen Gould, PhD understood the importance of Perspective when he stated;
"Data does not interpret itself."

Two lawyers often begin with the same data but with opposing Perspectives, and each argues to the court that their Perspective is the only correct one.

To the author, who was inspired by Dr. Missler;
"Persistence and Perspective are two sides of one coin"
– each as necessary as the other to come to the proper understanding of life. The writings of Moses in the ***Torah*** consistently provide fundamental 'timeless' Perspectives.

When anyone reads any document, the reader always begins with a particular mindset or Perspective. Perspectives that readers begin with will influence the meaning and relevance of all ***Torah*** instruction.

What **Moses** might write in a Preface, if he were alive today

I did not authorize this biography of my life, nor the commentary on my writing. After all, I thought the 'Five Scrolls' I wrote ≈3,500 years ago turned out very well, especially considering I used the inspiration of the LORD to guide my writing. These 'Five Scrolls' contained my complete autobiography. I began life in good health. Due to a death decree pronounced against Hebrew male babies, my parents floated me down the Nile in a basket. Pharaoh's daughter found me and hired my mother to nurse me. As a youth, I had a good education and I wore the finest clothes. As a young man, I commanded an army and I was being groomed for a high position in Egyptian government. I was also in position to marry into high society. I had it all, yet I still felt there was something lacking in my life. After I saw an Egyptian abusing a Hebrew, I got very angry and I killed the Egyptian. I guess letting my anger get the best of me was one of my worst faults. When I found out I was being sought for murder, I had to flee to Midian. In Midian, I had time to gather my thoughts, as I tended the sheep of my father-in-law, Jethro. But, I guess I got a little ahead of myself, didn't I, because I couldn't have had a father-in-law without first having a wife. My wife's name was Zipporah. She was a fine woman. It was also in Midian that my two sons were born. My times in Midian were some of the best times of my life. In Midian, I pondered some of life's great questions, such as: How did the world come to be?; Why am I alive?; Does God exist?; and What did I want to do with my life? One day I got some answers, when I saw a bush in the desert burn for the longest time without being consumed. When I went to investigate the burning bush, I met God. At the burning bush, I realized that I needed to go back to Egypt and redeem my Hebrew brethren from their bondage of slavery. However, I felt inadequate for the task; after all, I was only one unarmed man. It was then that God showed me the sign of my staff turning into a snake and then back into a staff. Well, I went back to Egypt with the LORD's prompting and after the Ten Plagues, the Hebrews and I exited Egypt for Midian. On our journey to Midian, the LORD showed us several miracles, including parting the Red Sea. In Midian, I went back to Mt Sinai, where I first met God at the burning bush. On Mt. Sinai, I received the Ten Commandments and I put down a rebellion and I tried to encourage the Hebrews to follow God. I guess you can lead a horse to water, but you can't make him drink, because except for Joshua and Caleb, the Hebrews did not choose to walk with the LORD. After receiving wise counsel from my father-in-law, Jethro, I led the Hebrews for forty years in the wilderness, as I instructed the Hebrews in the ways of the LORD and wrote the ***Torah***. The world can be a wonderful place full of potential and promise, but the world is also full of pitfall, problem and peril. I urged the Hebrews to be wise as a serpent, yet to walk as innocent as a lamb. When I was 120 years old, I still had the good health, good vision, and energy to climb Mt. Pisgah (aka – Nebo) and behold the glorious Promised Land before I died and I again met my LORD. I felt my autobiographical portion of the ***Torah*** as well as the rest of the commandments, ordinances and judgments were very self-explanatory. Everything was clear to me when I wrote it. Before my Scrolls, health was poorly defined. Some people gave little thought as to what was healthy, and they just lived life for the day. Other people that were seeking health and long life came to vastly different conclusions as to what was and what was not appropriate. I wrote the Scrolls to clear up these health questions and teach principles of health that would have broad and lasting applications. Though the Scrolls have been a best seller since they were first published, I now see that many people have misinterpreted and misunderstood the Scrolls. I also see that some people continue to use the Scrolls for their personal gain and self-interests. I suppose a commentary like *Moses, The First Author of Health* will be helpful to many people. By necessity, some of the explanation in this commentary on the Scrolls deals with moderately technical subjects, so a little thinking or reflection on the part of the reader will also be necessary. I hope this commentary on the Scrolls will be well read, will be understood, and will encourage people to wake up to truth, and to the importance of the health issues discussed in the ***Torah***.

ברוך השם אדני	***Baruch HaShem Adonai***,	Blessed be the Name of the LORD,
מ שׁ ה	***Moshe***	**Moses**
(L←R morf werbeH)	(English Transliteration)	(Translation to English)

Hebrew Alphabet and the *Torah* Text

The original Hebrew ***Torah*** text contained only consonants: no vowels, those were understood. Period-like (.) 'word dividers' separated words. Most Hebrew words begin as a three-consonant root, although some consonants may be dropped and/or other consonants added to make new words. In ≈900 AD, Masorites first added vowels to the ***Torah*** and the ***Tanakh***, producing the Masoretic text. Today, all ***Torah*** Scrolls add vowels beneath, beside or above consonants to pronounce words. (see pg 42-43) In ≈1,200 AD, chapters and, in ≈1,600 AD, verses were added to the ***Torah***, ***Tanakh*** and New Testament. English-transliterated Hebrew words constructed from a 'three-consonant' root with vowels added, such as ***Torah***, are used in Strong's Concordance and are printed in **bold**-*italic* type in this book. Hebrew words and sentences read from right to left (←), while English reads from left to right (→). Translation of a foreign word involves producing its accurate meaning in a domestic language. Transliteration makes a new domestic language word that 'sounds' like the foreign language word. ***Manna*** is a transliterated word that is taken from Hebrew 'without rendering its proper meaning'. The Hebrew word מצה is transliterated ***matzah*** or ***matsah*** and is translated 'unleavened bread'. Translation of words, phrases and sentences often involves both translation and interpretation. Context, idiom and genre are critical to translation, while a paraphrase includes much interpretation.

∗ **No *Torah* verse can mean today what Moses did not intend it to mean when he wrote it.**

∗ **As in all literature: one goal of *Torah* study is to identify the Perspective of the author, Moses, and grasp the mindset of a typical 15th century BC reader, such as Caleb or Joshua.**

In ≈250 BC, the ***Tanakh*** (Hebrew Bible), including the ***Torah***, was first translated into Greek as the *Septuagint*. The ***Torah*** was originally written on animal skins (parchment) and rolled into a 'Scroll'.

#	consonant	print	final (see pg 12)	number	keyboard	*transliteration*	Hebrew consonants as they sound in English.				
01	Aleph	א		1	(a)	ʼ	{glottal stop}	{silent}	space for vowel sound		as in ***'eretz***
02	Bet	ב		2	(b)	*b*	as in boy	(***Negeb*** – ***Negev***)	or	*v*	as in vow
03	Gimel	ג		3	(g)	*g*	as in gold	[גפר]	also	*g*	as in ***gopher***
04	Dalet	ד		4	(d)	*d*	as in dog	[דבש]	also		as in ***devash***
05	He(h)	ה		5	(h)	*h*	as in hat	[יהוה]	also	*h*	as in ***Yahweh***
06	Vav	ו		6	(v)	*v*	as in van	(or HolemVav as the vowel 'o' – as in ***tov***)	or	*w*	as in ***YHWH***
07	Zayin	ז		7	(z)	*z*	as in zip		also		as in ***zayith***
08	CHet	ח		8	(x)	*ch*	as in ***lechem***	{guttural}	also		as in ***CHanukkah***
09	Tet	ט		9	(u)	*t*	as in top	[טוב]	also		as in ***tov***
10	Yod	י		10	(y)	*y*	as in ***Yahweh***	[יהוה]	also		as in ***Yisrael***
11	Kap(h)	כ	ך	20	(k – ;)	*kh*	as in ***Tanakh***	{ka-au-f}	or	*k*	as in kettle
12	Lamed	ל		30	(l)	*l*	as in law	[***'Elohiym***]	also		as in ***chalav***
13	Mem	מ	ם	40	(m – ,)	*m*	as in ***manna***	[מן]	also		as in Mariners
14	Nun	נ	ן	50	(n –])	*n*	as in Noah	[נח]	a.k.a. – ***Noe***		a.k.a. – ***Noach***
15	Samek	ס		60	(c)	*s*	as in song	[סדם]	also	*s*	as in ***Sodom***
16	Ayin	ע		70	(i)	ʻ	{glottal stop}	[עץ] { ***'ets*** }	silent	'h'	as in honest
17	Pe(h)	פ	ף	80	(p – [ )	*p*	as in pot	{***gopher***	or	*ph*	as in photo}
18	Tsade	צ	ץ	90	(j – /)	*tz*	as in ***tzadik*** and	***matzah***	or	*ts*	as in ***tsara'at***
19	Qop(h)	ק		100	(q)	*q*	as in ***qibbutz***	{ca-oh-f}	also	*k*	as in ***kibbutz***
20	Res(h)	ר		200	(r)	*r*	as in run	[תורה]	(***Torah***		Tav-HolemVav-Res-He)
21	Sin | Shin	שׂ | שׁ		300	(s | w)	*s*	as in sip	{***Moshe***	or	*sh*	as in ship }
22	Tav (Taw)	ת		400	(t)	*t*	as in tin and	***Torah***	or	*th*	as in thin

An ordinary Hebrew 'three-consonant' root can be modified to: make a new word; or change a word's tense or its part of speech. The three-letter 'root' HeYodHe, ***hyh***, (היה) is the verb '*to be*'. A variation of ***hyh*** is the Tetragrammaton (יהוה) ***YHWH***, meaning '*I Am That I Am*', or more literally, '*He Is That He Is'*, which is the covenant name of God, and is transliterated to English as ***Yahweh***. To respect the LORD, the Tetragrammaton is often transliterated by Rabbis without vowels as ***Y-hw-h***, so no one can speak the Tetragrammaton in disrespect and violate the 3rd Commandment. (Ex 20:7)

∗ **In *Torah* study precise meanings of words may be crucial to the proper understanding of the text.**

Shofar and *Yad* and Ashkenazic *Torah* Scroll

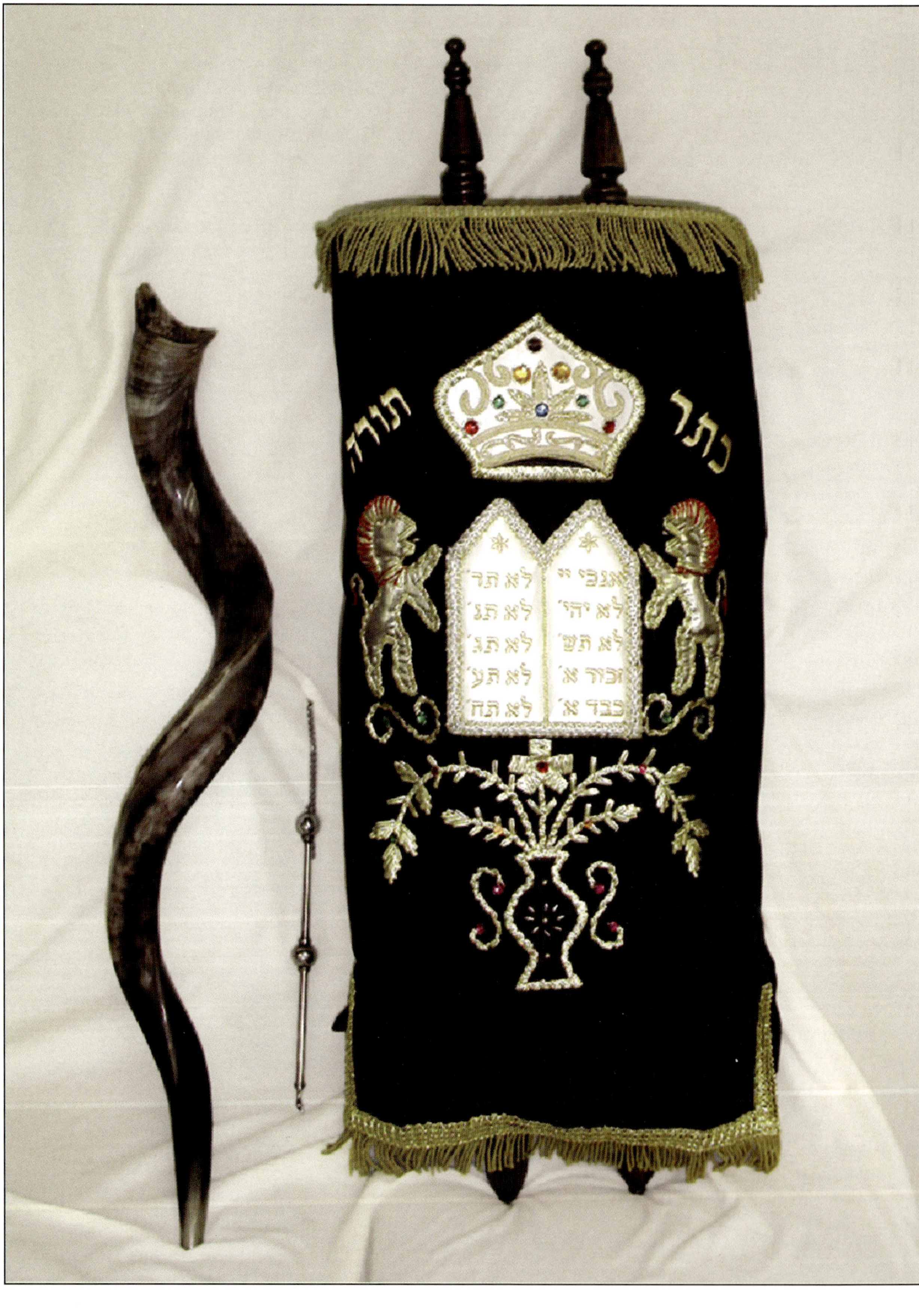

Worship the LORD

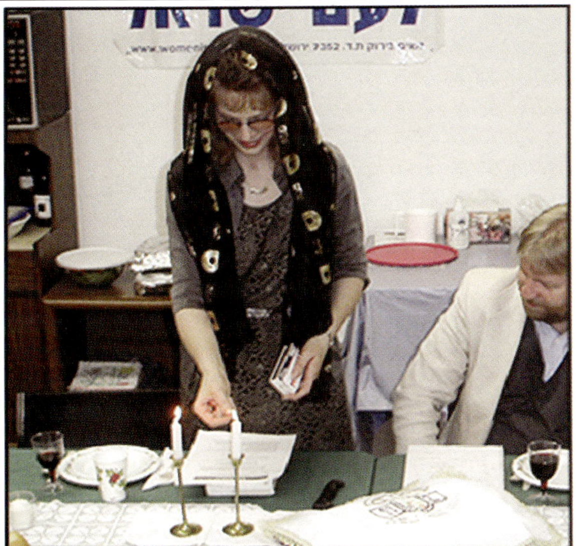
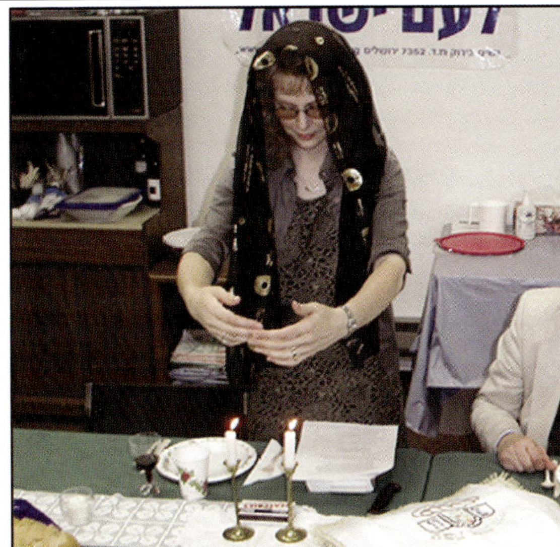

Susan Richardson lights the ***Shabbat*** candles and prays the prescribed blessing to the LORD.

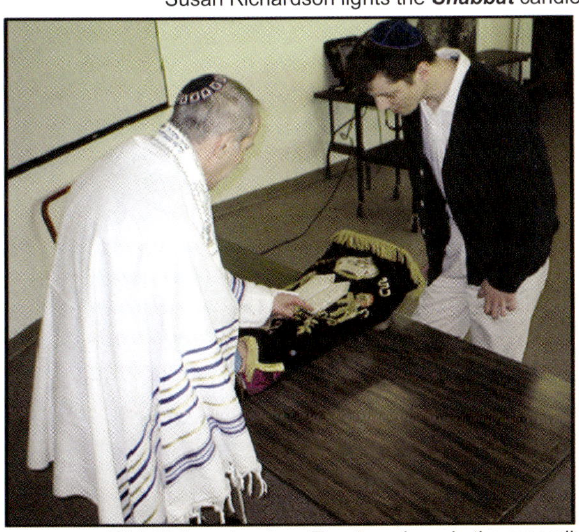
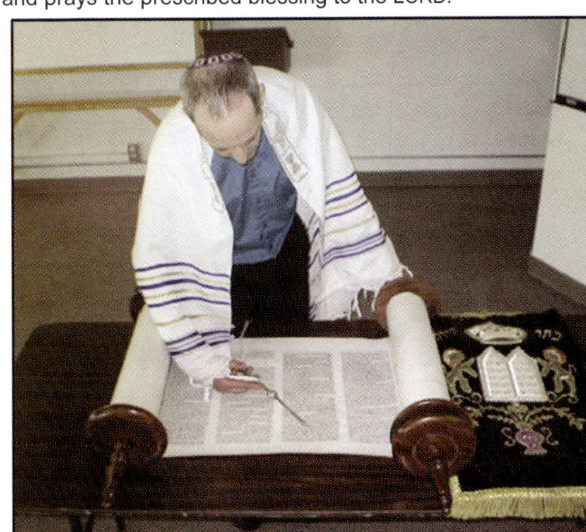

Rick Hebron teaches ***Torah*** and reads the prescribed weekly portion of the ***Torah*** during ***Shabbat*** ser

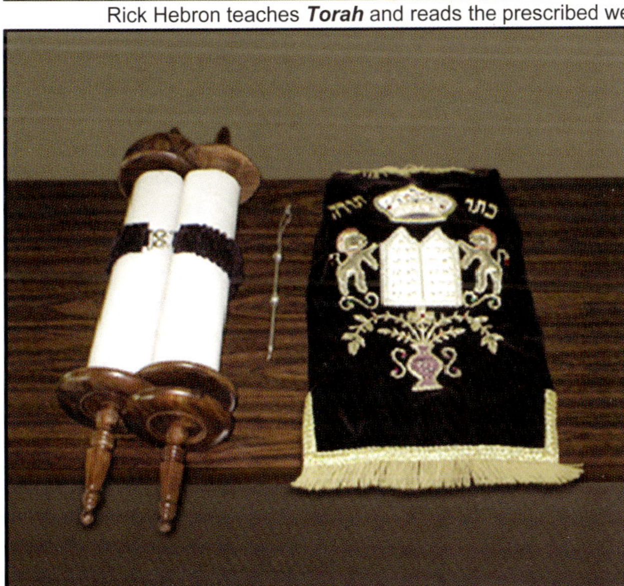

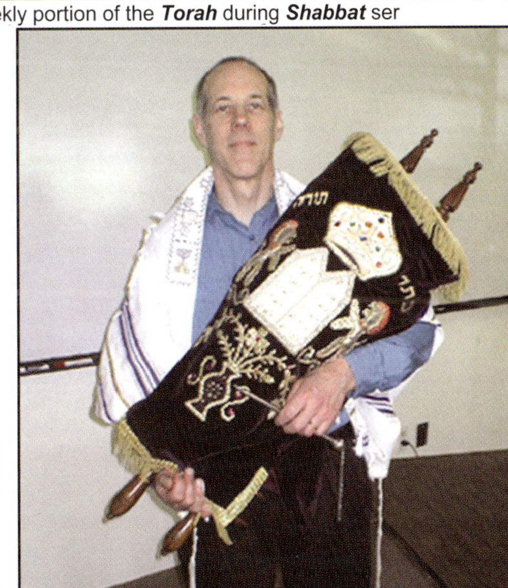

∗ The 5 Scrolls of Moses are powerful unto salvation for anyone who practices *Torah*.

Sephardic *Torah* Scroll – closed and opened

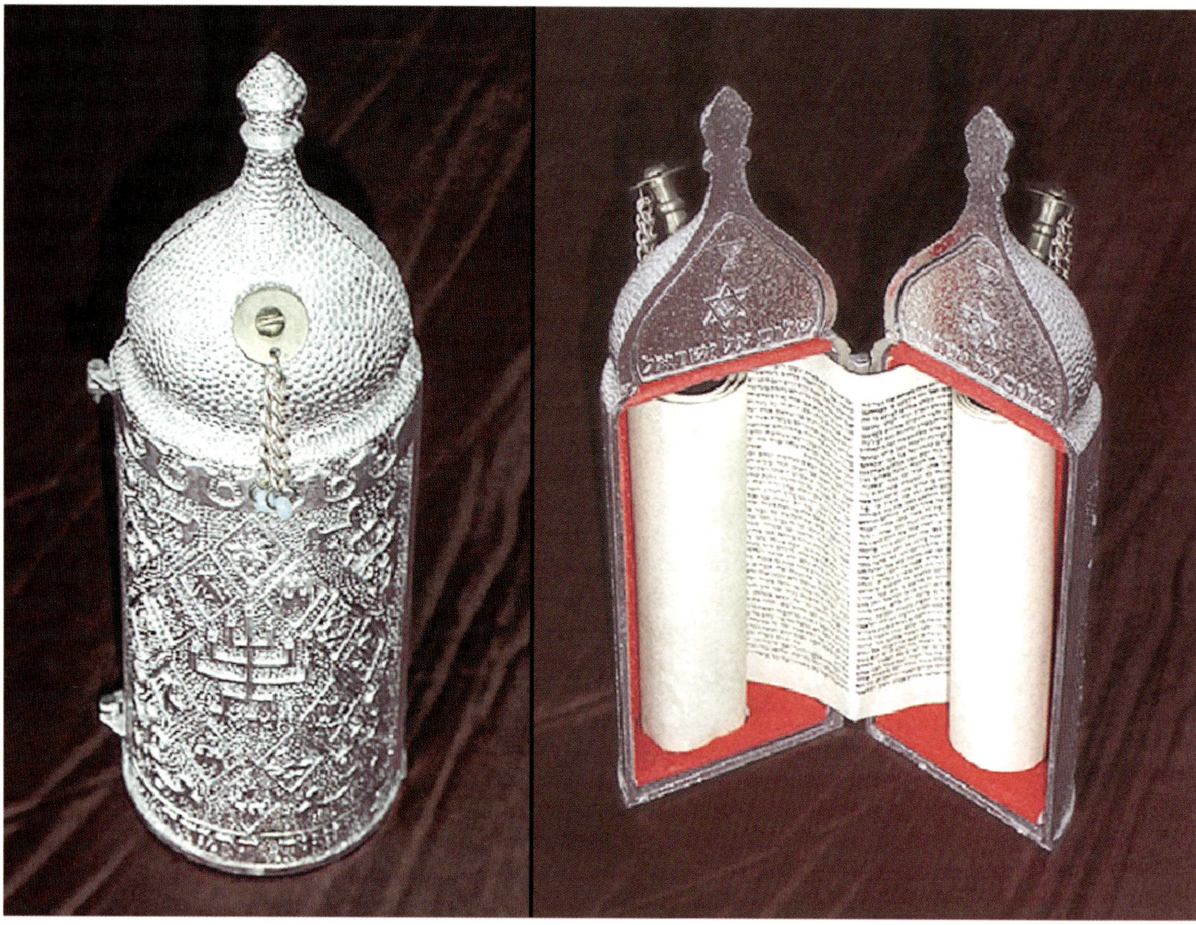

Shofar and ***Yad*** and ***Torah***

A ***Torah*** Scroll contains the five scrolls of Moses, which are sewn together as one ***Torah*** Scroll. Each of Moses' five books that make up the ***Torah*** Scroll is known by a Hebrew name that is based on a word used early in the Scroll and by a Greco-Latin name that is based on the theme of the Scroll.

Hebrew name	word (<u>underlined</u>)	Greco-Latin	theme – meaning
Beresheit	when [God] <u>began</u>	Genesis	in the beginning
Shemot	the <u>names</u> of the sons of Israel	Exodus	leaving from Egypt
Vayikra	the LORD <u>called</u> unto Moses	Leviticus	laws of Levitical Priests
Bamidbar	in the <u>wilderness</u>	Numbers	numbering of the Hebrews
Devarim	these are the <u>words</u>	Deuteronomy	second giving of the Law

A ***Torah*** Scroll is rolled onto two wooden poles called the ***Ets CHaim*** — meaning 'Tree(s) of Life'. ***Yad*** is a silver pointer that is used, while reading the ***Torah***, to keep place without touching the Scroll. ***Shofar*** is a Ram's horn that is used to call the Hebrews to assembly and announce specified events. Just like a bugle, various prescribed sequences of ***Shofar*** articulations convey specific messages. ***Keter*** (כתר) is the 'crown' or covering for the ***Torah*** (תורה) Scroll, which is made of cloth or metal. *Ashkenazic* (European) Jews use cloth for the ***keter*** (כתר), while *Sephardic* (Spanish) Jews use metal.

Shabbat – Sabbath

The 7th day of the week, Saturday, is the Hebrew ***Shabbat*** – a day to worship the LORD and to rest. All Hebrew days begin at sunset. ***Shabbat*** begins at sunset Friday and continues till sunset Saturday.

JPS Gen 1:5(b) And there was evening and there was morning, one day.

Shabbat is the 1st of 8 'Holy Convocations' (sacred assemblies) prescribed by Moses in the ***Torah***. Every ***Shabbat*** service begins with a woman lighting two candles and praying a prescribed blessing. During ***Shabbat*** service, the entire ***Torah*** (Gen 1:1 to Deut 34:12) is read in one year in weekly portions.

POSSIBLE LOCATIONS OF EDEN

MAP 20

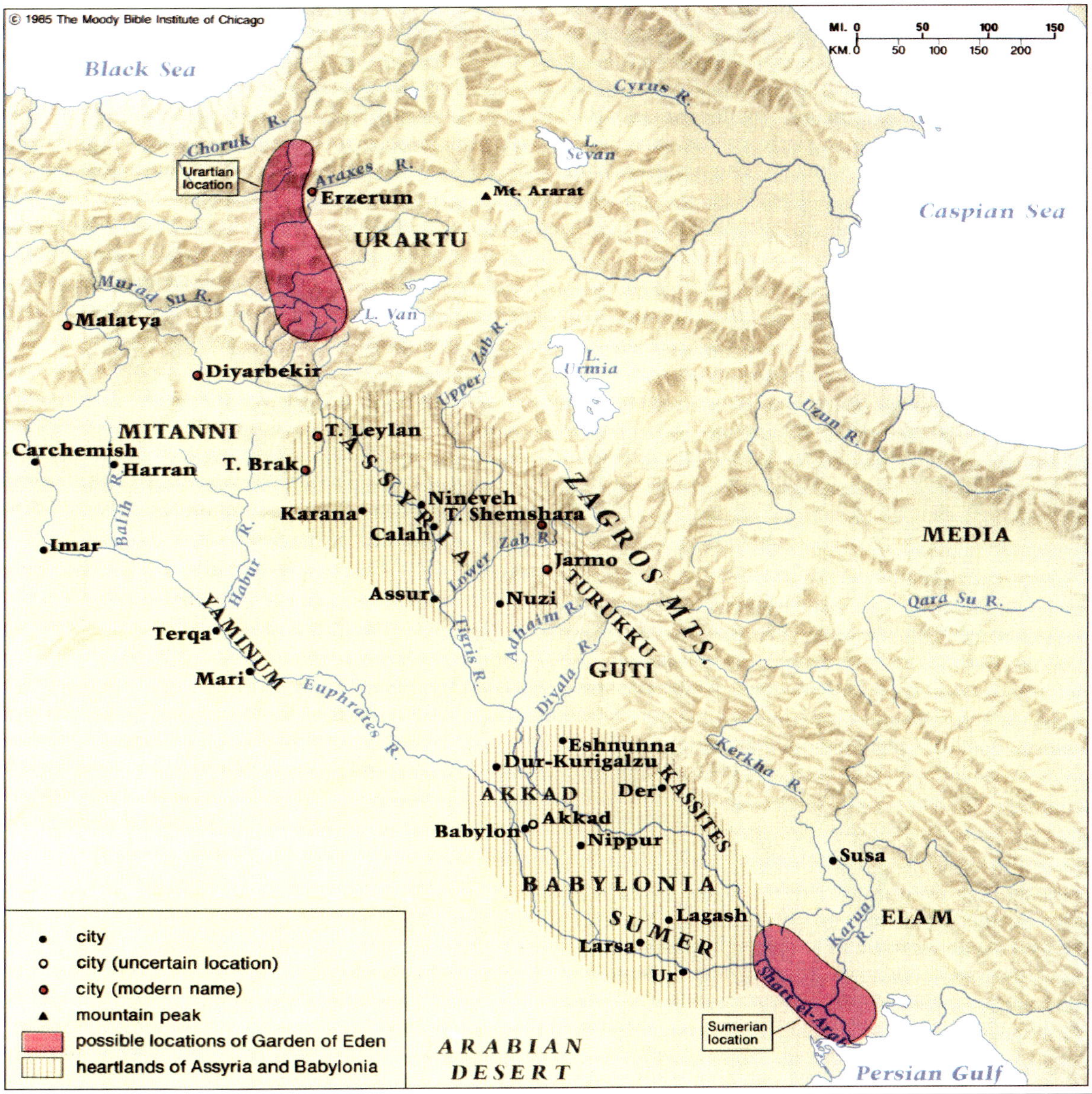

The Moody Atlas of Bible Lands

The Physical Geography of the Holy Land

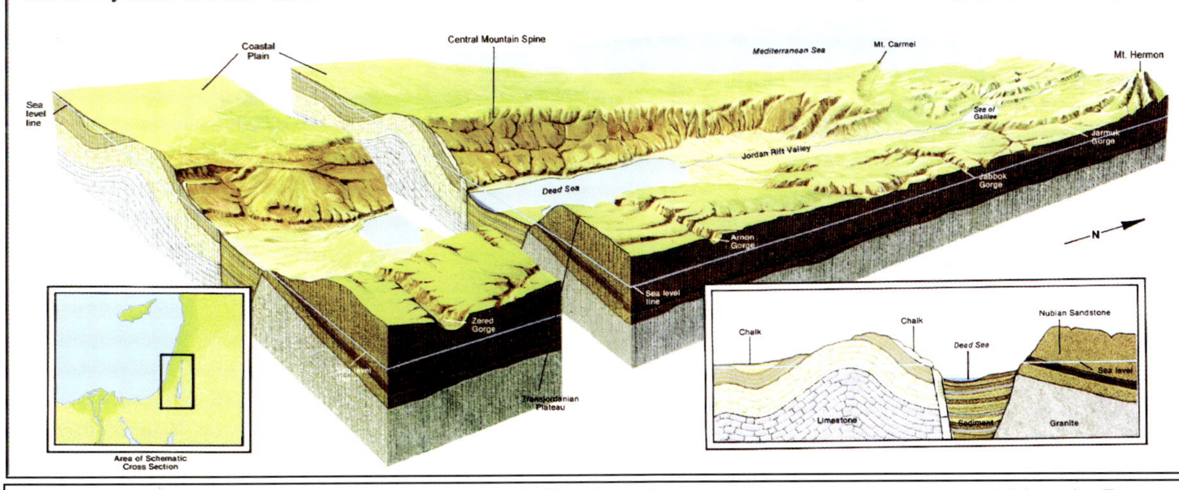

All maps in this book from Moody Atlas of Bible Lands and used with permission of Moody Press.

– Part of Map 16 – plus – Map 25 – Israel's Exodus from Egypt to Canaan – pt 1

Important Places in Egypt from Map 16

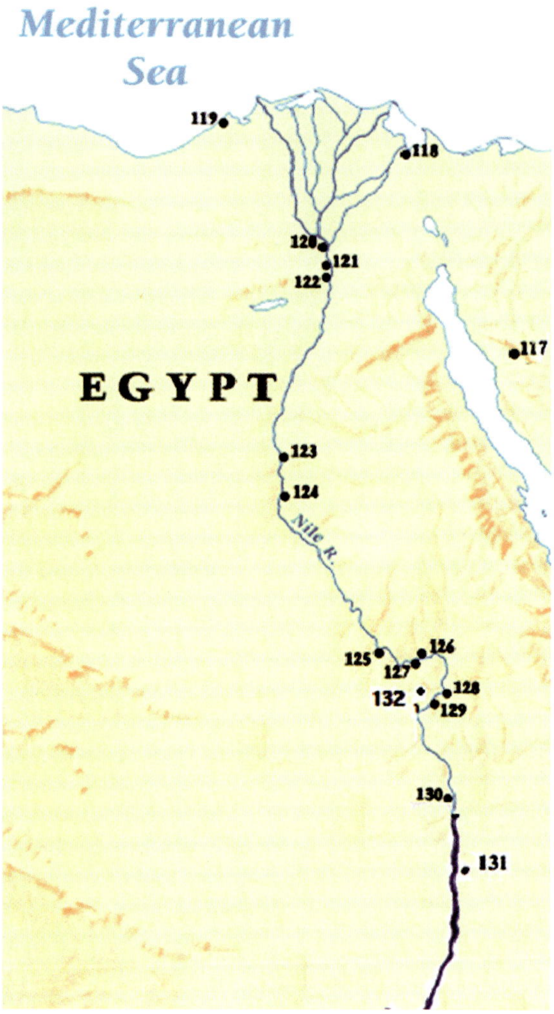

118 Tanis (and nearby Rameses) Likely were built by Hebrews.
119 Alexandria Library City built by Alexander the Great.
In ≈250 BC, the *Septuagint* was translated in Alexandria.
120 Giza Great Pyramid & Tomb of Pharaoh Cheops
121 Saqqara Step Pyramid built by Imhotep (aka - Joseph?)
122 Memphis (aka – Noph) Early capital of ancient Egypt.
128 Karnak Temples to Egyptian gods and Pharaohs
129 Luxor (aka – Thebes) Later capital of ancient Egypt.
Central trade city that joined Upper Egypt to Lower Egypt.
(aka – City of the Living) (aka – City of 100 Entrances)
132 City of the Dead and Valley of the Kings, where vandalized tombs of many Pharaohs, such as Ramses II, were found.
In Nov 1922, Howard Carter found King Tut's intact tomb here.
131 Aswan Sehel Island and site of the Famine Stela

Israel's Exodus from Egypt to Canaan

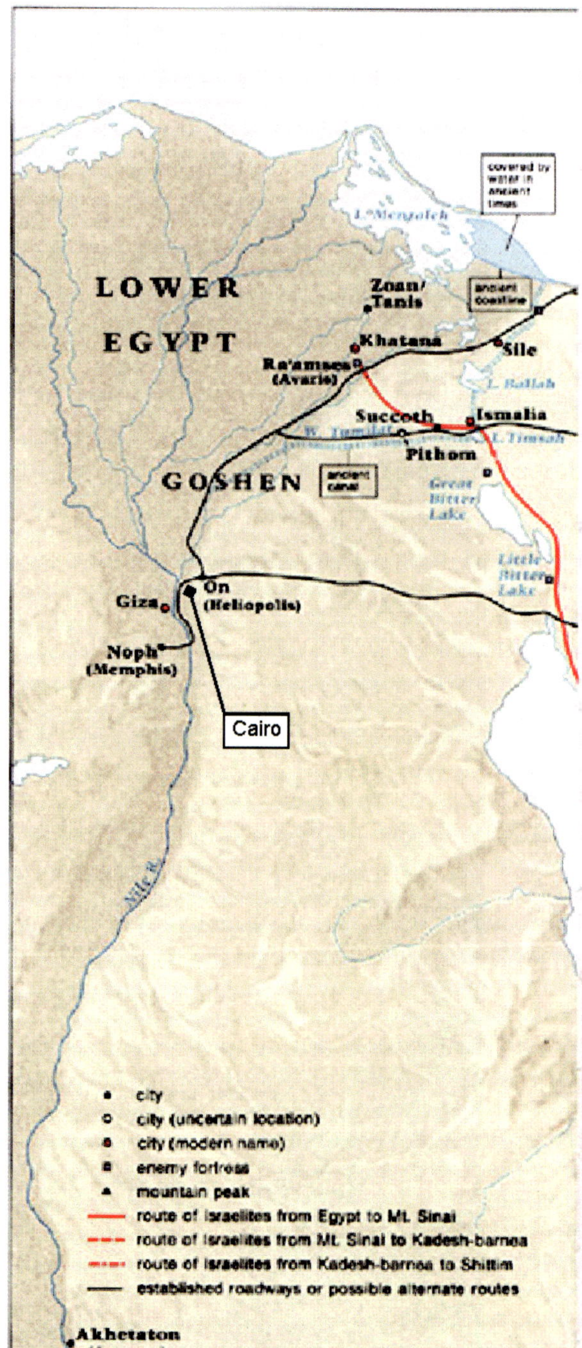

Since all Hebrew words begin with a consonant, words whose first sound is a vowel always begin with an ***aleph*** or ***ayin*** that have no sound. The Hebrew word ארץ is translated 'land' and may be transliterated ***'eretz***. (עץ is translated 'tree' & is transliterated ***'ets*** & is usually written as ***ets.***) {When 5 Hebrew letters are used at the end of a word, their shape is changed to their 'final form'.} For ease/simplicity, apostrophes that may begin Hebrew transliterated words are usually dropped. The 'Promised Land' that the Lord God promised to the Hebrews is often written as – ***Eretz*** Israel.

Map 25 – Israel's Exodus from Egypt to Canaan – pt 2

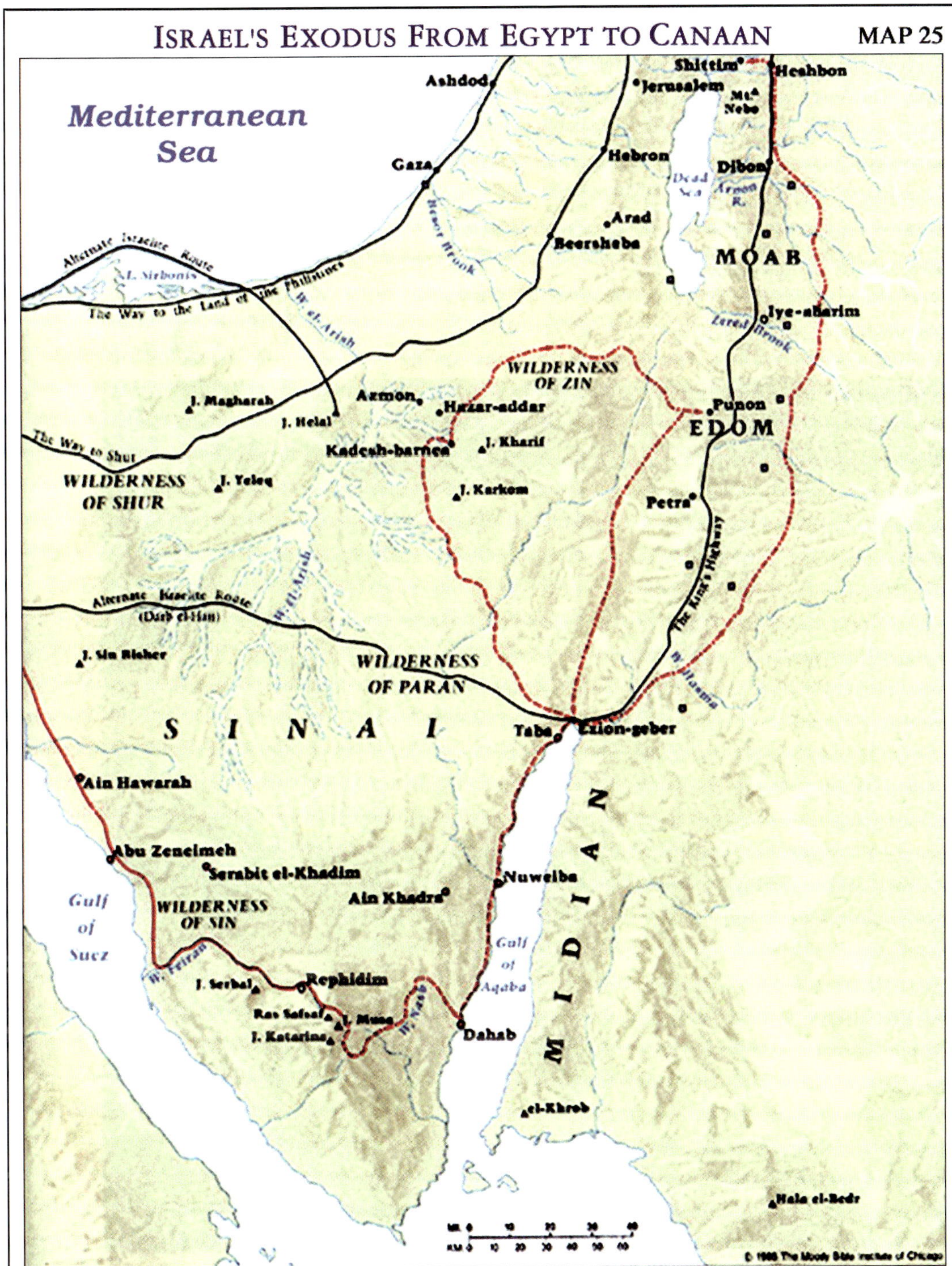

The principle of 'First Mention' or 'First Usage'

The principle of 'first mention' in ***Torah*** study indicates the pattern of defining a term in the verse in which the term is first used, to assist in the proper interpretation of the same term later in Scripture. Leaven (***seor***) is first used as the item to be removed from the Hebrew household prior to the Exodus.

JPS Ex 12:15 ... howbeit the first day ye shall put away leaven (***seor***) out of your houses;

Leaven has a primary meaning: yeast. (Leaven is killed in bread baking before it destroys the dough.) But in Scripture, leaven also has a consistent secondary spiritual meaning – a 'principle of evil'. (pg 180)

The Step Pyramid

The pyramid at Saqqara (aka – Sakkara) is called the Step Pyramid because of the 6 'step-like' platforms or levels rising from the desert sand. Egyptians considered Pharaohs to be like living gods. Pharaohs were buried in large elevated tombs called *mastabas* that were often made of mud bricks. The Step Pyramid was the first *mastaba* to be built of stone, to better withstand time and weather. The Step Pyramid at Saqqara is considered by many Egyptian scholars to be Egypt's oldest Pyramid. The Step Pyramid was built for Pharaoh Djoser (aka – Zoser) by Djoser's chief chancellor, Imhotep. The Step Pyramid after several additions is 460 ft long (E to W) – 387 ft wide (N to S) – and 197 ft high. The Step Pyramid has 35-45 ft high outer stone walls and 13 false doors, but only one true entrance. The Step Pyramid complex may have been patterned after Memphis, Egypt's capital city at that time. Ron Wyatt and Mary Nell Wyatt discuss that Imhotep was very likely an Egyptian name for Joseph. Imhotep means 'the voice or mouth of *Im*'. No Egyptian god was named '*Im*'; but later, Moses at the burning was given 'I AM" as the name of God. Did Joseph also use "I AM' as the name of his God? Imhotep (aka - Joseph?) may have meant 'the voice or mouth of the I AM God'. Joseph had an Egyptian name 'Zaphnath-paaneah', which may be translated 'the God lives or the God speaks'. (Gen 41:45) Imhotep is mentioned several times on inscriptions including the description of him a 'self-made man', which indicates he was likely not from Egyptian royalty. Pharaoh's advisers were often close relatives. One writing calls Imhotep priest of Heliopolis (aka – On). Since Joseph married Asenath, the daughter of Potipherah, the priest of On, it is likely that Joseph inherited the position of the priest of On from his father-in-law. (Gen 41:45) Other references discuss Imhotep as a wise man, physician and architect. These Egyptian references to Imhotep are similar to the titles and attributes of Joseph in the ***Torah***. Writing on rock: the 'Famine Stela' on Sehel Island, below the 1st cataract on the Nile, names Imhotep as Djoser's chancellor, but several earlier inscriptions about Djoser on clay jars don't mention Imhotep. This suggests that Imhotep was not Djoser's chancellor early in Djoser's reign, which fits the account in Genesis of Joseph becoming chancellor of Egypt after interpreting pharaoh's dreams. (Gen 41:40) The Famine Stela is a copy made in ≈400 BC by Egyptian priests of a document that Pharaoh Djoser wrote ≈1,200^{+} yrs earlier. The Famine Stela writing includes: references to a dream of Pharaoh Djoser that Imhotep interpreted; to a time of Plenty; to 7 years of Famine; and the collection of grain as tax. Inscriptions on the Famine Stela are legendary, elevate Imhotep to Pharaoh-like royalty and made him appear mythical rather than historical, especially since no gravesite for Imhotep has ever been found. No Egyptian grave fits with Joseph's bones being carried out of Egypt during the Exodus. (Ex 13:19) In 1926 AD, when excavations at the Step Pyramid found Imhotep's name as 'Builder' and 'Sculptor' and Imhotep's titles 'Chancellor of the King of Lower Egypt', 'Chief under the King, and 'Administrator of the Great Palace' on the base of a statue of Djoser, then scholars recognized Imhotep as historical. Biblical and Egyptian evidence that Imhotep and Joseph were the same person is only circumstantial. The South Tomb area has 11 large pits that could have been used to store grain and distribute grain. The author believes that Joseph (Imhotep) used the large South Tomb pits as one grain storage site. In ≈1670 BC, prior to the 7 years of Plenty, is when the author estimates the 11 Grain Pits were built. In 1928 AD, when the Step Pyramid complex was excavated, a few kernels of grain were found in the pits in the South(ern) Tomb area. Many Egyptologists suggest that this grain was part of a burial ritual. Ahmed Fakhry in his book *The Pyramids* discussed that the pits may not have been burial chambers.

> "The name 'Southern Tomb' was applied when this building was discovered in 1928, but we have no proof that it [the pit(s)] was ever intended to be a tomb, or was used as such." – [R28] pg 31

From the only entrance, the long corridor leading to a courtyard was ideal for exchanging gold or silver to buy grain; allowing a buyer to obtain grain from the large pits and discretely leave via the only exit. Foreign payments for grain during the 7 years of Famine likely added significantly to Egypt's wealth. The Step Pyramid at Saqqara was ideally located near farmlands of the Nile delta to collect grains and it was near enough to Egypt's capital city, Memphis, to easily transfer the wealth to Pharaoh's palaces. Gold from the sale of grain was likely used by the Egyptians for afterlife artifacts in Pharaoh's tombs. King Tut's tomb was one of 20 tombs built for Egypt's Pharaoh's. None of the artifacts from the other 19 tombs has been recovered. As the author understands Egyptian mineralogical resources, there weren't enough gold mines in Egypt to furnish similar artifacts for the other 19 tombs. The author theorizes: Much of the gold for the Pharaoh's tombs likely came from grain sales during the Famine. Please e-mail information/comments to Moses5in1Torah@msn.com

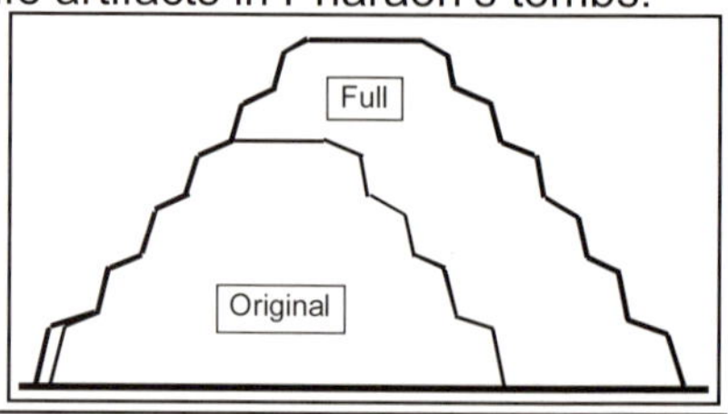

The South Tomb of the Step Pyramid was ideally designed for grain strorage during the 7 year Famine. Imhotep was likely an Egyptian name for Joseph, who oversaw the collection and sale of Egypt's grain.

Step Pyramid Complex and Grain Pits – plus – Famine Stela

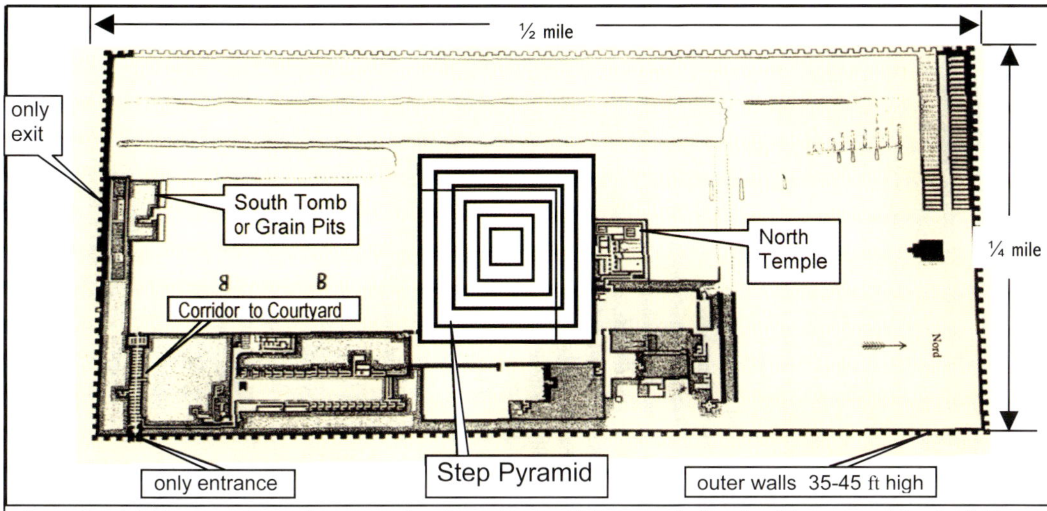

Step Pyramid of Djoser
460 ft long
387 ft wide
197 ft high
– original Pyramid dimensions
≈400 ft long
≈300 ft wide
≈175 ft high
within light rectangle on the SE corner –

Joseph might have enlarged the existing Step Pyramid for use during the '7 years of Plenty' & '7 years of Famine'.

Step Pyramid

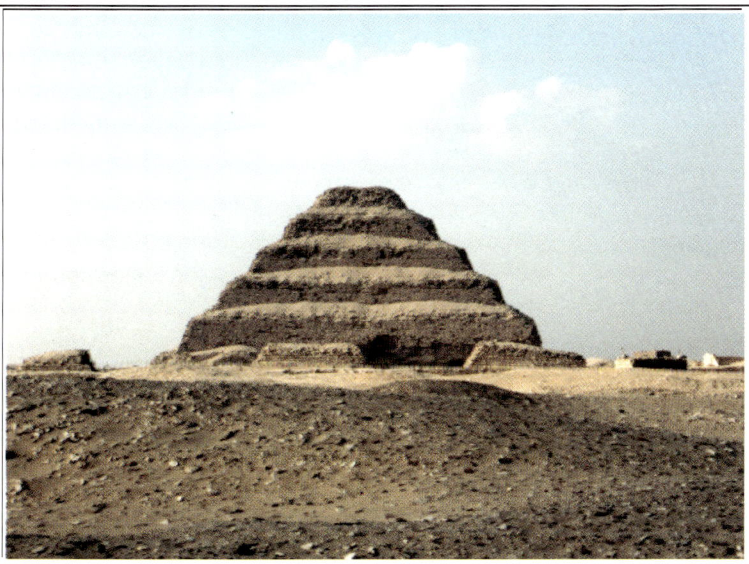

Famine Stela

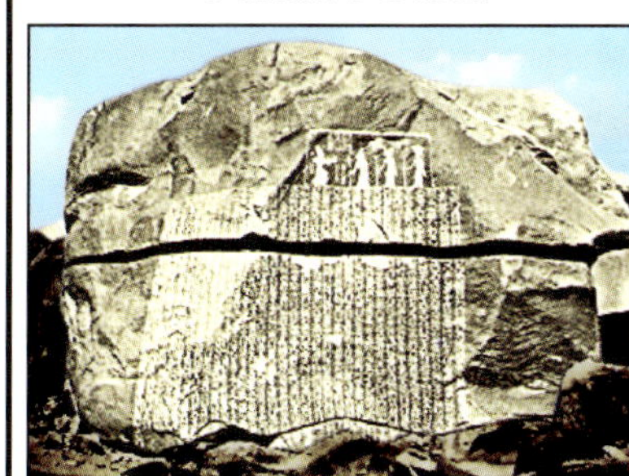

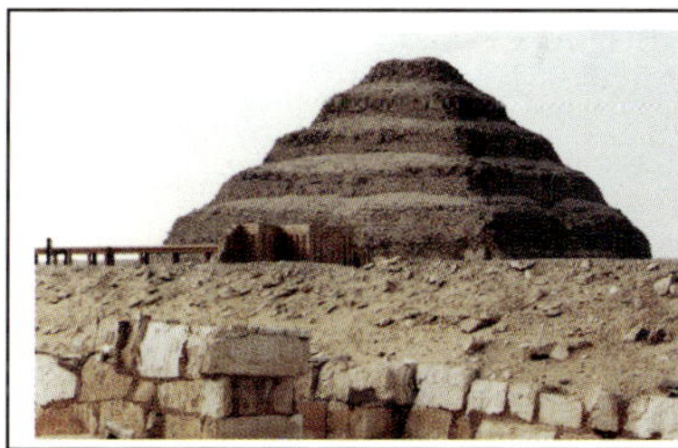

'Grain Pits'

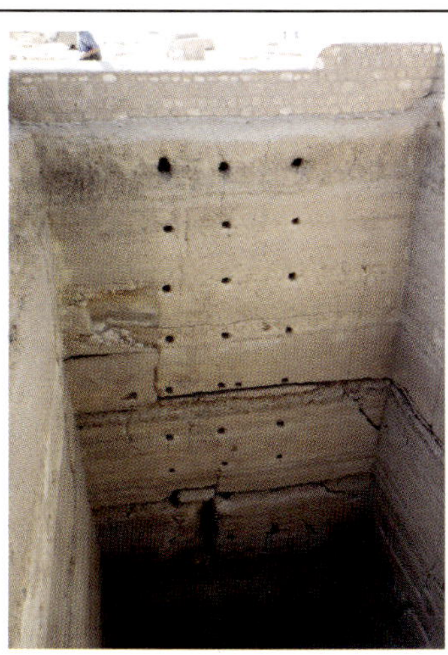

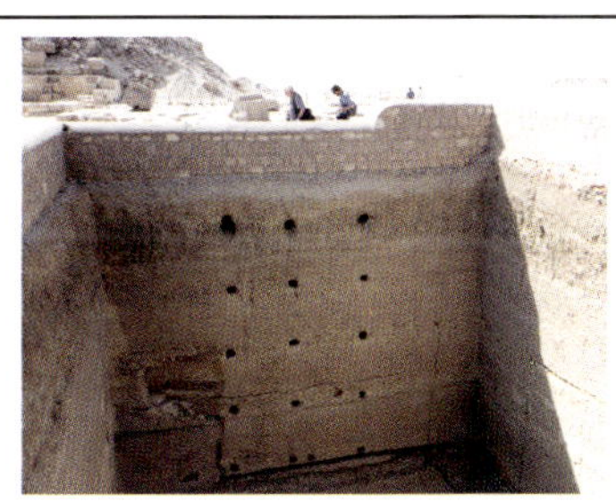

These photos suggest the strong likelihood that the pits were used by Joseph to store grain during the '7 years of Plenty'; and, during the '7 years of Famine' in Canaan, to sell the grain for gold and silver.

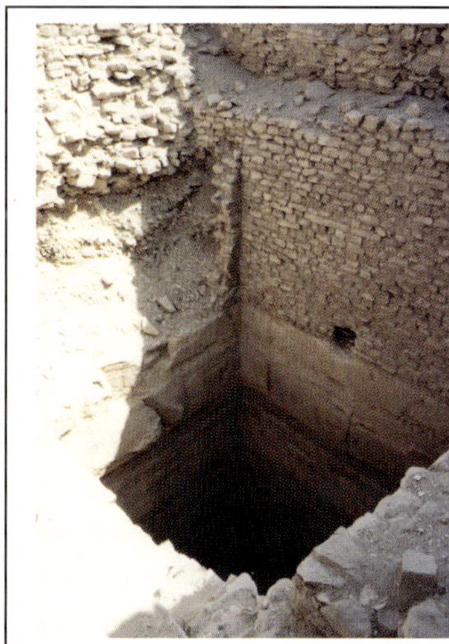

photos of Step Pyramid and of Grain Pits used with permission of Wyatt Museum – www.wyattmuseum.com

MOSES
THE FIRST AUTHOR OF HEALTH
by Jay Nelson, OD

Table of Contents

www.Mosesfirst.com **www.Mosesfirst.org** **www.Mosesfirst.net**
internet website
Moses5in1Torah@msn.com e-mail address

MOSES THE FIRST AUTHOR OF HEALTH
Table of Charts, Drawings, Illustrations, Images, Maps, Photos, Pictures & Sketches

Modern Translations and the *Torah*

Torah study may be influenced by the translation of the Scripture being read, since every translation also involves some interpretation. The 1917 AD, Jewish Publication Society (JPS) and the 1611 AD, King James Version (KJV) often render the most accurate translations of the ***Torah***. Phraseology and meanings of words may change with time, so common language for King James translators may be antiquated today. In Exodus 30:18, 'laver of brass' (KJV) is understood more easily as 'brass washing bowl' in the 1978 AD New International Version (NIV). In Leviticus 14:14, blood on the great toe may not seem relevant today unless it is understood that the 'great toe' is often symbolic of a person's walk with the LORD or their manner of life, while the 'blood of sacrifice' signifies forgiveness for their sins. Henry Morris, PhD has good advice for every ***Torah*** student.

"When the plain sense of Scripture makes common sense, seek no other sense."

Modern ***Torah*** translations attempt to update verbiage, add clarity and make reading easier but they may do so at the expense of adding interpretation to translation, which may unintentionally reduce the literal meaning of the ***Torah*** passage and/or subtly alter the original intent of a passage.

In Genesis 7:1 the verb ***bow*** is translated 'come' into the Ark (KJV) (NKJV) (JPS), but 'go' (NIV). ***Bow*** could be translated as either 'come' or 'go', but the 'feeling' of the language is lost in the NIV. The requirement for Noah to enter the Ark is the same, however the original Hebrew language intended to convey an invitation to 'come' and experience intimacy with the LORD inside the Ark. This is similar to a parent calling a child to 'come' into the house for a special time with the family, rather than harshly telling a child to 'go' into the house as discipline, when the family is outside.

Idiom is a unique word syntax or figure of speech used to express a concept, thought or idea. In the phrase, Jay Nelson is 'a man who wears many hats', hats could refer to items worn on the head, or hats could be used metaphorically to represent the diverse activities a person performs. Either meaning could be true, as the author owns many hats to wear and performs many tasks. Moses often intended a double meaning for a ***Torah*** verse, as 'crossing over the Jordan' refers to both physically possessing the 'Promised Land', and spiritually entering the 'presence of the LORD'. 'Groves' in the ***Torah*** are often places of spiritual defilement, where Canaanites worshipped idols.

Genre is the literary form, such as poetry, narrative or legal document, each of which must be interpreted differently. The genre of a ***Torah*** passage may be an area of honest scholarly debate. For the ***Torah*** to be understood as Moses intended Caleb to read it, it must be interpreted literally! If the genre is poetry, such as the song of Moses, it often contains much metaphorical language. If the genre is historical narrative of people, places or events, then descriptive terms may be used. If the genre is a legal contract, such as the Ten Commandments or the Abrahamic Covenant, then the proper interpretation of the passage may depend upon the technical meaning of words/phrases. In the first several chapters of Genesis there is a mixture of narrative with the use of metaphors, which causes considerable difficulty in determining the proper genre and the proper interpretation.

∗ No ***Torah*** passage can have a primary meaning today that is inconsistent with what Moses intended it to mean when he wrote it, or what a 15th century BC reader, such as Caleb, would be expected to understand when he read it. There may be secondary meanings to the ***Torah*** today that are also legitimate, but these must never negate, confuse or contradict the primary meaning.

The proper mindset is needed to understand a play by Shakespeare or a fantasy by Tolkien or a Sherlock Holmes mystery or a narrative/story by Mark Twain or the ***Torah*** by Moses. To deny that Moses wrote the ***Torah***, you may as well also deny that Mark Twain wrote Huckleberry Finn.

The ***Mizpah*** involves the final parting of Jacob and his father-in-law, Laban. (Gen 31:49-50)

KJV Gen 31:49 And Mizpah: for he [Laban] said, (b) The LORD watch between me and thee when we are absent one from another. vs 50 If thou shalt afflict my daughters, or if thou shalt take other wives beside my daughters, no man is with us; see God is witness between me and thee.

Today, the ***Mizpah*** is often <u>isolated</u> and <u>misused</u> on jewelry as indicating a 'term of affection' between lovers or close friends who are planning to part-company for a short while. (Gen 31:49b) In reality, the relationship between Jacob and Laban was one of distrust and deceit for 20 years. Jacob married uncle Laban's two daughters, Leah and Rachel. The ***Mizpah*** is really a covenant that Laban imposes on Jacob to be faithful to his wives, even when Laban is not present to insist upon their fair treatment. Laban called upon God as a witness to insure Jacob's fidelity. (Gen 31:50) The ***Mizpah*** as a 'term of affection' is the ultimate misuse of the ***Torah***, which happens by isolating a verse from its context, to impute a meaning that Moses never originally intended the text to mean.
∗ Every ***Torah*** verse must be read and studied within its context, to understand its proper meaning!

Genre, idiom, context and circumstance are always important in understanding the ***Torah*** properly.

Hebrew Myth and Hebrew History

Early chapters of Genesis include stories of: the Creation of the Universe; the Garden of Eden; Adam and Eve eating the 'forbidden fruit'; Cain murdering Abel; Methuselah living to 969 years; the LORD destroying the wicked world with a Flood; Noah building an Ark to preserve man and animals; Nimrod building the Tower of Babel; Sodom and Gomorrah being destroyed with fire and brimstone; and Abraham and his son, Isaac, traveling to Mt. Moriah, where Abraham planned to sacrifice Isaac, before God intervened and provided a substitutionary lamb for sacrifice – this is *THE **Ahkidah*** event. Charlton Heston stated in his video series *Charlton Heston Presents the Bible* that these stories from Genesis were told and retold around campfires and in Hebrew dwellings throughout many centuries. During the Exodus, Moses wrote the ***Torah*** and recorded these stories plus other events as history.

Elizabeth Vandiver, PhD in her lecture series *Classical Mythology* (parts I & II) defines myth. [R1]

"Myths are traditional stories a society tells itself that encode or represent the world-view, beliefs, principles, and often fears of that society." [R1A] (Greek 'myth' usually concerns stories about their 'gods'.)

"Legend refers to traditional stories rooted in historical fact, describing the (greatly exaggerated) adventures of people who actually lived, such as Robin Hood or George Washington." [R1B]

(The famous story of George Washington chopping down a cherry tree as a youth, and then 'not telling a lie' is likely 'legend'.)

Fable or Folktale refers to stories that are primarily entertaining, often concerning clever fictional characters and often involving animals, such as: Goldilocks and the Three Bears, or Santa Claus. [R1]

∗ Almost by definition, a myth is a cultural story whose historicity cannot otherwise be documented. Myth may also be used collectively for any story containing elements of myth, legend and/or fable. ** Myths were common in all ancient societies. Myths were especially important in cultures prior to the development of written language (pre-literate civilization), as the only means of preserving what was perceived by that society as truth, and passing the truth from one generation to the next generation. Myths may have several functions, including religious (ritual), scientific, historical and psychological. Myths help a culture make sense of the confusing world or justify an existing social system. [R2] Myths may not have well-defined origins since myths often begin orally rather than by being written. Almost by definition for the culture that develops a myth, the myth is spoken of as accurate history; while people from outside cultures, when they hear the same story, often discuss the story as fiction. (Moses was literate from his upbringing in Pharaoh's palace, Levitical Priests learned literacy during the Exodus, while Hebrew literacy became common between the Babylonian exile and the Greek occupation {≈550 to 250 BC}.)

Abraham and Isaac were historical figures. The story of *THE **Ahkidah*** – the binding of Isaac on Mt. Moriah – is central to the development of Hebrew culture. In all the Canaanite cultures surrounding the Hebrews, child/infant sacrifice to some 'god' was a ritual that was part of their religious practice. *THE **Ahkidah*** <u>prevented</u> the Hebrews from practicing child/infant sacrifice. [R7] *THE **Ahkidah*** story was told as Hebrew history from one generation to the next to teach a healthy reverence for life. [R7] Abraham and Sarah were the first Hebrews. The story of Sarah's miraculous conception of Isaac by Abraham in her old age teaches the healthy principle of trusting in the LORD to fulfill His promises.

In 620 AD, Mohammed, the prophet of Islam, had a 'night journey' vision where he was mystically transported from Mecca in Arabia to the Hebrew (Jewish) Temple Mount on Mt. Moriah in Jerusalem and then he ascended to heaven. This vision is important to Islam, as there are no other stories that Mohammed ever visited Israel. This legendary story along with the story that Ishmael, the father of the Arabs, rather than Isaac, went with Abraham to Mt. Moriah to be offered are the only stories upon which Islam bases its claim that Mt. Moriah and the Temple Mount area are sacred sites to Islam. [R6]

Definite elements of myth are apparent within several stories from the early chapters of Genesis. ∗ The question is: Are these stories from Genesis 'only myth' or are they also accurate human history? Today, many people consider Noah's story of a great Flood and an Ark as pure myth, yet a version of this story is common in many civilizations worldwide and many cultures treat the story as history. Noah had three sons: Ham was the father of Egyptian culture, Shem was the father of Hebrew culture and Japheth was the father of Greek culture. (Gen 10) These three cultures had very different myths. Egyptian myth and culture was preoccupied with death, as indicated by the pyramids, mummies and afterlife artifacts. Rah, the sun god, was supreme. Egyptian myth viewed Rah as traveling in a chariot each morning from the east to bring on day. Egypt's ruler, Pharaoh, was treated as a Rah-like god. Greek myth and culture often concerned sex and power struggles between their gods and goddesses. Hebrew myth and culture focused on one God, ***Yahweh***, who was viewed as the omnipotent Creator. Hebrew myth was preoccupied with life and teaching practical lessons about their one God, ***Yahweh***. ∗ Greek and Egyptian myths are now seen as fable, while Hebrew myth is often recognized as history.

∗ How the early chapters of Genesis are interpreted influences how all Scripture is interpreted.

Garden Eden | ***Torah*** **Timeline – Eden to the Flood** | pg 1 | 300 yrs ≈ 1 computer inch

4,000 BC · 3,700 BC · 3,400 BC · 3,100 BC · 2,800 BC · 2,500 BC · 2,300

|----- 3,988 to 3,058 BC -------------------- Adam ------------| 930 yrs

Enoch - 3,366 to 3,001 BC |--------- Enoch ------| 365 yrs — **Flood 2,332 BC**

Methuselah - 3,301 to 2332 BC |--------------------- Methuselah -- 969 yrs ----------------------

Noah - 2,930 to 1,980 BC = 950 yrs |-- Noah -- 600 yrs (preFlood) ----------------------------------

Shem -2,430 to 1,830 BC ≈ 100 (preFlood) + 500 (postFlood) ⟶ Shem ⟵ 99 yrs (preFlood) |-------------------------

Chronology of the *Torah*

Date	Event – age at death	Scripture
≈ 4,000 BC	Creation of the Earth that is fit for habitation	Gen ch 1
≈ 4,000 BC	Adam and Eve inhabit the Garden of Eden	Gen ch 2-3
≈ 4,000 BC	1st sin by mankind – God's curse on the Earth (*Gen 3:17)	Gen ch 3
	Cain – 1st son – murders younger righteous brother, Abel	Gen 4:1-9
	Adam, 1st man, from birth to death – age 930	Gen 5:1-5
	Enoch was translated prior to the Flood – age 365	Gen 5:21-24
	Methuselah died the year of (prior to) the Flood – age 969	Gen 5:25-27
ca 2332 BC	Noah survived the Flood for 370 days in the Ark	Gen ch 6-9
	Noah lived 350 yrs after the Flood – (600 + 350) = age 950	Gen ch 6-9
ca 2320 BC	Noah and sons Shem, Ham & Japheth begin postFlood life	Gen 10:1-29
	Japheth is the father of the Europeans and Asians	Gen 10:2-5
	Ham is the father of the Africans and Canaanites	Gen 10:6-20
	Shem father of Hebrews and Arabs – (100 + 500) = age 600	Gen ch 10-11
ca 2206 BC	Earth was divided during the days of Peleg	Gen 10:25
ca 2080 BC	Nimrod builds Tower of Babel – language is confused	Gen 11:1-9
ca 2000 BC	Abraham, Sarah, Terah and Lot leave Ur of the Chaldees	Gen 12:1
ca 1880-1450 BC	Hebrews dwell in Egypt-Canaan for 430 years – Gen 15:13 to	Ex 12:40-41
ca 1870 BC	Sodom and Gomorrah destroyed by 'fire and brimstone'	Gen ch 19
ca 1874-1872 BC	Abraham visits Melchizedek - King of Salem and Priest of God	Gen 14:18-20
ca 1835 BC	Abraham and Isaac – the ***Ahkidah*** on Mt. Moriah	Gen ch 22
ca 1791 BC	Abraham buried with Sarah in Cave of Machpelah – age 175	Gen 25:7-10
ca 1686 BC	Isaac dies in Canaan-buried in Cave of Machpelah – age 180	Gen 35:29
ca 1641 BC	Jacob dies in Egypt - buried in Cave of Machpelah – age 147	Gen ch 49-50
ca 1667-1660 BC	Joseph rules in Egypt during '7 years of Plenty' – 30 yrs -	Gen 41:40-47
ca 1660 BC	'Great Famine lasting 7 years' comes upon Egypt & Canaan	Gen 41:54
ca 1658 BC	Jacob heads 70 Hebrews living in Egypt after2 yrs of Famine	Gen ch 46
1530 BC	Moses – adrift in the Nile – raised in Pharaoh's court	Ex 2:1-10
ca 1490 BC	Moses kills an Egyptian and flees to Midian	Ex 2:11-15
ca 1490 BC	Moses marries Zipporah – Jethro's daughter –40 yrs -	Ex 2:15-21
	Moses finds the LORD at the 'burning bush' on Mt. Sinai	Ex ch 3
1450 BC	Moses delivers 10 Plagues against Egypt –80 yrs -	Ex ch 5-12
1450 BC	Passover – Exodus – and crossing of the Red Sea	Ex ch 12-14
ca 1449 BC	Hebrews came to the bitter waters of Marah	Ex 15: 22-24
	Hebrews camp at the Oasis of Elim with 12 wells	Ex 15:27
	Moses strikes the rock to provide water at Rephidim	Ex 17:1-7
	Hebrews defeat the Amalekites in battle at Rephidim	Ex 17:8-16
	Jethro visits Moses and the Hebrews at Rephidim	Ex ch 18
	Moses receives the Ten Commandments on Mt. Sinai	Ex ch 20
ca 1449-1448 BC	Moses directs Tabernacle and Ark of Covenant to be built	Ex ch 26-40
	Moses institutes Levitical Priesthood and worship of the LORD	Lev ch 1-27
	Joshua and Caleb lead 12 spies into the Promised Land	Num ch 13
	Korah's rebellion during 40 years of 'wilderness wandering'	Num ch 15
ca 1430 BC	Moses strikes the rock twice to bring water at Kadesh	Num ch 20
ca 1425 BC	Hebrews defeat the Amorites and Bashanites in battles	Num ch 21
ca 1420 BC	Balaam and Balak entice Hebrew sin at the Plains of Moab	Num ch 22-23
ca 1415-1410 BC	Moses recounts the Law to the Hebrews – ≈115-120 yrs -	Deut ch 1-33
1410 BC	Moses climbs Mt. Pisgah – views Promised Land – age 120	Deut ch 34
ca 1409 BC	Joshua leads the Hebrews across the Jordan	Josh 3:14-17
ca 1409 BC	Joshua leads the Hebrews to defeat Jericho	Josh ch 6
ca 1408 BC	Joshua leads the Hebrews in the Long Day battle	Josh ch 10
ca 1403 BC	Joshua conquers most of the Promised Land – age 110	Josh 24:29

The ***Torah*** TimeLine dates are all based on assuming 1,450 BC for the Passover/Exodus and then calculating the lives of the Patriarchs based on Abraham's 430 years promise. (Gen 15:3)

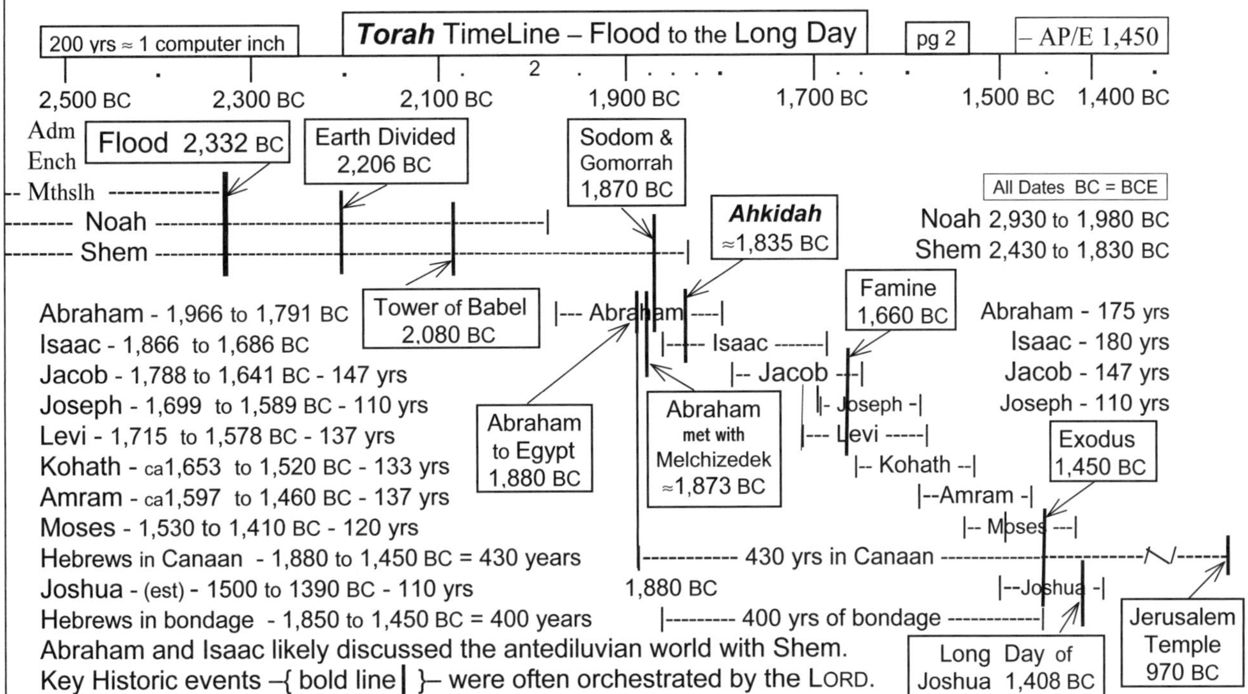

	T - Noah lived 350 yrs after the Flood	– age 950	
2430 to 1830 BC	T - Shem lived ≈500 yrs after the Flood	– age 600	
AP - 1880 BC	AP-TC 1880 to 1450 BC = 430 yrs - Hebrew bondage in Canaan/Egypt		Ex ch 1
2080 BC	Ham begat Cush – Cush begat Nimrod – Nimrod built Tower of Babel		Gen 10:6-8
ca 1891 BC	T - Abraham leaves Haran when he was	– age 75-	Gen 12:4
1880 BC	T - Abraham is given '430 years Promise' ****	– age 86-	Gen 15:13
ca 1880 BC	E - Abraham goes to Egypt – Sarah takes Hagar as handmaid		Gen 16
1880 BC	T - Ishmael is born to Abraham by Hagar	– age 86-	Gen 16:16
1866 BC	T - Isaac was born when Abraham was 100 years old		Gen 21:5
ca 1835 BC	E - ***Ahkidah*** when Isaac was ≈ age 30 – Abraham was ≈ age 130-		Gen 22
1826 BC	T - Isaac marries Rebecca – age 40 – {Jacob & Esau born later}		Gen 25:20
1686 BC	T - Isaac died (before Joseph is sold to Egyptian slavery)	– age 180	Gen 35:28
ca 1658 BC	T - Jacob came to Egypt – 2 years into the Famine – age 130-		Gen 47:9
1658 to 1641 BC	CT- Jacob spend 17 years in Egypt before he died	– age 147	Gen 47:28
1703 BC	T - Joseph, the 11th son of Jacob, is born by Rachel		Gen 30:24
ca 1690 BC	T - Isaac dies before Joseph is sold into Egyptian slavery		Gen 35:28
1686 BC	T - Joseph is sold into Egyptian slavery	– age 17-	Gen ch 37
1673 BC	T - Joseph is prime minister 12 yrs after coming to Egypt	– age 30-	Gen 41:46
1660 BC	T - Great Famine begins		
ca 1658 BC	T - 7 yrs of Plenty plus 2 years of Famine – Jacob to Egypt	– age 39-	Gen 45:6
ca 1658 BC	C - Joseph lives ≈65 years after Jacob comes to Egypt		
1593 BC	T - Joseph dies in Egypt	– age 110	Gen 50:26
ca 1 658 BC	T - 70 Israelites went to Egypt – a multitude left Egypt in the Exodus		Gen 46:27
ca 1715 to 1578	E - Levi is born a few years before Joseph	– age 137	Gen 29:34
ca 1653 to 1520	E - Kohath born about when Joseph dies	– age 133	Ex 6:16
ca 1597 to 1460	E - Amram – father of Aaron, Miriam and Moses	– age 137	Ex 6:18
1530 to 1410 BC	TC – Moses' life 40–40–40 is calculated from Passover	– age 120	Gen 34:7
ca 1500 to 1390	E - Joshua took Promised Land 7+ yrs after Moses died	– age 110	Josh 24:29
970 BC	T - The Jerusalem Temple was begun 480 years after the Exodus.		1 Kings 6:1

dates/ data AP - Assumed Passover 1,450 BC T - ***Torah–Tanakh*** C - calculated E - estimated

All dates in the ***Torah*** TimeLine are based on the assumed 1,450 BC Passover/Exodus date and are likely accurate to within 2 years, due to Hebrew chronicling of any part of a year as a full year. A 1,450 BC, Passover/Exodus date requires that the Jerusalem Temple was begun in 970 BC, which is consistent with later records for when Solomon began Temple construction. (1 Kings 6:1)

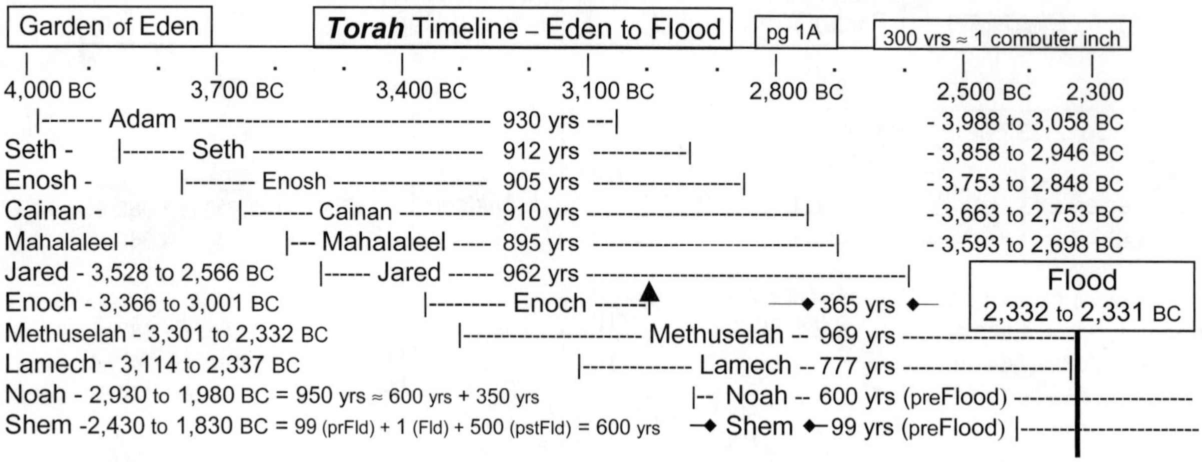

3,988 BC	T – Adam was created by the LORD from 'dust of the Earth'		Gen 1:26 - Gen 2:19
3,858 BC	T – Adam was 130 yrs when his 3rd son, Seth, was born	– age 903	Gen 5:1-5
3,753 BC	T – Seth was 105 yrs when Enosh was born {Seth lived till}	– age 912	Gen 5:6-8
3,663 BC	T – Enosh was 90 yrs when Cainan was born	– age 905	Gen 5:9-11
3,593 BC	T – Cainan was 70 yrs when Mahalealeel was born	– age 910	Gen 5:12-14
3,528 BC	T – Mahalealeel was 65 when Jared was born	– age 895	Gen 5:15-17
3,366 BC	T – Jared was 162 yrs when Enoch was born	– age 962	Gen 5:18-20
3,301 BC	T – Enoch was 65 yrs when Methuselah was born	– age 365	Gen 5:21-24
3,001 BC	T —— Enoch walked with the LORD and was taken to heaven without		dieing! --------
3,114 BC	T – Methuselah was 187 yrs when Lamech was born	– age 969	Gen 5:25-27
2,332 BC	T —— Methuselah died in the same year as the Flood but prior to the		Flood! --------
2,930 BC	T – Lamech was 182 yrs when Noah was born	– age 777	Gen 5:28-31
2,430 BC	T – Noah was 500 yrs after which Shem, Ham & Japheth were born		Gen 5:32
Gen 10-11	TE – Shem ≈99 yrs before Flood & 1 yr during Flood & ≈500 yrs after		Flood = 600 yrs

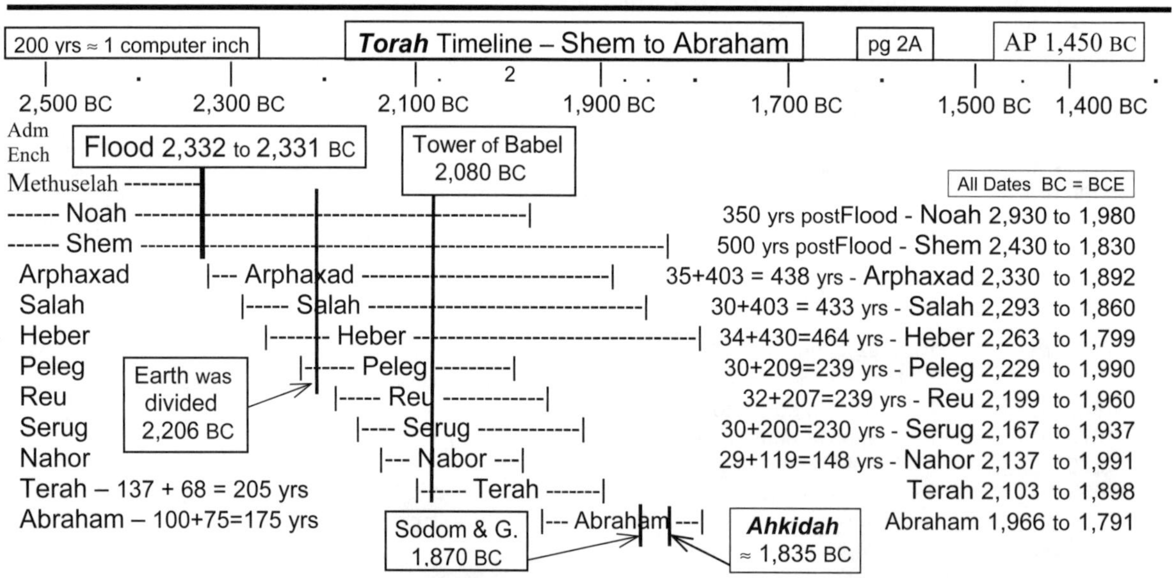

2,430 BC	T - Shem was 100 yrs when Arphaxad was born	– age 600	Gen 11:10-11
2,330 BC	T - Arphaxad was 35 yrs when Salah was born	– age 438	Gen 11:12-13
2,293 BC	T - Salah was 30 yrs when Heber (Eber) was born	– age 433	Gen 11:14-15
2,263 BC	T - Heber was 34 yrs when Peleg was born	– age 464	Gen 11:16-17
2,229 BC	T - Peleg was 30 yrs when Reu was born	– age 239	Gen 11:18-19
2,199 BC	T - Reu was 32 yrs when Serug was born	– age 239	Gen 11:20-21
2,167 BC	T - Serug was 30 yrs when Nahor was born	– age 230	Gen 11:22-23
2,137 BC	T - Nahor 29 yrs when Terah was born	– age 148	Gen 11:24-25
2,103 BC	TCE -Terah was 130+ when Abraham was born	– age 205	Gen 11:26-32
1,598 BC	TE - Terah died in Haran – (before Abraham left Haran)		Gen 11:31-32
1,966 BC	T - Abraham was 75 yrs when he left Haran (after Terah died)		Gen 12:4-5

Jewish scholars calculate that as of Sept 2003 human history began on Rosh Hashannah 5764 years ago. This book uses AD & BC dates, which are historically equal to BCE & CE dates used by Jewish scholars.

Torah Timeline – Abraham (Abram) and Moses

In a short time span after his father, Terah, died, Abraham's life was greatly changed when he: left Haran and went to Canaan; left Canaan and went to Egypt; in Egypt took Hagar, as handmaid to Sarah, who bore him Ishmael; returned to Canaan to dwell in the hills overlooking Sodom; received from the LORD – the promise of a son from Sarah and the covenant of circumcision; rescued Lot after a war; met with Melchizedek to give him a tithe and partake of bread and wine; met with the three messengers of the LORD who insisted that Lot be rescued from Sodom prior to its destruction; witnessed the destruction of Sodom and Gomorrah and the cities of the plain by fire and brimstone; experienced the LORD's promise in fulfillment when Sarah bore their son Isaac; and was instructed by the LORD to sacrifice his son, Isaac, on Mt. Moriah — known as the ***Ahkidah.*** The substitutionary sacrifice of the lamb during the ***Ahkidah*** was *THE* defining event in early Hebrew culture. (Many reliable ***Torah*** scholars chronicle that Isaac was ≈30 yrs and Abraham was ≈130 yrs during the ***Ahkidah***.)

Abraham and Isaac, had ample time to interact with Shem and gain reliable firsthand knowledge of the pre-Flood world; and the antediluvian history of events and people would have been passed on as oral (myth) stories for another 400$^+$ years until Moses wrote them as history in Genesis. (Several reliable ***Torah*** scholars conclude that Shem and Melchizedek were two names for the same person.)

Since Terah began to have sons when he was 70 yrs old and Abraham is listed first, some scholars conclude that the sons were triplets and were born to Terah at age 70 yrs. (Genesis 11:26) Most reliable ***Torah*** scholars conclude Abraham was listed first because he was first in importance. (In the case of Joseph's sons, Ephraim is often listed first, even though Manasseh was born first.) Most reliable ***Torah*** scholars conclude that Haran was born first, when Terah was 70 – and Nahor was born later, when Terah was ≈100 yrs – and Abraham was born when Terah was 130 years old. Abraham left Haran for Canaan at age 75 yrs, and likely after Terah died at age 205 yrs. (205 – 75 = 130) Haran was a very busy crossroads trade city, and it was here that Abram likely became wealthy. Haran, Terah's first son, was likely named after Haran the city where Terah and Abraham dwelt.

FIRST: a ***Torah*** Chronology and ***Torah*** Timeline must discuss the events and lifetimes in the ***Torah*** so all events and lifetimes are internally consistent with one another – and SECOND: the events/people must be related to other events/people from the ***Tanakh*** and from all human history. Historical records are often sparse/unreliable during the ***Torah*** and till the time of David/Solomon. Egyptian writing does not confirm the Exodus, as it is likely that Egyptians wanted to forget that it happened rather than record the devastation for their history. The evidence of Egyptian culture is: near the Passover/Exodus time, their once dominate civilization fell into drastic decline without another civilization claiming military victory. This fact supports, but doesn't confirm, the Exodus. Many events in the ***Torah*** are specified in relationship to other events, such as the LORD's promise to Abraham of 430 years being fulfilled in the Exodus, while other dates are educated estimates. As human civilization advanced, there is reliable evidence that Hebrew history from the ***Tanakh*** is accurate in describing names, dates, places and events that are common to other civilizations. While no outside writing confirms Joshua's conquest of Canaan in the 1400s BC, there is reliable Babylonian writing to confirm Nebuchadnezzar's destruction of the Jerusalem Temple in 587 BC. After Sennacherib's siege of Jerusalem in 701 BC, nearly all ***Tanakh*** TimeLines are in agreement.

The author constructed the ***Torah*** Timeline by assuming 1,450 BC as the Passover/Exodus date and calculating events and peoples lives backward to the Garden of Eden. Other TimeLines have the Exodus as early as 1,525 BC. This TimeLine should be used as a general time reference.

This TimeLine takes the position that genealogies in the ***Torah*** are 'tight' and without gaps. Tight genealogies allow for a meaningful dating of people and events in the ***Torah*** and elevate the ***Torah*** as a key document that can be used to help date people and events in other civilizations. If gaps exist between Seth and Noah or between Shem and Terah, and real people were omitted from ***Torah*** genealogies, how could Caleb be certain that Isaac was born to Abraham and Sarah?

∗ If Moses wrote the *Torah* for Caleb to read as accurate history, then tight genealogies are important. Allowing gaps in ***Torah*** genealogy forces using outside records to confirm ***Torah/Tanakh*** history, rather than using the ***Tanakh*** as the primary reference to date/authenticate outside historical events.

While plotting lives of people in the ***Torah,*** and the Long Day, Exodus, Famine and Sodom events, the author noticed the events occurred roughly on a 42 year cycle. The author adjusted the events to exactly fit a 42 year cycle and then placed the Babel, Division and Flood events on the TimeLine to fit a multiple of 42 year pattern.

Torah TimeLine indicates that 7 events in the ***Torah***/Joshua may have occurred on an interval of 42 years.

Flood	Division	Babel	Sodom	Famine	Exodus	Long Day
2,332 BC	2,206 BC	2,080 BC	1,870 BC	1,660 BC	1,450 BC	1,408 BC

The ***Torah*** TimeLine with events on 42 year multiples is based on the historic 360 days/year Hebrew calendar.

Hebrew Health and Egypt and *Eretz* Israel

Abraham, the first Hebrew, was a herdsman, as were Isaac, Jacob and Joseph, and Moses. From sheep, goats and cattle the Hebrews occasionally ate meat, and got milk, curds and butter for everyday food. When Joseph was sold into Ishmaelite slavery, he was taken to Egypt. In Egypt, Joseph interpreted Pharaoh's dream that warned of 7 years of great Famine, after which Pharaoh advanced Joseph to the position of Prime Minister. When the great Famine occurred throughout Canaan and Egypt as foretold, Jacob brought his entire extended family, 70 Hebrews in all, to Egypt. (As Prime Minister, Joseph likely stored grain at the Step Pyramid near Saqqara – the grain was sold during the great Famine.)

The Nile delta region of Egypt has some of the richest soil for farming in the world, and it was the 'breadbasket' of the Mediterranean. Joseph asked Pharaoh that his tribe of 70 people be allowed to settle in Goshen. Goshen, being near the Nile River delta, was ideally suited for the herds of cattle, sheep and goats that the Hebrews shepherded. ∗ Egyptians often preferred beer with meals. [ch 21-R50] ∗ Keeping herds of clean ruminant animals was a tremendous health advantage for the Hebrews. ∗ Milk and dairy products are discussed by many nutritionists as the best dietary sources for calcium. The author theorizes: Hebrew dependence upon milk from clean ruminant animals may have been a huge competitive edge in terms of fertility, health and longevity for the Hebrews over the Egyptians. From 'the Famine to the Exodus' the 70 Hebrews became a great multitude in ≈210 years. When a new Pharaoh, who knew not Joseph, came to power ≈130 years after the Famine, he felt threatened, since the Hebrews had become very numerous; so, he ordered all male Hebrew babies to be killed.

The Nile River, which the Egyptians worshipped as a 'god', picked up sediment throughout its 600^{+} mile long course through Egypt to the Mediterranean Sea. Every year from July to October the Nile overflowed its banks, spreading fertile, mineral-rich silt over many miles of Nile delta soil. The flooding of the Nile with silt and sediment was a continual renewal process for the soil, and the Nile's waters were essential to water crops. 'Upper Egypt' used the Nile for irrigation; 'lower Egypt' relied on the annual flooding; while the rest of Egypt was often barren. In most farmland areas of the world, the more crops that are grown on the land, the less productive the soil becomes, as more and more minerals and organic elements are removed from the soil by each successive harvest. Since the flooding of the Nile acted to continually enrich, renew and fertilize the soil, the farmland remained productive, and a very advanced society capable of specialization of skills was possible. In other societies of the day, people often devoted much energy to growing, producing, harvesting or gathering food, and few people had the opportunity to develop specialized, sophisticated skills. The ease of growing crops, such as wheat, barley, beans, onions and clover (for animals) from October to April, and cotton, tomatoes, corn, rice and potatoes from March to November made farming near the Nile delta very productive, and helped Egyptian society become rich and powerful.

Eretz Israel, the Promised Land that the LORD promised to Abraham and Isaac's descendants, and that Joshua and the Hebrews conquered was a rich land 'flowing with milk and honey'. ***Eretz*** Israel included the Jordan River valley, across rocky central mountains to the Mediterranean Sea, and from the Sinai Peninsula–Negev desert to the Golan Heights. ***Eretz*** Israel has a tremendously varied topography and climate from: the 3,000 ft of the Golan Heights and 9,232 ft Mt. Herman; to the Sea of Galilee at 686 ft below sea level; to the Jordan River that flows into the Dead Sea at 1,300 ft below sea level (the lowest point on Earth); to the Jezreel Valley that joins the great plains of Megiddo to bisect the central mountains; to the Mediterranean coastal plains of Sharon; and to the Negev desert. The moist, cool Golan Heights and the Hula valley region are ideal for apples; the Mediterranean plains are ideal for citrus; the great plains of Megiddo are ideal for many grains; the central mountains are ideal for grapes and olives; the sub-tropical below sea level Jordan River valley is suitable for bananas; while the arid Negev is sparsely vegetated. Much of ***Eretz*** Israel is suitable for cattle. The Mediterranean Sea, Sea of Galilee and Gulf of Aqaba(h) are ideal for fishing. Migratory flight paths annually bring flocks of clean game birds to ***Eretz*** Israel. In 1,400 BC, the Promised Land may have been greener and received more rain than today. Northerly winds bring the 'early' winter rains of November to ***Eretz*** Israel, and rain persists through the 'later' rains of May, while hot southerly ***sharav*** winds dominate the dry summer. This two-season climate of ***Eretz*** Israel is ideal for agricultural diversity; yet crops failed without the required winter rain and the summer sun at just the proper times, and for this the Hebrews were dependent upon the LORD. The diverse topography, temperature and rainfall of the Promised Land allow an incredible variety of climate within a geographically small area, which gave the Hebrews in ***Eretz*** Israel a huge health advantage over their neighbors, and should have made the nation of Israel the envy of all nations.

The deck was stacked in favor of the Hebrews to become the dominant society on Earth. All the Hebrews needed to do was play their cards properly – obeying the 'Law of Moses' in the ***Torah.***

Havdala

Badal means 'separation' — as in the separation of light from darkness on day one. (Gen 1:4). The principle of 'first mention' in ***Torah*** study indicates the pattern of defining a term in the verse in which the term is first used, to assist in the proper interpretation of the same term later in Scripture. ***Havdala*** has since come to include the ***Torah*** concept of the Hebrews separating themselves from the often idolatrous practices of their neighbors and dedicating themselves unto the LORD their God. Abraham and Sarah moved from Ur to practice ***havdala*** well in Haran, but they practiced ***havdala*** poorly during a brief stay in Egypt, after which they settled in Canaan to practice ***havdala*** very well. For ≈210 years, the Hebrews from the Famine to the Exodus maintained a distinct, unique ***havdala*** identity from their Egyptian neighbors. However, the Hebrews exited Egypt as a 'mixed multitude' – and maintaining ***havdala*** unto the LORD, while wandering in the wilderness, was continually difficult. After 490 years of ruling the 'Promised Land', some Hebrews eventually lost all respect for ***havdala*** as they copied the Ammonite practice of child sacrifice on a fiery–hot brass image of god: Moloch. In 606 BC, the nation of Babylon took the nation of Judah captive for 70 years — the 1st dispersion. After returning from Babylonian captivity, the Jews {Hebrews} never again sacrificed children to a god, while each prophet encouraged the Jews to abandon some pagan practice and to rekindle ***havdala***. In 70 AD, a 2nd global dispersion — the ***Diaspora***, began. Today, as always, maintaining a Hebrew ***havdala*** identity includes eating kosher, keeping ***Shabbat*** and observing the Feasts of the LORD. Today, followers of the LORD also seek to practice ***havdala*** in work, family, community and worship.

--------- References for Preface and Introduction – Hebrew Myth - pg 19 & TimeLine - pg 20-23 ---------

[R1] Classical Mythology (audio&book)\ by Elizabeth Vandiver, PhD; Fable /[R1A] pg 4 Myth /[R1B] pg 6 Legend
(Myth may refer denotatively only to myth; or myth may refer connotatively to myth, fable and/or legend.) (pg 90)

[R2] The New LaRousse Encyclopedia of Mythology; pg v reasons/rational for Myth

[R3] Text of the Old Testament\ by Ernst Wurthwein; pg 12 Mazorites = Jewish scholars // pg 21 chapter & verse

[R4] The Power of Myth (audio)\ by Joseph Campbell & Bill Moyers – (tape 2 – side 1) – Genesis 3 as only myth

[R5] Don't Know Much About the Universe (audio)\ by Kenneth C. Davis; Egyptian myth tape 1 – 2nd half

[R6] Understanding Islam (audio)\ by Thomas W. Lippman (tape2 – side1) 'night journey' – Koran (Surah XVII – 1)
"In effect, Mohammad made a distinction between the religious teachings of Judaism, which he professed to admire, and the actions of the Jews who lived around him, to which he responded with violence." – (tape2 – side2)

[R7] How the Irish Saved Civilization (BDD audio + book)\ by Thomas Cahill – (tp1-sd1) + pg 55-67 – Augustine on Gen 3

[R8] The Battle for God (audio+book)\ by Karen Armstrong – (tape1 – side1) In all religions, '*mythos*' looks to the past to explain the world; while '*logos*' looks to the future including science & technology for solutions to problems.

[R9] A History of God\ by Karen Armstrong; ***Ahkidah*** (***Akedah***) story prevented Hebrew child sacrifice

[R10] Prophet of Doom & Tea with Terrorists (w3.prophetofdoom.net)\ by Craig Winn; 9-11+ Moslems, Jews & Christians

[R11] The Bible and Its Story (Vol II)\ by Prof. Charles F. Horne; plate II-15 painting – Moses in the Desert

[R12] Knowing Scripture (audio+CD+VHS+book)\ by R. C. Sproul, DrS; (#6) Gen 3 & Num 22 as history (1-800-435-4343)

[R13] Genesis A Living Conversation\ by Bill Moyers views Genesis as myth – not history

[R14] Illustrated Map of Bible History\ of Bishop Usher; first biblical chronology + young history of Earth

[R15] Catastrophism and the Old Testament\ by Donald Patten; catastrophism + young history of Earth

[R16] Time Line of the World & Bible Lights Time Line (Internet) people/events + young history of Earth

[R17] Creation Seminar (videos & booklet)\ by Kent Hovind, PhD; creationism + young history of Earth

[R18] Strong's Comprehensive Concordance of the Bible\ by James Strong, STD, LLD

pg 587	law / teaching	# 8451 (#3384)		H pg 123	the ***Torah***		Deut 33:2 - Josh 1:1
pg 855	Sabbath	# 7676		H pg 112	***Shabbath***	***Shabbat***	Ex 16:23 & Ex 16:25
pg 538	Jehovah יהוה	# 3068	***YHWH***	H pg 47	***Y-hw-h***	***Yahweh***	Ex 6:3
pg 1074	tree or trees	# 6086		H pg 90	***'ets***	***ets***	Gen 3:22
pg 581	land	# 776		H pg 17	***'eretz***	***eretz***	Gen 12:1
pg 269	divided – separated	# 914		H pg 19	***badal***		Gen 1:4
pg 591	leaven	# 7603		H pg 111	***seor***		Ex 12:15

Apostrophies Frequently Deleted - pg 12

[R19] The Genesis Flood\ by John Whitcomb, PhD and Henry Morris, PhD; Flood + young history of Earth

[R20] What's in the Bible\ by R. C. Sproul, DrS and Robert Wolgemuth; overview + young history of Earth

-- References for the Step Pyramid --

[R21] The Pyramids and Cities of the Pharaohs (video) – Step Pyramid at Saqqara

[R22] The Exodus (video)\ by Ron Wyatt – grain pit photos at the 'South Tomb'

[R23] Wyatt Museum (website/newsletter) – www.wyattmuseum.com

[R24] Step Pyramid of Djoser (website) – http://interoz.com/egypt/steppyram.htm

[R25] Step Pyramid at Saqqara (website) – Mastaba – w3.crystalinks.com/stepr.html

[R26] Famine Stela (websites) – Famine Stela at Sehel Island – writing is ≈3 ft by 3 ft

[R27] The Pyramids\ by Miroslav Verner – pg 108 Step Pyramid schematic & photo

[R28] The Pyramids\ by Ahmed Fakhry – pg 23 Famine Stela / pg 28 schematic / pg 31 South Tomb

(painting)

Moses in the Desert

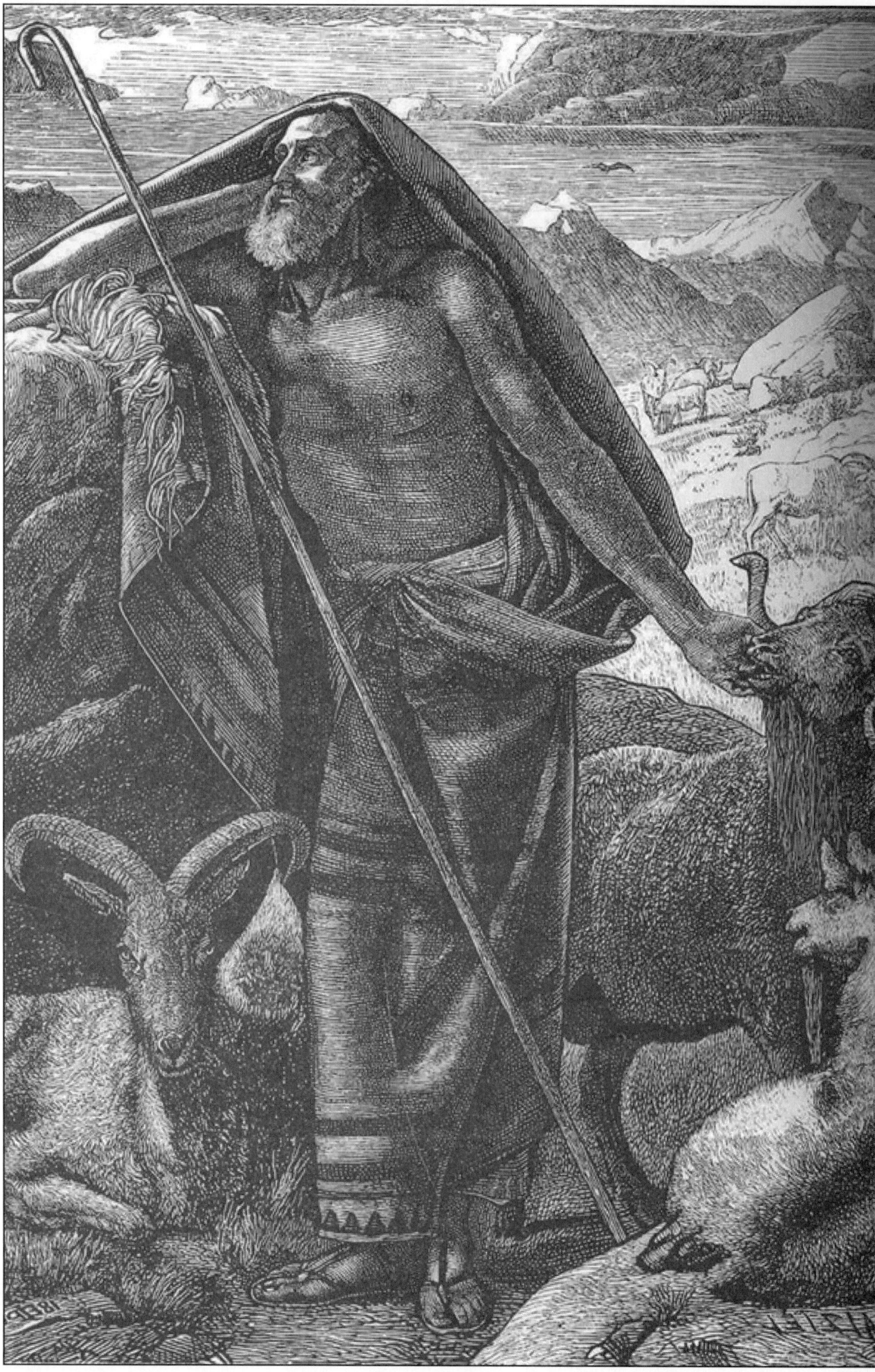

Section I: MENTAL HEALTH
Chapter 1 Moses
Moses and the *Torah*

Moses wrote five scrolls – Genesis, Exodus, Leviticus, Numbers and Deuteronomy – which contain early human history and instructions from God concerning how man should live on Earth. The five scrolls of Moses are called the ***Torah,*** which is Hebrew for the 'Teachings' or the 'Law'; and are placed at the beginning of the Hebrew Scriptures, called the ***Tanakh***. As the first five books of the Bible, which is Greek for 'The Book', these writings are also called the *Pentateuch*.

Genesis describes: the creation of the Universe in six days and calls it very good; the fall of man and the need for a Redeemer; the world overcome by sin that necessitated Noah's Flood; Abraham as the father of faith; the lives of the Patriarchs; and the Hebrews' journey to Egypt.

Exodus describes: the 70 Hebrews in Egypt becoming numerous; Moses escaping from Egypt as a fugitive to find shelter and family life in Midian; Moses encountering God at the burning bush; Moses delivering the Hebrews from bondage through The 10 Plagues; the Hebrews crossing the Red Sea; Moses receiving 'The 10 Commandments'; and the Hebrews defeating the Amalekites.

Leviticus describes: the implications of 'The 10 Commandments' as a Covenant between the LORD and the Hebrews; the need for a Priesthood between a sinful mankind and the righteous LORD; and what is meant by keeping oneself sanctified, clean and holy, just as the LORD is holy.

Numbers describes: the Hebrew's failure to understand the nature of the Covenant as they fail to exercise faith, fail to enter the Promised Land, and wander in the wilderness for 40 years; Korah's rebellion against the LORD; and the Hebrews victory over the Amorites and Bashanites.

Deuteronomy describes: Moses re-establishing God as LORD; recounting the dietary laws and 'The 10 Commandments'; the final words of advice to the Hebrews, who will follow Joshua into the Promised Land; warnings for failure to keep the Covenant with the LORD; and the death of Moses.

The life of Moses is a familiar story made famous by legend, book, song and several movies: *The Ten Commandments*, *Moses* (TNT) and *The Prince of Egypt*.

Born a Hebrew, at birth Moses was saved from a death decree, when by faith his mother placed him in a basket and left him hidden in the reeds of the Nile River (Ex 2:3);
Moses was found and raised by Pharaoh's daughter, who named him Moses, which means 'drawn out from water' (Ex 2:5-10);
Moses left Egypt and fled to Midian after killing an Egyptian (Ex 2:15);
Moses dwelt in Midian, where at age 40 he married Zipporah and tended Jethro's sheep (Ex 2:20);
Moses was commissioned by God on Mt. Sinai (Horeb) from the burning bush to deliver the Hebrew people from Egyptian slavery (Ex 3:8);
Moses returned to Egypt at age 80 to pronounce 10 Plagues against the Egyptians, culminating with the Passover (Ex 7 to 12);
Moses parted the Red Sea, so the Hebrews could cross over on dry ground (Ex 14:22);
Moses led the Hebrews in a victorious battle against the Amalekites (Ex 17:8-15);
Moses received the 10 Commandments from the LORD on Mt. Sinai (i.e. – Horeb) (Ex 20:1-17);
Moses directed the Hebrews as they built the Tabernacle of the LORD (Ex 40);
Moses led the rebellious Hebrews for 40 years of wandering in the wilderness (Num Ch 1 to 36);
Moses led the Hebrews to victories in war over the nations of the Amorites (Num 21:21-32) and the Bashanites (Num 21:33-35); and
Moses died on Mt. Pisgah (i.e. – Nebo) after viewing the Promised Land when he was 120 years old; yet Moses' eyesight was not dim, nor was his natural stamina and strength lost (Deut 34:7).

When reading of executives today whose careers are highlighted by such achievements, frequently major health setbacks are the price they pay for success. What kind of man was Moses that he could gain the respect of the Hebrew nation so they would follow and obey him? What allowed Moses to maintain his perfect health and vitality through all he accomplished? How did Moses maintain his great vision until he was 120 years old?

As a Doctor of Optometry I have studied and examined the health of eyes for over 25 years. I know that 'the eye reveals the health of the body'. Ocular diseases such as: glaucoma, cataracts, and macular degeneration; and systemic diseases including diabetes and high blood pressure often cause decreased vision. I wanted to understand what was different about Moses, so after reading *None of These Diseases* by S. I. McMillen, MD, and *God's Key to Health and Happiness* by Rev. Elmer Josephson, in 1987, like Paul Harvey, I began researching: 'The Rest of the Story'!

Develop a Good Character

The success of Moses can be attributed to the healthy character traits he developed:

Compassion and Understanding concerning the feelings of his brethren, as when Aaron failed to offer the sacrifice and eat the sacrifice after his sons were killed for offering strange fire.

NIV Lev 10:20 And when Moses heard this he was satisfied.

Confession: as Moses confessed the nation's sins as his sins.

KJV Ex 34:9 O LORD, let my LORD. I pray thee, go amoung us; ...
... pardon our iniquity and our sin and take us for thine inheritance.

Contentment to accept whatever position God wanted for him.

KJV Ex 2:21 Moses was content to dwell with the man [Jethro].

Courage and willingness to stand up for the rights of others;

NIV Ex 2:17 Some shepherds came and drove them [Jethro's daughters] away but Moses got up and came to their rescue and watered their flock.

Humility of heart and Worship for the LORD God:

KJV Ex 34:8 And Moses made haste, and bowed his head toward the earth, and worshipped.

Leadership to his brethren.

JPS Ex14:13 And Moses said unto the people: fear ye not, stand still, and see the salvation of the LORD,

Logical thinking – In Numbers 14:13-19 the Hebrews had rebelled against the LORD again.

The LORD was ready to disinherit the Hebrews, until Moses interceded, and convinced the LORD to keep His covenant with the Hebrews for the sake of His oath. (Ps 105:42 & Ps106:23)

Love of God, and of self and of his brethren {discussed later*}

Meekness as a man of God and a way of life; (Meekness is strength under control.) [R14]

KJV Num 12:3 Now the man Moses was very meek, above all men that were on the face of the earth.

Obedience to the LORD.

JPS Ex 40:16 Thus did Moses; according to all that the LORD commanded him, so did he.

Prayer to the LORD for direction in his life.

NKJV Ex33:13 .... I pray, if I have found grace in Your sight, show me Your way, that I may know You and that I may find grace in Your sight.

Resourceful in bringing together materials and skills necessary to build the Tabernacle.

JPS Ex 36:7 For the stuff [materials for the Tabernacle] they had was sufficient...

JPS Ex 39:32 Thus was finished all the work of the tabernacle ...

Righteous indignation (disdain) toward idolatry and toward disobedience of the LORD.

JPS Ex 32:19 ... he [Moses] saw the calf and the dancing; and Moses' anger waxed hot.

Trust in the LORD.

JPS Ex 15:2 The LORD is my strength and song, and He is become my salvation.

Truth is exemplified when one lives his life according to the standards he professes. Moses wrote the ***Torah*** and he lived his life by the statutes of the LORD God, which he wrote.

* Truth in the life of Moses is evident from the statutes he wrote concerning the love of God, the love of neighbor, and the love of oneself; and how he practiced and demonstrated this love. 'The ***Shema***', which means to 'hear and obey', is likely the most often read and most frequently quoted verse in Hebrew Scripture, and it contains the requirement to 'love the LORD'. (Deut 6:4)

JPS Deut 6:4 HEAR, O ISRAEL: THE LORD OUR GOD, THE LORD IS ONE.

{***Shema Yisrael, Adonai*** (יְהוָה) ***Eloheinu, Adonai*** (יהוה) ***Echad***}

vs5 And thou shalt love the LORD thy God with all thy heart, and with all thy soul, and with all thy might.

KJV Deut 6:4-9 Hear, O Israel: The LORD our God is one LORD. vs5 And thou shalt love the LORD thy God with all thy heart, and with all thy soul, and with all thy might. vs6 And these words, which I command thee this day shall be in thine heart: vs7 And thou shalt teach them diligently unto thy children, and shalt talk of them when thou sittest in thine house, and when thou walkest by the way, and when thou liest down, and when thou risest up. vs8 And thou shalt bind them for a sign upon thine hand, and they shall be as frontlets between thine eyes. vs9 And thou shalt write them upon the posts of thy house, and on thy gates.

Moses also wrote about loving one's neighbor and loving oneself.

JPS Lev 19:18 Thou shalt not take vengeance, nor bear any grudge against the children of thy people, but thou shalt love thy neighbor as thy self: I am the LORD.

*** Love the LORD, love thy neighbor and love thyself are lofty standards for anyone to follow.**

Love the LORD

The British Medical Journal 'Lancet' once noted:
"By far the most significant discovery of mental science is the power of love to protect and to restore the mind." [R11]

Similarly, Hans Selye, MD, a noted stress specialist, wrote:
"It is not the person of the frustrating boss who will get ulcers, hypertension and heart disease. It is the one who hates or the one who permits himself to be frustrated.
'Love thy neighbor as thy self' is one of the sagest bits of medical advice ever given." [R12]

Dr. Erich Fromm, a psychoanalyst, wrote:
"The injunction, 'Love thy neighbor as thyself,' is the most important norm of living and ... its violation is the basic cause of unhappiness and mental illness ... Whatever complaints the ... patient may have, whatever symptoms he may present, are rooted in his inability to love – if we mean by love a capacity for the experience of concern, responsibility, respect and understanding of another person and an intense desire for that other person's growth." [R4]

Whenever this principle of health is violated, unhappiness and ill health soon follow. [R3-7]

The first issues within the Ten Commandments deal primarily with mans relationship to God and are in agreement with the statute from the ***Shema*** of Deuteronomy 6:5: "Thou shalt love (***ahab***) the LORD thy God with all thy heart, soul and might." The second issues within the Ten Commandments primarily deal with man's relationships to his fellow men and are in agreement with the instruction from Leviticus 19:18: "Thou shalt love thy neighbor as thyself." In this sense these two principles of love are interwoven within the Ten Commandments (also known as – 'the Decalogue') and within all the rest of the 613 statutes, ordinances, and judgments of the Law.

The love that Moses had for the LORD God was expressed by doing everything that the LORD commanded him to do and in his prayers to the LORD. (Ex 40:16)

KJV Ex 34:8-9 And Moses made haste, and bowed his head toward the earth, and worshipped. vs9 And he said, If now I have found grace in thy sight, O LORD, let my LORD I pray thee, go amoung us, for it is [we are] a stiffnecked people; and pardon our iniquity and our sin, and take us for thine inheritance.

Moses acknowledges his sin, acknowledges the iniquity of his brethren and prays to God. Love and respect for God begin with confession of sins and prayer to the LORD for forgiveness. Love of the LORD is manifested in lives by obedience to following the LORD's commandments.

Love Your Neighbor

The love that Moses showed for his brethren is best documented by the conversation between Moses and the LORD after Moses' Hebrew brethren worshipped the golden calf.

KJV Ex 32:10 & 13-14 [God said to Moses] Now therefore let me alone that my wrath may wax hot against them [the Hebrews] and that I may consume them and I will make of thee [Moses] a great nation. ...[Moses said to God] Remember Abraham, Isaac and Israel thy servants, to whom thou swarest by thine own self and said unto them, I will multiply your seed as the stars of heaven and all this land that I have spoken will I give unto your seed and they shall inherit it forever. And then the LORD repented of the evil which he had thought to do unto his people [the Hebrews].

The grace of God spared judgment on the Hebrews only after Moses showed his love for his brethren. First Moses convinced the LORD God to give the Hebrew nation a stay of execution. Then after removing from the camp of Israel those men that stood against the LORD God, Moses made another extraordinary request unto the LORD on the part of his Hebrew brethren:

KJV Ex 32:33 Yet now, if thou wilt forgive their sin--; and if not, blot me, I pray thee, out of thy book which thou hast written.

Moses asked God to forgive the sins of his brethren or to blot out his name from His book of eternal life (***cepher chaim***). It is rare love that will cause someone to offer to sacrifice his earthly life for his brethren. It is extraordinary love that would cause someone to offer his eternal position with God in heaven as ransom for the forgiveness of the sins of his brethren. Only as a result of this incredible love did God graciously spare the Hebrew nation. Moses' love also caused his brethren to follow Moses in war, in work and in worship of the LORD, and while wandering in the wilderness.

Truth is defined: When the word and deed become as 'one'. Truth fits the life of Moses well.

*** Follow Moses and the LORD to become part of the solution, rather than part of the problem.**

Love Yourself and Love Summary

Leviticus 19:18 also calls for a man of God to love himself. Many important people become so tied up in the entanglement of daily duties that they forget this necessity of personal health. Moses demonstrated 'love of self' when he accepted the wise counsel of his father-in-law, Jethro, and appointed judges to help settle people's grievances and relieve excess duties that he had taken upon himself. [R23] Moses continued to delegate responsibility to capable men. (Deut 1:13) Later, Moses recognizes his responsibilities are still too great and he asks the LORD for help. Then, God instructs Moses to appoint 70 elders of Israel to help support Moses. (Num 11:11-17) (In ≈330 BC, during Greek occupation, 70 elders became the basis for the Jewish *Sanhedrin* Council.)

NIV Ex 18:13 The next day Moses took his seat to serve as judge for the people, and they stood around him from morning till evening. vs18 [Jethro's advice] You and these people who come to you will only wear yourselves out. The work is too heavy for you; you cannot handle it alone. vs25 He [Moses] chose capable men from all Israel and made them leaders of the people, officials over thousands, hundreds, fifties and tens.

Certainly, Moses loved God, loved his neighbor, and loved himself: three very important steps to follow for perfect health and peace of mind. Truth in a man's life is defined when word and deed become as 'one', which leads to perfect Mental Health. The life of Moses documented that his words and writings and actions were in agreement with one another. ∗ Perhaps no one else for hundreds of years before Moses, or after Moses, more perfectly lived his life in such truth.

Health truly begins in the mind. The mind and the will of man through his brain direct the activities of the entire body. The beginning of Mental Health is learning faith and trust rather than doubt and worry. Through faith in God, Moses accepts the will of God for his life. After 40 years of wandering in the wilderness, the entire rebellious Hebrew generation has died, and the new generation is ready to enter the Promised Land. Moses is allowed to see the land of his dreams from the top of Mt. Pisgah (i.e.- Mt. Nebo), but is told by the LORD that he will not cross the Jordan River to enter the land. (Deut 31:12) Moses knew it was the LORD's will that he would soon die, and he needed to commission Joshua to be the new man-of-God to lead the nation. (Deut 31:14)

JPS Deut 34:7 And Moses was a hundred and twenty years old when he died; his eye was not dim, nor his natural strength abated. vs 9 And Joshua the son of Nun was full of the spirit of wisdom; for Moses had laid his hands upon him;

As chronicled earlier (pg 1), the entire life of Moses was directed by God with one purpose in mind: to lead the Hebrew nation to this land of milk and honey, which God had promised to their father Abraham. Now, when Moses was so close to the Promised Land to see it, the LORD told him he could see it, but wouldn't make the final few steps into the Promised Land.

Outdoorsmen often climb mountains for enjoyment, accomplishment and the love of nature. After years of planning, training and practicing for a major climb, and after overcoming obstacles during the completion of the climb of a lifetime of dreams, if God said, "Go no farther, you are near the summit, you can see the summit, but you can not go all the way to the top". Most people would become disappointed, upset, angry, and start complaining! Moses responded quite differently; he made sure this was the LORD's will for his life and then accepted it as God's will.

Trust in the LORD undoubtedly led to a great peace of mind and Mental Health for Moses.

Finally, Moses, being mighty in 'word and deed', exhorted his brethren to trust the LORD, to have courage and not fear: for if the LORD be for thee, who can be against thee?

KJV Deut 31:6 Be strong and of a good courage, fear not, nor be afraid of them, for the LORD thy God, he it is that doth go with thee; he will not fail thee, nor forsake thee.

At the burning bush when Moses received his commission to deliver the Hebrews from Egyptian bondage, his answer to the LORD was ***hinnehni***. ***Hinnehni*** means 'here I am' or ask anything of me and I'll do it. Today, this must be the attitude of everyone who follows the LORD.

JPS Ex 3:4 … And he [Moses] said: 'Here am I' (***hinnehni***).

The life of Moses measures up very well against the standard of 'love' that he wrote about in the ***Torah***, as should all people who are implementing the LORD's principles into their lives.

When challenging circumstances arise today, ask yourself: **What Would Moses Do?** or **W W M D ?**

---------------------------------- References Ch 01 Moses -------------------------------

[R1] Moses A man of Selfless Dedication\ by Chuck Swindoll, PhD (Insights for Living 1-800-772-8888)
[R2] None of These Diseases\ by S I McMillen, MD; pg 129 - love thy neighbor as thyself
[R3] None of These Diseases Revised\ by McMillen, MD and David Stern, MD; pg 2 - love
[R4] None of These Diseases Revised and Updated\ by McMillen, MD and Stern, MD; pg 167-223 stress
[R5] Liberated to Love (6 audio tapes)\ by Charles Stanley, PhD (In Touch 1-800-323-3747)
[R6] Teaching on the Torah\ by Rev. Chuck Smith (Calvary Chapel 1-800-272-WORD)
[R7] Teaching on the Torah\ by Chuck Missler, PhD (Koinonia House 1-800-KHOUSE1)
[R8] Teaching on the Torah\ by J. Vernon McGee, PhD (Through the Bible 1-800-65-BIBLE)
[R9] Moses\ TNT // [R9A] The Price of Egypt // [R9B] The Bible\ by John Huston CBS/Fox (movies)
[R10] The 10 Commandments\ by Cecil B. DeMille // [R10B] Moses\ on History Channel (biography)
[R11] Mental Health and Spiritual Values\ by Geoffrey Vickers; (Lancet 12 Mar 1955; pg 524)
[R12] How to Avoid Harmful Stress\ by J D Radcliff; Today's Health July 1970; pg 43
[R13] Life: How Did It Get Here?\ (both R11 & R12) \by The Watchtower Society of Penn
[R14] The Jewish Way in Love and Marriage\ by Rabbi Maurice Lamm; pg 43 meekness
Judaism teaches that if you are not in control of yourself, you are not a human being.
[R15] Stress without Distress\ by Hans Selye, MD; pg 118-125 the power of love
[R16] The Pentateuch in Its Cultural Environment\ by G. Herbert Livingston, PhD
[R17] Heaven Help Me to Love (audio tapes 2000)\ from Discover the Word (radio program)
[R18] Strong's Comprehensive Concordance of the Bible\ by James Strong, STD, LLD

pg 486	hear and obey	# 8085	H pg 118	***shema***	Deut 6:4
pg 526	Israel	# 3478	H pg 53	***Yisrael***	Deut 6:4
pg 617	LORD יהוה	# 3068	H pg 47	***Yahweh*** ⇒ ***'Adonai***	Deut 6:4 & Deut 6:4
pg 399	our-God	# 430	H pg 12	***'Eloheinu*** – ***Eloheinu***	Deut 6:4
pg 749	one	# 259	H pg 10	***'echad*** – ***echad***	Deut 6:4
pg 637	love	# 157	H pg 9	***'ahab*** – ***ahab***	Deut 6:5
pg 397	God-Creator	# 430	H pg 12	***'Elohiym*** – ***Elohiym***	Gen 1:1
pg 398	God	# 410	H pg 12	***'El*** – ***El***	Gen 14:18
pg 220	the council	# 4892	G pg 69	*Sanhedrin*	Matt 5:22
pg 479	here – behold	# 2009	H pg 33	***hinneh***	Ex 3:4
	here am I	(from #2009)		***hinnehni***	
pg 135	book	# 5612	H pg 84	***cepher***	Ex 32:32
pg 601	life	# 2421	H pg 39	***chayah*** – ***chaim***	Ex 32:32
pg 200	come – go	# 935	H pg 19	***bo*** – ***bow***	Gen 7:1
pg 692	Moses – drawn out of water	# 4872	H pg 73	***Moshe***	Ex:10
pg 685	Miriam – bitter – (root of Mary)	# 4813	H pg 72	***Miriam***	Ex 15:20
pg 005	Aaron – (origin - unknown)	# 175	H pg 9	***Aharon*** – ***Aharown***	Ex 4:14
pg 1210	Zipporah – {little} bird	# 6855	H pg 101	***Zipporah*** – ***Tzipporah***	Ex 2:21
pg 545	Jethro – his excellence	# 3503	H pg 54	***Yithro*** – ***Yithrow***	Ex 3:1
pg 551	Joshua – ***Yahweh*** saved	# 3091	H pg 48	***Yehoshua***	Num 14:6
pg 159	Caleb – attack {as a dog}	# 3612	H pg 55	***Kaleb***	Num 14:6
pg 269	divided – separated	# 914	H pg 19	***badal***	Gen 1:4
	– the separation	(from #914 ⇔ bet – dalet – lamed)		***havdala***	
	– 'binding' (of Isaac) עקדה	{pronounced – Ah-key-dah}		***Ahkidah*** or ***Akedah***	Gen 22

Apostrophes that begin transliterated words are frequently deleted. (see - pg 12)

**Jethro was a Priest of Midian, and a descendant of Abraham by his wife, Keturah. (Gen 25:2)
The birthright often carried the responsibility of being the priest (spiritual leader) of the household.
[R19] Studies in the Pentateuch\ by W. R. Newell // [R20] First Love\ by Bill Bright, PhD
[R21] Antiquity of the Jews\ by Flavius Josephus – life of Moses – Book II & III & IV
[R22] Dust to Glory (30 audio tapes)\ by R. C. Sproul, DrS from Ligonier Ministries (1-800-435-4343)
[R23] Wisdom of Counsel\ by R. C. Sproul, DrS (#WIS02AI) Moses & Jethro - Exodus18 (01-01-03)
[R24] Moses The Servant of Yahweh\ by Dewey M. Beegle, PhD
[R25] Moses The Servant of God\ by F.B. Meyer, BA
[R26] All That Really Matters\ by Sheila Walsh {Dick Staub interview 2003} Love God & neighbor & self

Moses is transliterated ***Moshe***. Moses means 'drawn out of the water'. (Moses' sons: Gerhom & Eliezer.)
Aaron is transliterated ***Aharon***. Origin of Aaron is unknown – has come to reference Levitical Priesthood.
Miriam is already a transliterated. ***Miriam*** means bitter and, when translated to English, is Mary.
Jethro, the father-in-law of Moses and priest of Midian, is likely a title and is transliterated ***Yithro***. (Ex 3:1)
Reuel is likely the personal name of Moses' father-in-law. ***Reuel*** means friend of God. (Ex 2:18)
Tzipporah was married to Moses, and since her father, Jethro, was a Midianite, so was she.
Miriam and ***Aharon*** were unhappy with Moses for marrying a Cushite woman. (Num 12:1)
Cushites were dark-skinned descendants of Cush (great-grandson of Ham), who lived in Ethiopia.
Either, Moses married a second wife at an unspecified time that is not mentioned in the ***Torah*** or,
Jethro married a Cushite woman and their daughter, ***Tzipporah***, was both Cushite and Midianite.

{ The author believes that Moses' wife, ***Tzipporah***, was of both Midianite and Cushite descent. }

Love – is a process	* **Aspects of Love in the life of Moses**	**Aspects of Love in the readers life**

Love - is patient;
(is not anxious or impulsive),
(waits upon the LORD for strength and direction),
Love - is kind;
(considerate of the emotional needs of others),
Love - is content;
(not envious),
(has poise and inner peace),
Love - does not brag or boast;
(is polite),
Love - is not arrogant;
(is not proud),
(has a quiet spirit),
Love - does not act unbecomingly;
(is not rude or selfish),
(is well-mannered),
Love - does not seek its own;
(recognizes other people may have different opinions),
(may surrender or yield self rights),
(does not insist upon its own way),
(places expectations for all needs upon the LORD),
Love - is not provoked to anger or bitterness;
(does not provoke others to anger),
(stays emotionally calm despite circumstances),
Love - does not take into account wrongs suffered;
(need not 'even up' the score with others for mistreatment),
(is forgiving of others),
Love - does not rejoice in unrighteousness;
(does not gloat over other peoples' sins),
(does not take pleasure in retribution delivered upon others),
Love - rejoices in the truth;
(rejoices when word and deed become as 'one'),
(helps others to develop emotional maturity),
(rejoices with people when they triumph),
Love - bears all things;
(bears others' {emotional} burdens — protects against {emotional} trauma,
(is compassionate of other peoples' needs during tough times),
(grieves with people when they are in despair),
Love - believes all things;
(reaches a level of emotionally maturity to objectively evaluate others),
(recognizes character strengths/weaknesses and responds accordingly),
(accepts or acknowledges 'what is' as: 'what is'),
(believes the objectively discernible scenario to be 'what it is'),
Love - hopes all things;
(seeks to help make 'what is' better than 'it is'),
(looks to encourage others despite difficult situations),
(finds a silver lining in a dark cloud),
Love - endures all hardships;
(becomes strong through testing),
(never ceases to stop practicing the above),
Love - never fails;
(is always necessary in every situation and in every circumstance of life),
Love - prevails for all eternity.

---

* To love the LORD, love self, and love neighbor, become 'Moses-like'. A useful list that contains many attributes of love should be learned and lived (memorization may be helpful) and continually applied to daily life. [R5-17]

One goal of ***Torah*** study is to find examples of the character aspects of 'love' in the life of Moses.

(Envy refers to resenting talents or treasures that someone else has, that you don't have.)

(Jealousy refers to seeking respect that is rightfully yours – as parents require from children or – as the LORD requires from His followers.)

∗ Faith in the LORD and Hope in the promises of the LORD, as well as Love of the LORD, Love of self, and Love of neighbors are all vital elements of Mental Health.

Chapter 2 Teach and Learn
The 10 Commandments

Moses received his command from the LORD to teach the Hebrews while on Mt. Sinai. The Hebrews accepted Moses as their teacher, and Moses accepted the responsibility to teach them.

KJV Ex 24:12 And the LORD said unto Moses, Come up to Me in the mount and be there: and I will give thee tables of stone, and a law, and commandments which I have written; that thou may teach (***yarah***) them.

The Ten Commandments were part of the covenant between ***Yahweh*** (***Y-hw-h***) and the Hebrews. When the Hebrews agreed to the terms of the covenant, they established ***Yahweh*** as the one and only, true living God. As LORD of their lives, ***Yahweh*** alone was to be worshipped. Worshipping other gods (idolatry) and irreverent use of the name of God are agreed upon as not being the method to develop a personal relationship with God as LORD. Murdering, adultery, lying, stealing, gossiping and coveting were also agreed upon as not being a healthy way to treat one another. The terms of this covenant were set by the LORD, as being those that would lead to the health and well-being for all who entered the covenant with Him. The terms of this covenant also established Moses as the teacher of God's instructions. (Ex 24:3&7) Of course, teaching is not valuable without learning (***lamad***), and the Hebrews vowed to be diligent learners of the ***Torah***. The requirement to teach and learn is a mandate for mastery; not an excuse for ineptitude.

KJV Ex 24:3 And Moses came and told the people all the words of the LORD, and all the judgments: all the people answered with one voice, and said, All the words which the LORD hath said will we do. vs7 and he [Moses] took the book of the covenant, and read in the audience of the people: and they said, All that the LORD hath said will we do, and be obedient.

JPS Deut 4:10 ... before the LORD thy God in Horeb, when the LORD said to me: 'Assemble Me the people, and I will make them hear My words, that they may learn (***lamad***) to fear Me all the days of that they live upon the earth, and that they may teach (***lamad***) their children.'

The Ten Commandments were repeated a second time in the ***Torah*** because Moses wanted to establish obedience to the Law and emphasize the covenant nature of the agreement between the LORD and His chosen people. (Ex 20 – Deut 5 – Ex 34:10) <u>Repetition is a great teaching technique</u>. Repetition as a means of establishing the certainty and importance of a message from God is first explained by an example from the life of Joseph. Repetition is also vital in legal issues. (Deut 17:6)

NKJV Gen 41:32 And the dream was repeated to Pharaoh twice because the thing is established by God, and God will shortly bring it to pass.

The 10 Commandments were given twice by the LORD and were twice recorded in the ***Torah***. (Ex 20 and Deut 5) The Hebrews also twice agreed to adhere to the principles of the covenant. The importance of following the precepts of the 10 Commandments cannot be overemphasized. Moses warns and encourages God's chosen people many times to be not only <u>hearers</u> of the Word of God, but also to be <u>doers</u> of the Word and to <u>obey</u> the principles of the LORD. The phrase a 'heart to perceive, eyes to see and ears to hear' indicates that learning must be experiential and cumulative.

KJV Deut 13:4 Ye shall walk after the LORD your God, and fear him, and keep his commandments, and obey his voice, and ye shall serve him, and cleave unto him.

KJV Deut 29:4 … an heart to perceive, and eyes to see, and ears to hear, unto this day.

The most important requirement for any teacher/leader is to be of the highest possible moral character and integrity. As Chapter 1 documented, Moses was such a person. The best teacher must also be certain that his instructions are in agreement with all the principles from Scripture. The ***Torah*** records many times that Moses listened to the LORD directly for his instructions, ensuring that the words he taught would be in agreement with the heart, mind and will of the LORD.

KJV Ex 7:2 Thou [Moses] shalt speak all that I [the LORD] command thee.

KJV Ex 39:42 According to all that the LORD commanded Moses, so the children of Israel made all their work.

The best part of any teacher's job is to acknowledge or praise his disciples, children, or pupils when they do well by following instructions. Moses practiced this when he praised the Hebrews for their obedience in building the Tabernacle of the LORD, according to instructions. (Ex 39:42-43)

*** Teaching often seems to be unappreciated, but when lessons are learned the effort is worthwhile.**

Learn Lessons and Teach Lessons

Part of the reason the Hebrews successfully built the Tabernacle was that the skilled Hebrew craftsmen used their building skills on the Tabernacle and taught these skills to others. (Num 11)

JPS Ex 35:30-35 - vs31 And He [God] hath filled him [Bezalel] with the spirit of God, in wisdom, in understanding, and in knowledge, and in all manner of workmanship. vs34 And He [God] hath put in his [Bezalel's] heart that he may teach (***yaroh***), both he, and Oholiab ...

Once a person has learned skills or has learned wisdom through instruction from the LORD, the LORD desires this person to take on a new role of added responsibility as a teacher to others.

A less pleasant but equally important responsibility of a teacher is to criticize or to issue correction when students fail to follow instructions. Because Hebrew soldiers did not completely follow his orders, Moses rebuked them harshly when they returned victorious from battle. After the Hebrews worshipped the golden calf, Moses spoke frankly and harshly, yet honestly to them.

KJV Num 31:14 Moses was wroth [angry] with the officers of the host, with the captains over thousands, and the captains over hundreds, which came from the battle.

NKJV Ex 32:30 And it came to pass on the next day that Moses said to the people, "You have sinned a great sin. So now I will go up to the LORD; perhaps I can make atonement for your sin."

∗ **If teachers want students to learn, teachers must praise students when they do well.** (At first teachers may need to praise students, even when students only approximate doing well.) Teachers must guide wisely, with a spirit of encouragement, when students need improvement. Students learn best from 20 parts praise to 1 part correction. [R8] When discipline is necessary, it must be firm and just. Good teaching helps the student learn self-discipline and self-assessment. **All learning is sequential!** Good teachers always begin instruction with the most basic concepts. Gifted students learn basics quickly. Some pupils need time before advancing to higher concepts. Thomas Armstrong, PhD in his book *In their Own Way* discusses various aptitudes that people use to learn. Moses masterfully instructed the Hebrews using many teaching methods in the ***Torah***.

The LORD also knew that the tendency or inclination of mankind is to act independently of a teacher (authority): as when the Hebrews murmured and rebelled against their teacher Moses, and murmured and rebelled against the LORD, shortly after crossing the Red Sea to Midian.

KJV Ex 15:24 And the people murmured against Moses, saying, What shall we drink?

Murmuring and rebellion, which is as witchcraft, always leads to terrible consequences. (1Sam 15:23) Here, as is often the case, rebellion can be attributed to the mixed multitude of people who crossed the Red Sea with Moses. (Ex 12:38) Some of the mixed multitude sought to do the will of the LORD. A few people sought only to be disruptive and to encourage others to partake in their rebellion. Spiritually-minded people need to associate with one another, for the LORD knows that mankind is rebellious from a youth upwards and small rebellions unchecked often lead to bigger rebellions.

KJV Gen 8:21 ... for the imagination of man's heart is evil from his youth.

The sinful nature common to all people must be trained away if people are to be productive for the good purposes of the LORD. Training in the ways of the LORD should begin at home, and may include tough testing if lessons are to be learned. (Deut 6:4-9 & 21) Moses took special care to personally teach the laws of God to young Joshua, who would lead the nation after Moses died.

∗ **The value to Joshua of having Moses as mentor and role model cannot be overemphasized.**

KJV Ex 24:13 So Moses arose with his assistant Joshua and Moses went up to the mountain of God.

In 1985, when I studied nutrition with Bernard Jensen, DC, PhD, he told me: [R25]

"The master appears when the student is ready."

Moses has been the master for nearly 3,500 years, and his teachings are as old as the hills and yet as modern and up to date as the latest magazines, TV programs or the morning newspaper.

Moses is my role model. Moses is my mentor. Moses is my teacher. Moses is my leader.

Even memorizing all 613 commandments of the ***Torah*** does not guarantee teaching success. The teacher of moral principles must have a relationship with the student for the student to see the principles in action in the teacher's life. This results in changed lives and a teaching success. Joshua learned well from his teacher, Moses. ∗ **Rules without relationship result in rebellion.**

∗ When challenging circumstances arise today, ask: **What Would Joshua Do?** or **W W J D ?**

Meditation

Joshua understood that part of the process of teaching and learning the lessons from the ***Torah***, including the 613 commandments, statutes and judgments, was to meditate upon them.

KJV Joshua 1:1 ... the LORD spake unto Joshua the son of Nun, Moses' minister saying
vs 8 This book of the law (***Torah***) shall not depart out of thy mouth; but thou shalt meditate (***hagah***) therein day and night, that thou mayest observe to do according to all that is written therein: for then thou shalt make thy way prosperous, and then thou shalt have good success.

Today, society is faced with people who are encouraging the practice of different forms of meditation. Bill Bright, PhD and Ron Jensen, PhD discuss this in their book *Kingdoms at War*:

"Eastern forms of meditation encourage people to focus on nothing, or within themselves, or on a universal power or force, or on some seemingly meaningless word. The Biblical concept of meditation is the idea of 'chewing' as a sheep chews its cud. As we meditate on Scripture, we allow God's thoughts to so permeate our lives that they actually become our thoughts, resulting in new behavior patterns and changed lives." [R1]

The authors outline several key steps to follow to develop the practice of Hebrew meditation.

1. Select a time, preferably daily, to be alone so that you can concentrate.
2. Select a verse or passage, one that when internalized will help you in a specific area, such as a besetting sin, a weakness, an area you have selected for growth, or an issue in your work.
3. Study the passage in context.
4. Memorize. You do not have to memorize verses in order to begin meditation, but memorization will significantly aid the process of internalization.
5. Visualize – make the truth of the Scripture as vivid in your mind as possible.
6. Personalize the Scripture passage and make it a prayer to God.
7. Take time to be quiet, to listen to what God has to say to you.
8. Take action, applying the commands and principles of Scripture to your life.

(Another good way to meditate on the Word of God is from teaching on radio, TV, CD or cassette.)

Dr. Ron Jensen also discusses applying principles of biblical 'Meditation and Memorization' to people's lives in his book *Biblical Meditation: A Transforming Disciple*.

∗ Training and growth from Moses as a teacher and learning the ***Torah*** involves the M & M's: 'Meditate upon and Memorize' the instructions of the LORD God, so as to obey them.

The Hebrew practice of meditation (***hagah***) also leads to a heart relationship with the LORD. Meditation develops a bond between man and God, intertwining the thoughts of the LORD and the thoughts of man into a single purpose: like two strands of cord being twisted together to form one (***echad***) double-stranded rope. The thoughts of the LORD and the thoughts of man becoming like one is what allowed the Tabernacle to be designed by God, conveyed to Moses and built by men.

The teaching/learning method of meditating on Scripture also involves the exclusion of the extraneous, false, and anti-scriptural sources of information of the world from influencing the mind and thoughts of the serious ***Torah*** student. Since the ***Torah*** and all the Word of God is error-free, dwelling on the Scriptures assures the ***Torah*** student of saturating himself with truth. To the outsider this procedure may seem to present the diligent ***Torah*** scholar as being very intolerant, narrow-minded or self-centered. However, to the insightful ***Torah*** student, this Hebrew method represents the best way to learn 'truth' apart from any error. Once the Hebrew student knows, understands and practices truth from the ***Torah***, then he is in the best possible position to recognize 'error', when encountered from other sources. Error that is found must be ignored or dismissed or rebuked. Errors should also be pointed out to other serious ***Torah*** students.

∗ The Hebrew method of study has the huge advantage of beginning with truth from the ***Torah***. The Greek method of searching for truth begins by gathering all related material, sorting the data and then deciphering truth from falsity. Treasury Agents often use Hebrew study as they initially examine legal currency exclusively, and later they quickly recognize counterfeit money as fraud.

Moses knew that Meditation on and Memorizing the ***Torah***, and learning the principles from God's Word, were important first steps toward developing a mature relationship with the LORD. The LORD's desire is that people act according to the perfection of the instruction of the Word that is in their heart; then and only then will their witness to the world be what God wants it to be.

KJV Deut 30:14 But the word [of the LORD] is very nigh unto thee, in thy mouth, and in thy heart, that thou mayest do it.

∗ Meditation upon the *Torah* pays great benefits in youth and dividends throughout life.

Shema – Hear and Obey

Moses wrote a special instruction to the Hebrews, warning them that doing as every man felt was right in their own eyes would not be healthy behavior in the land that God would give them.

JPS Deut 12:8 Ye shall not do after all that we do here this day, every man whatsoever is right in his own eyes.

The Book of Joshua reveals times of military success and victory for the first generation of Israelites, who dwelt in the Promised Land. Although Joshua learned his lessons well from Moses: apparently, Joshua was unable to train anyone else as a leader to follow him; and he was unable teach the next generation to obey and have an attitude of reverence for the statutes of the LORD.

The Book of Judges begins to chronicle the repetitive historical pattern of the Hebrew nation. The Israelites often turned their hearts away from the LORD and each man did as he felt was right; which sounds like today's value relativism that produces rebellion, indifference, chaos or anarchy.

KJV Judges 21:25 In those days there was no king in Israel; every man did that which was right in his own eyes.

Many generations of Hebrews living in Israel collectively 'did as every man felt was proper', or followed idolatrous Canaanite practices: causing unrest, hardship or lack of ***havdala*** unto the LORD. Moses prohibited offering children as fiery sacrifice to Canaanite gods, such as Moloch. (Lev 18:21) Yet, King Josiah had to prevent re-occurrence of sacrificing Hebrew children to Moloch. (II Kg 23:10) Jeremiah, the prophet, chastised Hebrews who had sacrificed their children to Moloch. (Jer 32:32-35)

The Hebrew nation often followed a leader (Judge, Prophet or King) who called people to obey Mosaic Law and repent of a sin affecting the nation. While the Hebrews briefly followed the leader, abandoned their idolatry and repented of sins, they temporarily restored ***havdala*** in ***Eretz*** Israel.

Today, amidst the demands of day-to-day life, by allowing the writings of Moses in the ***Torah*** to teach the will of the LORD and by practicing healthy ***Torah*** principles, all of God's people can enjoy the desired benefits of a relationship with the LORD: good Mental Health and peace of mind.

Teachers should encourage creative thought. However, when creativity violates principles of health from the ***Torah***, especially concerning moral and spiritual issues in which the will of the LORD is clearly known, then the results are always unhealthy, unwise and inappropriate.

The ***Shema*** (Deut 6:7), and Deuteronomy 11:19 exhort the Hebrew father (***av horah***) and mother (***am horah***) to teach (***yarah***) all the statutes of the LORD God to the following generation.

∗ Lessons and instruction from the ***Torah*** are what Hebrew parents are required to teach their children.

KJV Deut 6:6 And these words, which I command thee this day, shall be in thine heart: vs7 And thou shalt teach them diligently unto thy children, and thou shalt talk of them when thou sitteth in thine house, and when thou walkest by the way, and when thou liest down, and when thou ristest up.

JPS Deut 6:6 And these words, which I command thee this day, shall be upon thy heart; vs7 and thou shalt teach them diligently unto thy children, and shalt talk of them when thou sittest in thy house, and when thou walkest by the way, and when thou liest down, and thou risest up.

JPS Deut 11:19 And ye shall teach them your children, talking of them, when thou sittest in thy house, and when thou walkest by the way, and when thou liest down, and when thou risest up.

By following the mandate to teach, lessons learned by one generation would be perpetually handed down to the next generation. A nation that achieved health and prosperity and worship of God would teach these principles to their youth to insure that the next generation achieved no less success. Hebrew children have always related to their parents as: my father–my teacher and my mother–my teacher. The Hebrew concept of teacher and parent are very closely related. Grandparents are like parents, since there is no Hebrew word for grandfather or grandmother. This is the basic healthy pattern of home education that the LORD always wanted for His people. This same pattern of teaching is also vital today. There are many opportunities for children to find wrong role models who act as teachers and after whom many children may pattern their lives. Since Moses wrote the ***Torah***, Hebrew children have had the added opportunity and advantage of allowing the Word of the ***Torah*** to also be their teacher. Should a Hebrew child not have a parent or extended family to teach them, then the ***Torah*** by itself could become like a teacher!

∗ Remember that the ***Torah*** and the entire Word of the LORD is inspired and is profitable for doctrine, instruction and teaching unto righteousness for the person who takes it to heart.

(The Patriarchs demonstrated good and bad examples of teaching as will be seen in Ch 3.)

∗ Teaching begins at home. The child who learns well at home will learn well everywhere.

---------------------------------- References Ch 02 Teach ---------------------------------

[R1] Kingdoms at War\ by Bill Bright, PhD and Ron Jensen, PhD; pg 75-76 meditate upon the 'Word'
[R2] Biblical Meditation: A Transforming Disciple\ by Ron Jensen, PhD
[R3] Our Father Abraham\ by Marvin Wilson; pg 154-155
[R4] Milestones in Exodus\ by Jack Hayford
[R5] Survivor's Guide to Home Schooling\ by Luanne Shackelford and Susan White (1-800-A-FAMILY) (F o t F)
[R6] Teaching on the Torah\ by Rev. Chuck Smith; (Calvary Chapel) (1-800-272-WORD)
[R7] Teaching on the Torah\ by Chuck Missler, PhD (Koinonia House) (1-800-K-HOUSE-1)
[R8] Teaching on the Torah\ by J. Vernon McGee, PhD (Through the Bible) (1-800-65-BIBLE)
[R9] Teaching Our Kids to Kill\ by LtCol. D. Grossman (08-18-99) (Truths that Transform) (1-800-229-WORD)
[R10] The Ten Commandments\ by Laura Schlessinger, PhD and Rabbi Stewart Vogel
[R11] Lecture at Hidden Valley Ranch (in 1985)\ by Bernard Jensen, DC, PhD; master and student
[R12] Basic Institute in Life Principles\ by Bill Gothard; teaching life principles begins at home
[R13] Is Public Education Really Necessary?\ by Samuel Blumfield
[R14] Turning Point (Dec 97 or Jan 98 and 29 Dec 98)\ by David Jeremiah, PhD; fill a vessel – full vessel
[R15] Explore the Bible for Yourself\ from Discover the Word/ by Robinson, Matthews and DeHann
[R16] How to Read the Bible for All It's Worth\ by Doug Stewart and Gordon Fee
[R17] Ben Yehuda's Pocket Dictionary/ (English to Hebrew) (Hebrew to English)\ by Ehud Ben Yehuda

pg 197	parent	father-teacher	{ab}	***av horah***	\\ and David Weinstein
pg 197	parent	mother-teacher	{***am***}	***a(i)m horah***	

[R18] Strong's Concordance\ by James Strong, STD, LLD ***Rabbi*** means ***Torah*** teacher.

pg 466	hear	# 8085	H pg 118		***shema***	Deut 6:4
pg 668	meditation	# 1897	H pg 32		***hagah***	Josh 1:1
pg 748	one	# 259	H pg 10		***echad***	Gen 2:24
pg 590	learn/teach	# 3925	H pg 60		***lamad***	Deut 4:10
pg 999	teach/learn	# 3925	H pg 60		***lamad***	Deut 4:10
pg 999	teach	# 3384	H pg 52		***yarah***	Ex 4:12
pg 587	law/teaching	# 8451 (#3384)	H pg 123		***torah***	Deut 33:2 - Josh 1:1
pg 1000	teacher	# 3384	H pg 52		***yarah***	Hab 2:18
pg 1000	teacher	# 995	H pg 20		***biyn***	I Chr 25:8
pg 335	father-teacher	# 001	H pg 07	{***ab***}	***av horah***	Gen 2:24
pg 695	mother-teacher	# 517	H pg 13	{***am***}	***a(i)m horah***	Gen 2:24
pg 424	ground-land	# 127	H pg 8		***'adamah***	Gen 3:17

Tanakh or ***Tenakh*** includes the Law (***Torah***), Prophets, and Writings (Job, Psalms, Proverbs, Ecclesiastes)
Tanakh is an acronym for all Hebrew Scripture: ***T**orah* (Law), ***N**evi'im* (Prophets) and ***K**'tuvim* (Writings).
Adding vowels to the letters ***T N K*** results in the ***Tanakh***, which is also known as the Old(er) Testament.

[R19] The New Strong's Guide to Bible Words\ by James Strong, LLD, STD
[R20] Alexander's Hebrew Grammar\ by Ralph Alexander //to teach (infinitive) ***yaroh***
pg 77-79 he taught (3rd masculine singular) ***hora'ah*** (common three-letter root)
[R21] Interlinear Hebrew-English Old Testament\ by John R. Kohlenberger III
[R22] Theological Workbook of the Old Testament\ by Laird Harris, Glesson Archer, Bruce Waltke
[R23] A Survey of Old Testament Introduction\ by Glesson Archer, Jr
[R24] Hebrew and English Lexicon of the Old Testament\ by F. Briggs, S.R. Driver and C. Brown
[R25] The ***Shema*** (audio tape) (08-04-2001)\ by Rabbi Saul Wallach requirement to teach/learn
[R26] Rabbi Daniel Lapin (08-28-2001 audio)\ by James Dobson, PhD (Focus o t Family) biblical family values
[R27] 'Failing to Prepare means Preparing to Fail'\ quote by John Wooden
[R28] In Their Own Way\ by Thomas Armstrong, PhD; learning aptitudes – Moses used many methods
[R29] Nature, Nurture and the Power of Love (video)\ by Bruce Lipton, PhD; consequences of parenting
[R30] Analytical Key to the Old Testament – Vol 1 Genesis to Joshua\ by John Joseph Owens
[R31] Resentment (08-31-2004 audio)\ by Archibald Hart, PhD (Focus o t Family) like Cancer, destroys people from within
[R32] The Ultimate Guide to the Bible\ from Truth for Life (1-888-58-87884)
[R33] The Bible as History\ by Werner Keller // [R34] Closing of the American Mind/ by Alan Blum
[R35] Walk Through the Bible (The 7 Laws of the Learner)\ by Dr. Bruce Wilkinson
[R36] Education – Home School (09-03&04-02)\ by William Bennett, PhD; (Focus on the Family)
[R37] Home School Achievers (09-17to19-02)\ by Ballard brothers & Mike Ferris, PhD; (Focus on Family)
[R38] Children's Love and Limits (08-29&30-2001)\ with Bill Maier, PhD (F o t F) divorce – child growth
[R39] Every Child Can Succeed: (Making the Most of Your Child's Learning Style)\ by C. U. Tobias
The Way to Learn\ by Cynthia Ulrich Tobias (audio by James Dobson, PhD) (1-800-A-FAMILY)
[R40] Jars of Clay (4 audio cassettes)\ by Alistair Begg (Truth for Life) Caleb as a leader

(see pg 3 – COLOR Photos of 4 Vessels:) { Perceptive readers learn to: | read | – read between the lines. }

Chapter 2 – 4 Vessels (Jars) Demonstration/Teaching

A speaker brought out a large jar and several big stones. He put as many stones in the jar as the jar could hold. Then he asked the audience, "How many people think the jar is full?" Pause.

Then the speaker brought out some small rocks and put as many rocks in the jar as the jar could hold. Then he asked the audience, "How many people think the jar is full?" Pause.

Then the speaker brought out some tiny pebbles and put as many pebbles in the jar as the jar could hold. Then he asked the audience, "How many people think the jar is full?" Pause.

Then the speaker brought out a bag of fine gravel, and poured as much gravel in the jar as the jar could hold. Then he asked the audience, "How many people think the jar is full?" Pause.

Then he asked the audience, "What is the point of how the jar (vessel*) was filled?" Pause.

The speaker said, "You must put the big stones in the jar first. If you put fine gravel in the vessel first; you won't have any room for the big stones, small rocks and tiny pebbles later." [R14]

Then he asked the audience, "What lesson about life does this demonstration teach?" Pause.

The jar teaches the life principle that if the jar is analogous to human emotional makeup, then filling the jar with the largest, most important elements of Emotional Health first is paramount. Big stones may represent foundational aspects of Emotional Health: feeling loved, trust, respect for authority, discipline; small rocks may represent returning love, emotional control, self-esteem; tiny pebbles may represent safety, stability, security; and fine gravel may represent positive and negative interactions prompting growth from triumph and testing that promotes peace of mind. The vessel teaching helps explain the pattern of complete emotional development for all people. For the natural man who was taught or has learned these principles of life, his emotional makeup is complete and the vessel is as full as it can be. Unfortunately, nobody's vessel is ever perfectly formed or perfectly filled. The nearly filled jar/vessel represents many successful people today.

Trust and being loved begin as newborn–to–parent relationships and are models, so growing maturing children can develop the same sense of intimacy with the LORD and with other people. Everybody doesn't start with identical or perfect vessels, but all vessels need to be filled with the same elements if human development is to be complete. Unique vessels may necessitate some specialized programs to teach or develop essential emotional qualities. As a vessel is being filled, unfortunately, the vessel is also subject to damage. Vessels that are not well formed are also the easiest ones to damage. A vessel that is damaged through injury or disease is obvious, and demands immediate repair or attention. Damage to a human vessel that is not as obvious but is equally serious, is unseen physical, emotional or sexual abuse. All trauma/abuse can and must be healed before normal growth and development can proceed. A marred or broken vessel can be repaired with mortar or glue, but the repaired cracks may still be visible; just as even healed trauma from abuse frequently leaves emotional scars to the human vessel. Trauma that is not healed often leaves a jar fractured and not very useable. Trauma or abuse to people that is not healed may destroy people from within and/or cause people emotional problems throughout life.

∗ Learning and living lessons from the *Torah* will help everyone develop an emotionally full vessel.

Suppressed feelings of pain and anger from trauma may lead to a sense of bitterness and/or rage.
People afraid of more trauma learn not to express their true feelings, and learn to suppress pain.
Feelings of emptiness (problems without solutions) may lead to a sense of fear or hopelessness.
Life (a vessel) with emotional hopelessness + rage = the potential for self-destruction or suicide.
Life with emotional elements missing + many traumas = a potential for self-destruction or suicide.
Moses struggled with self-confidence, even though being described as 'mighty in word and deed'.

KJV Ex 4:10 And Moses said unto the LORD, O my LORD, I am not eloquent, neither heretofore, nor since thou hast spoken unto thy servant: but I am slow of speech, and of a slow tongue.

History is full of people whose lives do not include all essential elements of Emotional Health.
People unaware of their emotions may feel their jar is full, yet have a sense of lacking something.
People are often concerned with dressing up the outside of the vessel, rather than filling the inside.
A partly full vessel is often characterized by anxiety, fear, doubt, insecurity and/or low self-esteem.
Wise counsel from someone whose vessel is full, like parents, is essential to growth and healing.
Wrong counsel without attention to growth and healing may leave people empty and/or confused.
Filling the vessel as an adult and/or repairing trauma is difficult, painful and often requires help.
Adults with emptiness and trauma may wallow in despair or try to escape problems through drugs, alcohol, sex, sports, work, etc., rather than face reality and go through the painful, yet necessary growth/healing processes. ∗ Parents who fill their children's vessels earn a lifetime of respect. ∗

∗ A full vessel allows people to overcome obstacles. Obstacles destroy people with empty vessels.

Four Vessels – diagramed

(see pg 3 –
COLOR Photos of 4 Vessels:)

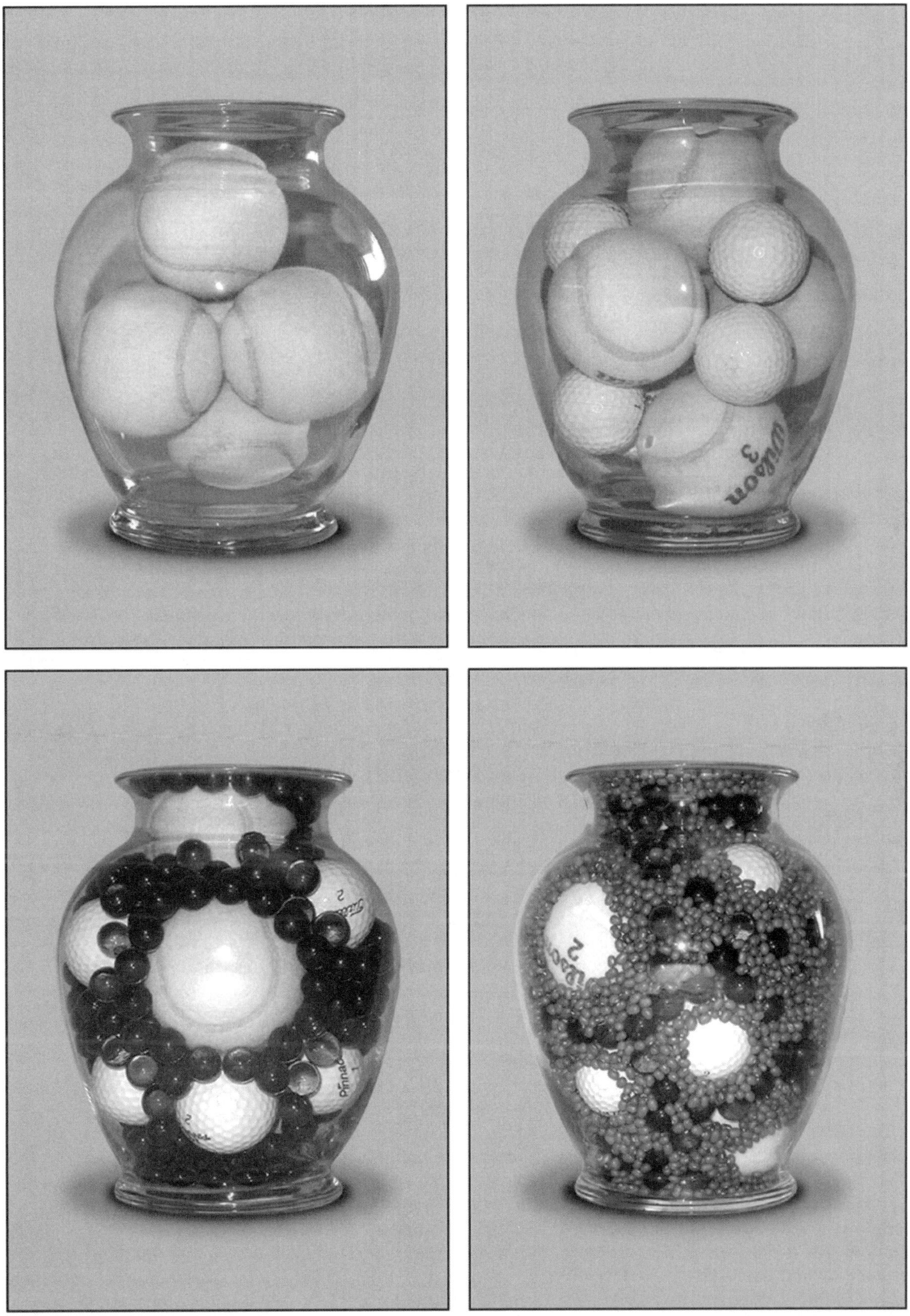

∗ Wise people often hunger and thirst to develop a full vessel, and they find fulfillment.

Chart 03 Patriarch Genealogy

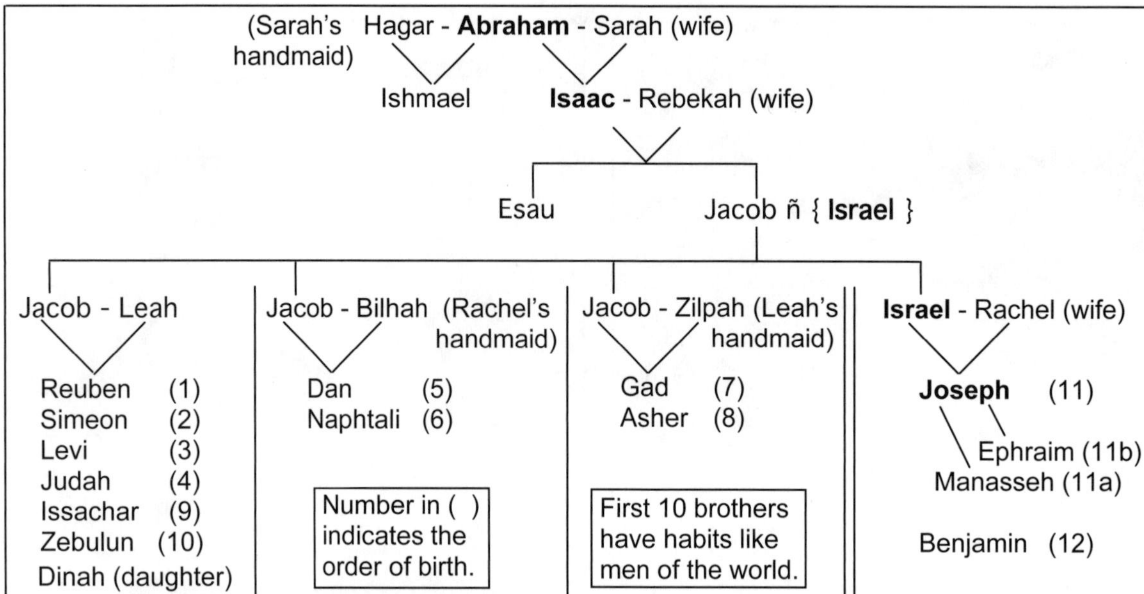

The twelve sons of Jacob {Israel} were conceived by two wives and two handmaids, and they became the twelve tribes of the nation of Israel. Joseph, by virtue of his righteousness and the failure of his brothers, inherits the double blessing of the firstborn. Joseph's two sons, Manasseh and Ephraim are each awarded the status of being the head of a tribe. When Levi becomes the tribe of the priesthood and is singled out for special consideration, twelve tribes apart from Levi can still be listed by separating Joseph into Ephraim and Manasseh; or the tribes can be listed as the original twelve by including Levi, and listing Ephraim and Manasseh together as Joseph. Though Manasseh was firstborn, Ephraim is consistently given greater blessings in the ***Torah***.

Abram means 'high father' and is the name by which Abraham was called in his youth.
Abraham means 'father of a multitude' and is transliterated ***Avraham***.
Eliezer, Abraham's trusted servant, means 'God of help' or 'God of Comfort' and is transliterated ***Eliyezer***.
Abraham is known as the first Hebrew. Hebrew means 'to cross over' or 'pass over' (as to cross a river).
Sarai is transliterated ***Saray***, and is the name by which Sarah was called in her youth.
Sarah is transliterated ***Sarah***. Sarah means mistress, lady, princess or queen.
Lot, Abraham's nephew, is transliterated ***Lot*** or ***Lowt***. Lot left Ur with Abraham and Sarah.
Lot's daughters each had an incest episode with Lot, and each bore a son from their incest with Lot.
  Moab, the son of Lot's firstborn daughter, became the father of the Moabite nation.
  Benammi, the son of Lot's younger daughter, became the father of the Ammonite nation.
  God cursed these nations, and they warred against the Hebrews during the Exodus from Egypt.
Isaac means laughter and sounds like laughter, and is transliterated ***Yitsak***, ***Yitzhak*** or ***Yitschak***.
  The ***Ahkidah*** – the 'Binding' of Isaac – prevented human sacrifice amongst the Hebrews.
Jacob means 'supplanter' {to supersede - especially by deceit} and is transliterated ***Yacov*** or ***Ya'akov***.
Jacob, after his redemption experience, when he wrestled with an angel, is called Israel. (Gen 32)
Israel means 'preservere or contend with God – (and prevail with God)' and is transliterated ***Yisrael***.
Joseph means 'increase' or 'add' and is transliterated ***Yoseph*** or ***Yowceph***.
Joseph was Israel's favored son, and Joseph wore a special coat or a 'coat-of-many-colours'.
Esau, Jacob's twin, means 'rough'. Esau is transliterated ***Esav***. (Gen 25:25)
  Esau was 'hairy' and 'red' or 'red-haired' man. {Esau was a man of the world: or a 'man's man'.}
  Esau moved east of the Jordan River to become the father of the Edomites.
  Amalek was a grandson of Esau, who became the father of the Amalekites.
  Amalekites continually confronted and often warred against God's chosen people: the Israelites.
Ishmael means 'God will hear' and is transliterated ***Yishmael***. (Gen 16:11-12)
Ishmael was a 'wild' man. {Ishmael was a tough-guy, and a don't-mess-with-me type man.}
Ishmael moved southeast to Saudi Arabia to become the father of the Arabs. (Gen 25:13)
  (The Hebrew language has no word for parent or grandparent or grandfather or grandmother.)

∗ In the ***Torah*** the meaning of a person's name(s) often reflects their origin, character and/or destiny.

Map 22 – Patriarch's Journeys

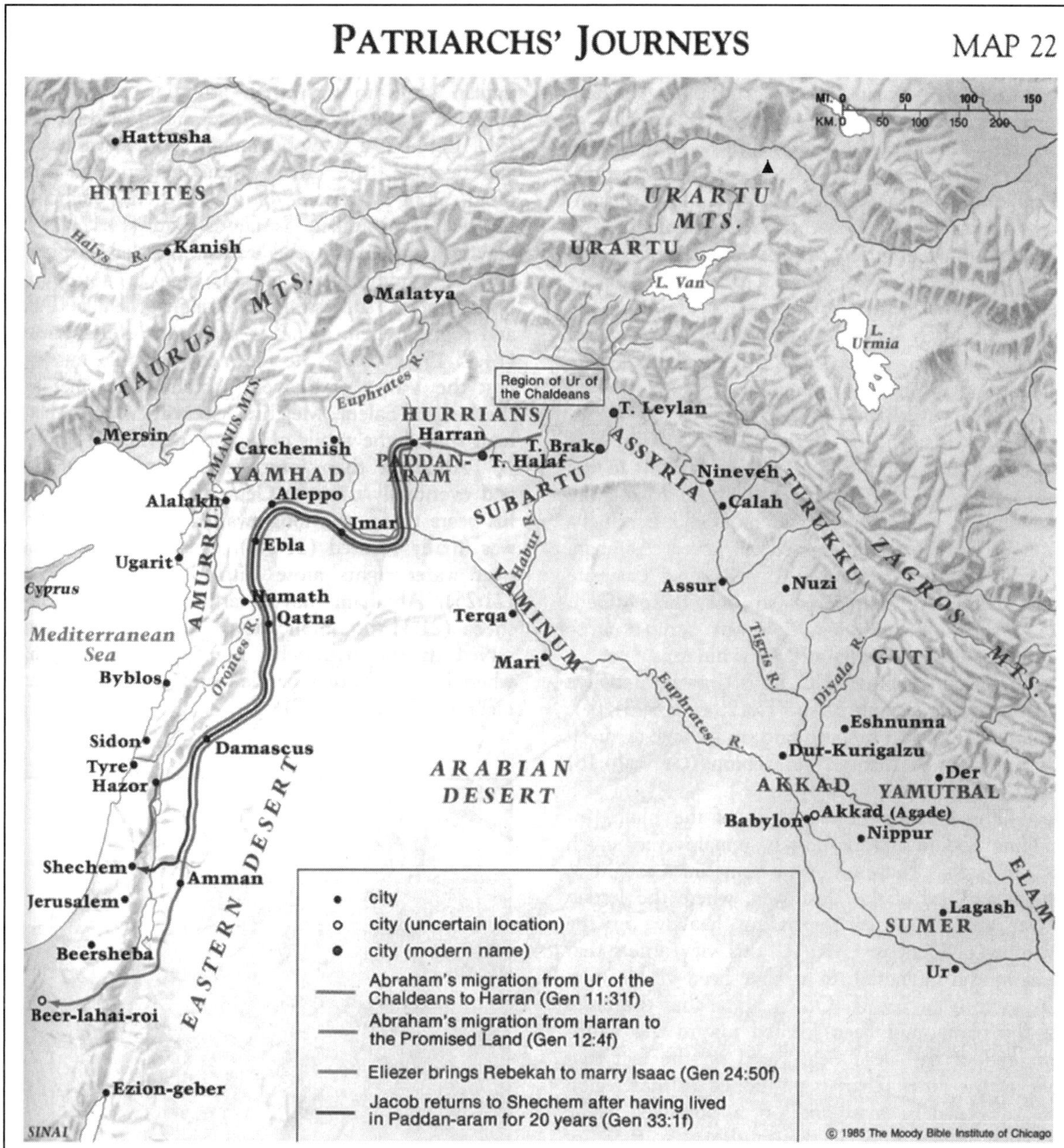

Much behavior in the ***Torah*** is descriptive – events are described they way they really happened. Descriptive behavior should not necessarily be considered ideal for following as a proper role model. Prescriptive behavior that is ideal to follow as proper role model is often exemplary of a principle that is discussed elsewhere in the ***Torah***. Isaac married Rebekah when they were virgins and they were faithful to one another throughout life, which is prescriptive of the marriage requirement. (Gen 3:16) Jacob married both Leah and Rachel, which describes what happened, but not what is prescribed as ideal by other instruction in the ***Torah***. Any behavior in the ***Torah*** may be evaluated as to whether it is appropriate or not by this same standard – whether it adheres to other instruction from the ***Torah***.

The ***Ahkidah*** was without precedence when it occurred, yet it established a standard that was to guide Hebrew culture for hundreds of years. The ***Ahkidah*** is evaluated to be prescriptive of proper behavior: by its comparission to the idolatrous Canaanite practice of child sacrifice to a god, Moloch, and by being exemplary of later Mosaic instruction in the ***Torah*** prohibiting child sacrifice. (Lev 18:21)

Map 23 – Abrahams Journey in Canaan and Egypt – pt 1

Abraham's Journey from 'Ur of the Chaldees' to Haran to Canaan to Egypt back to Canaan

Abraham's homeland was Ur of the Chaldees, where pagan people worshipped their false gods. In ≈1900 BC, Abraham, his wife Sarah, his father Terah, his nephew Lot and perhaps others left Ur. There are several cities in the region now called the 'Middle East' that were called Ur in Terah's day. Ur on the Euphrates River in modern Iraq is near a confluence with the Tigris River before the rivers enter the Persian Gulf, and it is discussed by many scholars as a likely site of Abraham's homeland. Ur on the Euphrates has been extensively excavated and Ur was a large advanced city in its time. Ur, a city in the Urartu region of modern Turkey, is another likely location for Abraham's homeland. Ur in the Urartu region in the plain of Cinar near Lake Van in southern Turkey is now known as Urfa. An inscription on a Temple to the god Khaldi discussed that Urarueans worshipped at least 63 gods and 16 goddesses called 'the Chaldees'; and life there likely wasn't conducive to genuine spirituality. From Ur, Abraham moved to Haran. Haran is near modern Turkey's southern border with Syria. Haran is one of the oldest continually inhabited cites. Abraham lived in Haran for perhaps ≈50 years. Since Abraham in Canaan was wealthy, it's very likely he became rich in the trade centers of Haran. Abraham likely remained in Haran until after the death of his father, Terah, who was 205 years old. When Abraham left Haran, he went directly to Shechem in Canaan, where built an altar to the LORD. Canaan is 'the land' that the LORD promised to Abraham, while Abraham was still living in Haran, and the land has since also been called the 'Promised Land'. Abraham undoubtedly had much of his wealth in the herds of cattle that he shepherded, and when there was a famine in Canaan, Abraham decided to leave Canaan and journey to Egypt.

In Egypt, Abraham went to Heliopolis (aka – On). In On, Abraham told Pharaoh that Sarah was his sister to avoid troubles with the Egyptians. In On, Abraham took Hagar as a handmaid to Sarah. According to the 'Code of Hammurabi', a very widely accepted legal handbook, a man could have a child by a surrogate handmaiden if his wife were barren. A son from a surrogate would be legal heir to his estate, and he could be treated as if he was born to the man's wife. In On, Ishmael was born to Abraham by Hagar, which caused strife between Sarah and Hagar. After Abraham returned to the Promised Land he dwelt in the plains of Mamre and the hills of Hebron, while Lot lived in Sodom. After a war Abraham met with Melchizadek from Salem. Abraham hosted three messengers from God and he negotiated the deliverance of Lot from Sodom prior to witnessing the destruction of Sodom and Gomorrah by fire and brimstone. Abraham received the promise of a son, later Sarah miraculously conceived and bore, Isaac. Abraham and Isaac traveled north from Hebron to Mt. Moriah to offer sacrifice — the ***Ahkidah***. Sarah was buried in the Cave of Machpelah. Abraham sent his servant, Eliezer, to Haran to find a bride of his own kin (Rebekah) for Isaac. Abraham remarried after Sarah's death and he had several more children. Isaac and Ishmael buried Abraham in the Cave of Mechpelah.

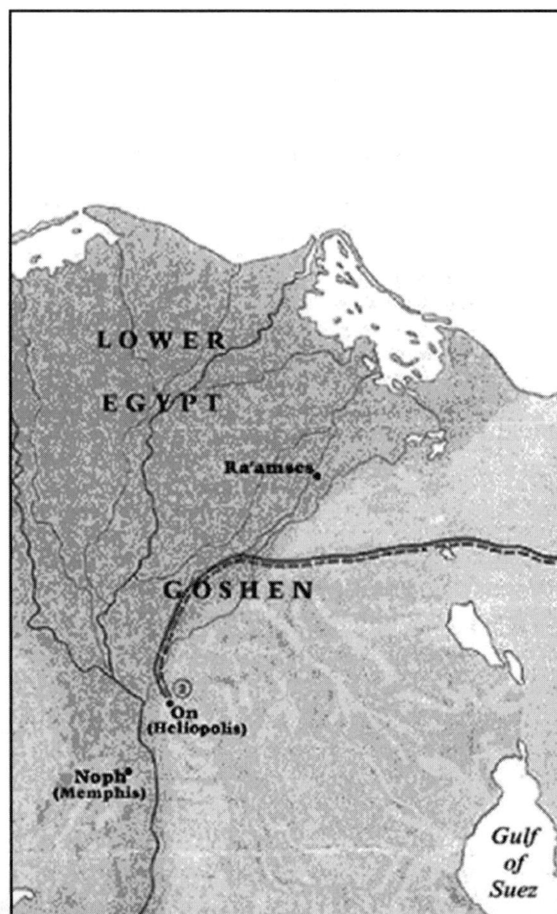

Genesis 1:1[+] with vowels and spaces between words.

בְּרֵאשִׁית בָּרָא אֱלֹהִים אֵת הַשָּׁמַיִם וְאֵת הָאָרֶץ׃ וְהָאָרֶץ
הָיְתָה תֹהוּ וָבֹהוּ וְחֹשֶׁךְ עַל־פְּנֵי תְהוֹם וְרוּחַ אֱלֹהִים

Map 23 – Abrahams Journey in Canaan and Egypt – pt 2

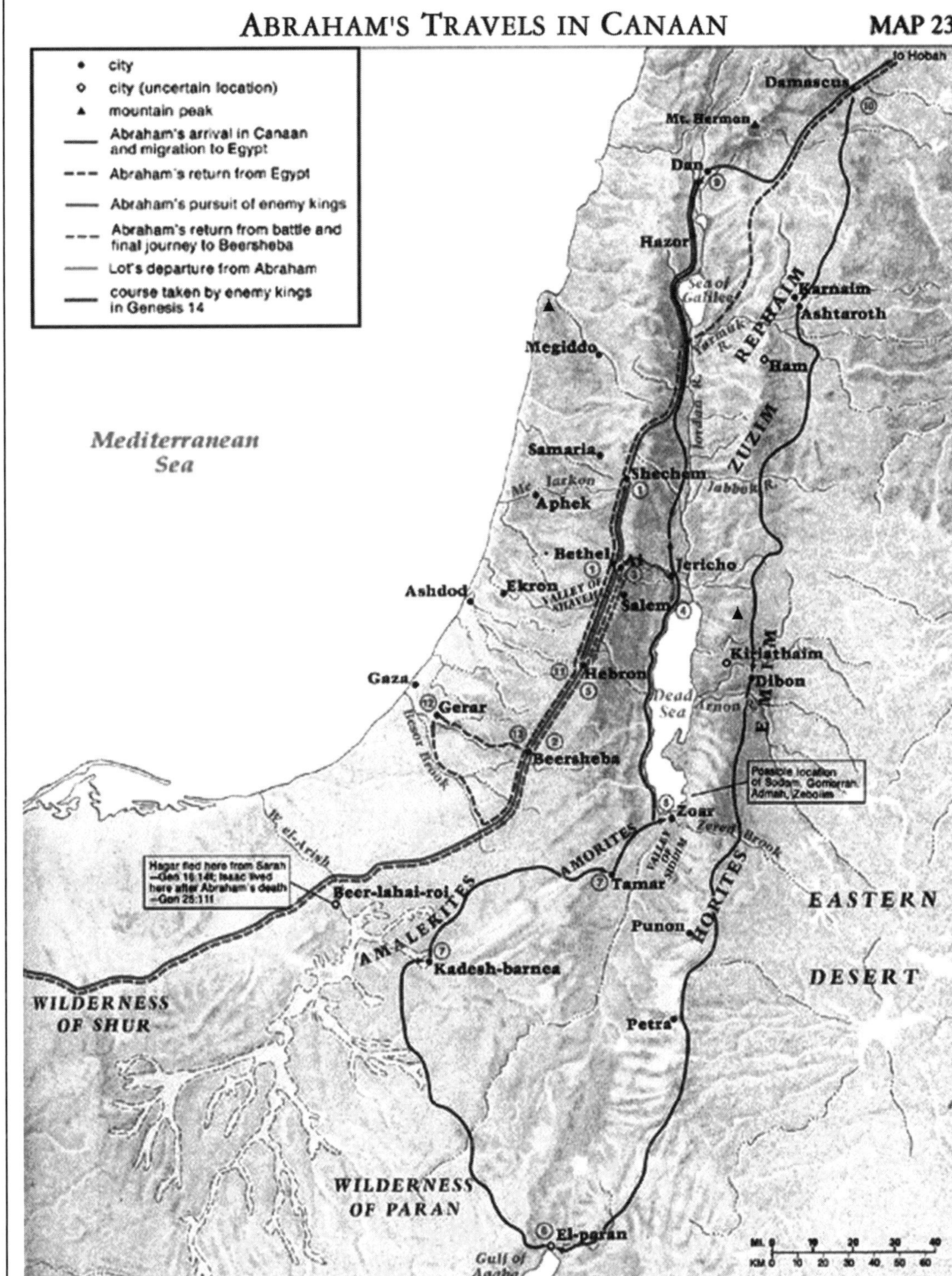

(א) בראשית.ברא.אלהים.את.השמים.ואת.הארץ:והארץ

(see pg 7) היתה.תהו.ובהו.וחשך.על-פני.תהום.ורוח.אלהים

Genesis1:1+ without vowels: with 'word dividers' (.) & ***silluq*** (**:**) to end a sentence.

Chapter 3 The Patriarchs:
Abraham, Isaac and Jacob; plus Joseph and his Ten Older Brethren
The *Ahkidah*

The lives of the Patriarchs: Abraham, Isaac and Jacob; as well as Joseph and his ten older brothers, provide interesting examples of faith and a lack of faith, and trust and a lack of trust.

By teaching principles of health, lessons learned by one generation would be perpetually handed down to the next generation. Thus, a family or a nation that achieved health and prosperity and worshipped the LORD, would teach these principles to their youth; to insure that the next generation would enjoy the same, if not greater health benefits and blessings from the LORD.

JPS Deut 6:6 And these words, which I command thee this day, shall be upon thy heart; vs7 and thou shalt teach them diligently unto thy children, and shalt talk of them when thou sittest in thy house, and when thou walkest by the way, and when thou liest down, and thou risest up.

The Patriarchs showed both good and bad examples of following the principle of the elder generation teaching faith and character to the next generation. God commanded Abraham to take his son Isaac, whom the LORD had promised would be the father of many nations, to Mt. Moriah. Here Abraham was told by God to bind Isaac upon an altar and offer his son, Isaac, as a sacrifice. This event is known as the 'binding' (***Ahkidah***). Isaac, being a man of ≈33 years old*^, could have resisted; however, both he and Abraham trusted the LORD and they both followed His instructions.

JPS Gen 22:2 And He [God] said: 'Take now thy son, thine only son, whom thou lovest, even Isaac, and get thee into the land of Moriah; and offer him there for a burnt-offering upon one of the mountains which I will tell thee of.'

Abraham was prepared to sacrifice his son, Isaac, on the altar until the LORD said, 'Stop'. Then, the LORD provided ('arranged' – or – 'saw to it') the lamb for Abraham to sacrifice.

When challenged by circumstances today, ask: **What Would Abraham Do?** or **W W A D ?**

KJV Gen 22:12-14 And he [God] said, Lay not this hand upon the lad, neither do thou any thing unto him: for now I know that thou fearest God, seeing thou has not withheld thy son, thine only son, from me. vs13 And Abraham lifted up his eyes and looked and behold behind him a ram caught in a thicket by his horns; and Abraham went and took the ram and offered him up as a burnt offering instead of his son. vs14 And Abraham called the name of that place Jehovah-jireh: as it is said to this day, In the mount of the LORD it shall be seen. {Jehovah-jireh is an impossibly poor transliteration – there is no 'J' sound in Hebrew. & Jehovah uses the vowels from ***A<u>do</u>n<u>a</u>i*** — (LORD) — with the consonants of ***YHWH***.} Either ***Y-hw-h-yireh*** or ***Yahweh-yireh*** are better transliterations.} {***Yireh*** means: see (as in – see to it –) [active verb] or provide}

As a role model, Abraham twice demonstrated a lack of trust in God's ability to keep him safe by telling a half-truth concerning the nature of his relationship with Sarah, his wife and also his half-sister: first to Pharaoh and again later to Abimelech. (Gen 12 & 20) Later, Isaac also mimicked Abraham's lack of trust when he dwelt in Abimelech's land with his wife, Rebekah. (Gen 26:6-16) ∗Isaac learned good habits from his father Abraham during the ***Ahkidah***, and Isaac also found out that the iniquity of the parents could be passed on to following generations. (Ex 20:5 & Num 14:18)

∗ Isaac learned both good and bad character traits from his father, Abraham.

Isaac went on to a long, prosperous life and he had twin sons: Esau, the elder, and Jacob, the younger. Jacob had twelve sons who prospered and multiplied, becoming the twelve tribes of the Israeli nation (also called the Hebrews and later called the Jews). Jacob's favorite son, Joseph, was betrayed by his brothers and sold into slavery in Egypt, where he eventually worked for Pharaoh. After the loss of Joseph, Jacob, although only one generation from Isaac, who demonstrated great faith on Mt. Moriah, found it difficult to believe that God would work all things together for good to those who trust in Him. The reason for Jacob's doubt may be traced to his upbringing. Jacob did not learn crucial faith lessons concerning the ***Ahkidah*** from his father, Isaac; on the contrary, Jacob learned deceit and trickery from his mother, Rebekah, and from his uncle, Laban.

JPS Gen 25:28 Now Isaac loved Esau, because he did eat of his venison; and Rebekah loved Jacob.

Symbolically, Esau and his descendants are consistently used to represent the physical or the worldly man. Before his redemption experience, Jacob often behaves like a man of the world; after redemption, when Jacob is renamed Israel, he is consistently representative of the spiritual man.

∗ Faith lessons learned by Abraham and Isaac during the Ahkidah weren't learned by Jacob and Esau.

Jacob

Rather than learning faith in the LORD from his father, Isaac, Jacob learned lying and trickery from his mother, Rebekah. After Jacob traded his birthright to Jacob for a bowl of lentil porridge, and Rebekah taught Jacob how to steal Esau's blessing by deceiving his father, Isaac.

JPS Gen 27:15 And Rebekah took the choicest garments of Esau her elder son, which were with her in the house, and put them upon Jacob her younger son.

Later, after Jacob fled to live with Rebekah's brother Laban, Jacob learned the same lesson. Here, Jacob contracted with Laban to marry Laban's younger daughter, Rachel. Later, when the wedding took place, Laban and Rachel and Leah tricked Jacob into marrying Laban's oldest daughter, Leah. Jacob then spoke to Laban the morning after Jacob's wedding to Leah.

JPS Gen 29:25 And it came to pass in the morning that, behold it [the woman Jacob married the night before] was Leah; and he [Jacob] said to Laban: 'What is this thou hast done unto me? Did not I serve thee for Rachel? Wherefore then hast thou beguiled me?

Many years later, when Jacob should have been accepting the apparent loss of his son, Joseph, as being the will of the LORD, he instead vowed to go down to the grave distrusting God.

JPS Gen 37:35 And all his sons and all his daughters rose up to comfort him [Jacob]; but he refused to be comforted; and he said: 'Nay, but I will go down to the grave to my son mourning.'

Moses knew well that **people retain what they learn from their elders**. Jacob was well-schooled in deceit and lying by the works of his mother and uncle; rather than having learned faith from his father, Isaac, and his father, Abraham. After Mt. Moriah Abraham is known as the 'father of faith'. ∗ **The faith of Abraham and Isaac are examples people should follow today.**

Jacob spent much time being miserable over Joseph's presumed peril when Joseph was actually quite safe. In fact, shortly afterward the Famine in Canaan, where Jacob lived, caused their whole family to move to Egypt, where there was still food. In Egypt, the LORD had elevated Joseph to the position of Prime Minister. ∗ Thus, Joseph, who was presumed lost, was actually quite safe and was used by God in a miraculous way to provide for the safety of his entire family.

KJV Gen 42:5-6 And the sons of Israel [Jacob] came to buy corn (***bar***) – [i.e. – grain] among those that came: for the famine was in the land of Canaan. vs6 And Joseph was governor [Prime Minister] over the land [Egypt]; and it was he [Joseph] that sold to all the people of the land.

Jacob had a part of his nature that was full of trickery, deceit, doubt and distrust, and yet Jacob also had a side of him that was very interested in spiritual matters. The name Jacob means supplanter. * [R3] Jacob resorted to deception and trickery twice: to take from his older brother, Esau, the spiritual privileges (birthright and blessing) that were rightfully Esau's according to the law. (Gen 25&27) It was after deceitfully stealing Esau's blessing that Jacob experienced an important spiritual event in his life at Bethel: the dream of the ladder from earth to heaven with angels ascending and descending. (Gen 28) The ladder is symbolic of a passageway from earth to heaven; ascending and descending angels may be symbolic of prayer and answers to prayer. Thus, Jacob had every expectation that prayer and answered prayer would be an important part of his life. Later, during Jacob's return to the Promised Land from Haran, Jacob wrestled with a 'man-of-God"** for control of his life. (Gen 31:13) At this time, Jacob's hip was pulled out of joint and he submitted to the LORD; and he had a change in character and his name was changed to Israel; *** and he received a blessing from the LORD. (Gen 32:24-30) [R4] After Jacob put away the idols in his life; then the LORD confirmed to Jacob the promise of a new name (Israel); and the LORD God renewed to Israel the promises He made to his {fore}-fathers. (Gen 35:2 &10-11) [R5]

∗ The man had two natures to his personality: an earthly or worldly nature by which he is first known — Jacob; as well as a spiritual nature by which he is later known — Israel.

∗ Wrestling with the LORD was part of Jacob's change in character and his redemption experience.
∗ This event shows the two natures within Jacob were wrestling with each other for control of his life.
* Jacob means: supplanter – to supersede, especially through deceit or treachery. [R13]
** possibly an angel of the LORD (Gen 23) *** Israel means: persevere/contend with God.
*^ Sarah was 90 years old when Isaac was born. (Gen 17:17)
Just after the ***Ahkidah*** (Gen 22:9) Sarah was 127 years old when she died. (Gen 23:1)
∗ Thus, Isaac was ≈33 years old at the time of the ***Ahkidah***. ∗

∗ Jacob's redemption experience was dramatic and is examplary for all people of all ages.

Joseph and his Testing

A careful study of the life of Joseph is needed to reveal how Joseph learned to have the faith and trust in God that he practiced so well while in Egypt. [R5] The life of Joseph compared to the lives of his 10 older brothers, shows the dual nature of the men and how this nature is reflected in their personalities. Joseph's coat was a status symbol of favored position within the tribe of Israel.

JPS Gen 37:3 Now Israel loved Joseph more than all his children, because he was the son of his old age; and he [Israel] made him [Joseph] a coat of many colors.

The life of Joseph demonstrates many examples the principles of Mental Health. Joseph's own brethren plotted to kill him, then threw him into a pit, and later sold him into slavery. (Gen 37) Joseph could have developed a bitter attitude: rage, anger, hate and a contentious spirit could have become the thought patterns of someone who wasn't trusting God. When in Egypt, Joseph became Potiphar's slave. Though Joseph may not have liked these circumstances, he didn't let them affect his relationship with God or his conduct with the people that God brought into his life. As a result of Joseph's continued application of the principles of proper Mental Health, he was the best witness for the righteousness of the LORD that he could be; and God continued to bless him.

* Today when circumstances are tough ask yourself: **What Would Joseph Do?** Or **W W J D?**

KJV Gen 39:3-4 And his [Joseph's] master [Potiphar] saw that the LORD was with him, and that the LORD made all that he did to prosper in his hand. vs4 And Joseph found grace in his sight, and he served him: and he made him overseer over his house, and all that he had he put into his hand.

Potiphar's wife saw that Joseph was a man of fine character, and she tried to entice him into a morally improper sexual relationship. When Joseph refused to get involved with Potiphar's wife, she unjustly accused him of rape and Joseph was thrown into prison for three years.

KJV Gen 39:21 But the LORD was with Joseph, and showed him mercy, and gave him favor in the sight of the keeper of the prison. vs22 And the keeper of the prison committed to Joseph's hand all the prisoners that were in the prison; and whatever they did there, he was the doer of it.

Once again Joseph found himself in unfavorable circumstances, despite having shown great restraint, by not doing what he knew was morally improper. Instead of Joseph immediately receiving some great reward from God for his restraint, he ended up in prison. Surely, this would have been cause for Joseph to be angry and upset, but once again he responded by doing the best that he could do in the circumstances in which he found himself. Today, the rewards of following a godly lifestyle may not be immediately apparent, but despite this, the sanctified morality is still the course of action that allows the LORD to bestow His blessings upon His people.

* It was because Joseph remained committed to do the will of his LORD, that the LORD blessed him.
* Joseph's commitment is why the LORD gave Joseph the interpretation of the prisoner's dreams.

KJV Gen 40:8 And they [the butler and the baker] said unto him, We have dreamed a dream, and there is no interpreter of it. And Joseph said unto them, Do not interpretations belong to God? Tell me them, I pray you.

After interpreting the dreams, Joseph had told the butler of his own unjust imprisonment and asked the butler to remember him. The butler was released from prison and restored to his former position as chief butler to Pharaoh, but he forgot Joseph. Joseph continued in prison for two more years, despite having been faithful to the LORD. This could have caused Joseph much mental distress, but Joseph continued to wait upon the LORD for renewed strength. Today, as well, if we endure hardships for doing what is right before the LORD God, this is commendable. Later, as the LORD established Joseph to be the second most important ruler in Egypt, he refused to give any credit for his success to himself; rather, he encouraged looking to the LORD for peace of mind.

Happiness depends upon the external circumstances in life; but love, joy and peace of mind come from the LORD and resides in the heart of a man. The special coat 'of many colours' or 'seamless coat' or 'coat with sleeves' was a symbol of this privileged relationship and privileged position that Joseph enjoyed with his father and his LORD. In the Scripture, the type of garment a person wears is often symbolic of his/her walk with the LORD; whether it be positive or negative.

KJV Gen 41:16 And Joseph answered Pharaoh, saying, It is not in me: God shall give Pharaoh an answer of peace.

∗ Testing can result in Triumph or Tragedy depending upon a person's preparedness.

Joseph and his Ten Older Brethren

When Joseph's brethren came into Egypt to buy grain, Joseph was in a position to repay his brethren with unkindness for the unkind, unlawful deeds they did unto him, but he refrained. Joseph, who was actually happy to see his brothers, could have immediately told his brothers that he was their brother, whom they had years before sold into slavery. Instead, Joseph chose to conceal his true identity for a short time, so he could arrange circumstances that would cause his brothers to come to admit their guilt before the LORD God and the law. Then after his brothers sought forgiveness for their sins, Joseph revealed himself to them. The activities of Joseph's older brothers also show the tremendous negative power of peer pressure in doing evil deeds. None of Joseph's brothers as individuals might have had the courage and the determination to consider murdering their brother or selling him into slavery, and then lie to their father about his whereabouts, but as a group, with their collective mischievous (evil) thoughts reinforcing one another, the plot against their brother seemed to be quite a reasonable course of action.

KJV Gen 44:16 And Judah said [to Joseph], What shall we say unto my lord? what shall we speak? or how shall we clear ourselves? God hath found out the iniquity of thy servants: behold, we are my lord's servants, both we and he also with whom the cup is found.

Joseph confronted his brothers and established 'boundaries' so their sin would not be repeated. Scripture reveals that after this confession, Joseph and his brothers went on to have the kind of relationship with one another that God intended. This attitude of forgiveness by Joseph was consistent with the writings of Moses, although the instructions were not yet written.

Forgiveness may be defined as giving up the right to hurt other people after they hurt you.

KJV Lev 19:18 Thou shalt not avenge, nor bear any grudge against the children of thy people, but thou shalt love thy neighbor as thyself: I am the LORD thy God.

While Joseph's life exemplifies the godly character traits of love, the undisciplined, unruly habits of his 10 older brothers suggests a lack of love and little peace of mind in their lives. This sharp contrast of character between Joseph and his ten older brethren suggests a sharp contrast in how they were raised. Jacob, in his early days as a father, may not have taken the time to instruct and discipline his sons properly; or the ten older brothers' behavior might be linked to the bickering and jealousy they learned from Jacob's two wives and their two handmaids; or Joseph may have been the only son who was interested in listening to the instructions of his father; or Israel may have only late in his life known enough about parenting to teach love to Joseph.

∗ Apparently, Jacob and his life style in Haran served as the primary role model for the 10 older sons; but Israel taught Joseph love. ∗ Thus, only Joseph developed a Godly character and only Joseph was used by the LORD to witness the power of the LORD to the ungodly Egyptian world. ∗ Righteousness is not something people are born with; righteousness is what people become when they seek to be obedient to the instructions of the LORD that Moses wrote in the ***Torah***.

The ***Torah*** also records that Moses lived his life according to the principle of love. (Ch 1) Anyone who is living his/her life as Joseph and Moses did (a moment-to-moment walk with God) knows instinctively from the spirit of the LORD, what is the proper behavior whether he/she had or had not read these instructions in the ***Torah***. Joseph's consistent acts of kindness toward his brethren led them to acknowledge their iniquity, when they returned to Joseph the second time. (Gen 43-45) The first step in repentance is often to examine one's own life before the law and to admit one's own failure to the LORD. Only after confessing one's sins, and repenting of the sins, and planning in one's heart not to do them in the future, and accepting that the LORD is able to forgive the sins; can true fellowship with the LORD and fellowship with one's brethren be restored.

∗ The life of Joseph and his brethren demonstrates well repentance and forgiveness.

God calls His people to set themselves apart (be sanctified – ***havdala***) from the behavior patterns of their heathen neighbors. (Lev 11:44; Lev 19:2; Lev 20:7-8; Lev 21:8,15,23: and Lev 22:9,16)

KJV Lev 20:7 Sanctify yourselves therefore and be ye holy: for I am the LORD your God.

∗ Joseph learned loving, godly personality traits from Israel after Israel's redemption experience, which allowed Joseph to be successful and respected, even though he often faced adverse circumstances in his life; while Joseph's 10 older brothers learned worldly personality traits from Jacob before his redemption event, which permitted their cruel, disorderly, inappropriate behavior.

∗ The LORD always desires followers who are striving to develop character traits like Joseph.

------------------------------------ **References Ch 3 Patriarchs** --

[R1] Back to Bethel\ by J. Vernon McGee, PhD – transformation & redemption of Jacob to Israel
[R2] Precepts (radio)\ by Kay Arthur; – health principles learned from lives of the Patriarchs
[R3] The Road to Redemption\ by Rabbi Burton L. Visotzky studies in Exodus
[R4] Study in Exodus (audio)\ by Bob Phillips (Come Up Higher 1-800-313-2202) Amalek battles Israel
[R5] The Constant Fight with Amalek (audio)\ by David Gurevich (Beit Tikvah 02-15-03) flesh battles spirit
[R6] Teaching on the Torah\ by Rev. Chuck Smith; (Calvary Chapel) (1-800-272-WORD)
[R7] Teaching on the Torah\ by Chuck Missler, PhD (Koinonia House) (1-800-K-HOUSE-1)
[R8] Teaching on the Torah\ by J. Vernon McGee, PhD (Through the Bible) (1-800-65-BIBLE)
[R9] Heroes of the Faith\ by David Jeremiah, PhD; (Turning Point) (July 2001); (1-800-947-1993)
[R10] Gleanings from Genesis\ by R. C. Sproul, DrS; (Renewing Your Mind) (1-800-435-4343)
[R11] Prodigal People\ by Woodrow Kroll ; Jacob (Back to the Bible) (1-800-811-2397)
[R12] Abraham – Jacob – Joseph (3 movies)\ by TNT
[R13] Webster's New World Dictionary (1966); pg 1465 supplant - supersede, especially by deceit/treachery
[R14] Genesis Commentary\ by George Bush; life principles from the lives of the Patriarchs
[R15] Commentary on the Torah\ by Richard Elliot Friedman
[R16] The Patriarchs and Prophets\ by Ellen G. White; discusses the lives of the Patriarchs
[R17] Nelson's Illustrated Bible Dictionary\ ed by Herbert Lockyer, Sr. – pg 666 Cave of Machpelah
[R18] Strong's Concordance\ by James Strong, STD, LLD – meanings of names

pg 12	Abram	# 087	H pg 8	***Avram***	high father	– childless for 100 years	(Gen 11:26)
pg 11	Abraham	# 085	H pg 8	***Avraham***	father of a multitude	– while still childless	(Gen 17:5)
pg 877	Sarai	# 8297	H pg 121	***Saray***	dominative (from #8269) – having rank or position		
pg 877	Sarah	# 8283	H pg 121	***Sharah***	mistress - female noble – lady, princess or queen		
pg 525	Isaac	# 3327	H pg 51	***Yitzhak***	laughter, mockery – ***Yitschak*** sounds like laughter		
pg 302	Eliezer	# 461	H pg 13	***Eliyezer***	God of help	– Abraham's trusted servant	(Gen 15:2)
pg 637	Lot	# 3876	H pg 59	***Lowt***	a veil or covering	– lived a checkered life	(Gen 12:5)
pg 310	Esau	# 6215	H pg 92	***Esav***	rough – {Esau = red or hairy or red-haired (Gen 25)}		
pg 534	Jacob	# 3290	H pg 51	***Yacov***	* heel-catcher - supplanter – to supercede by deceit		
pg 526	Israel	# 3478	H pg 53	***Yisrael***	*** who wrestled with God – will rule as or with God		
pg 550	Joseph	# 3130	H pg 48	***Yoseph***	let him add (Rachel desired God 'add' to her another son)		
pg 1208	Zaphnath-paaneah	# 6847	H pg 101	(may mean –	God lives/speaks or revealer of secrets)	– pg 16 Step Pyramid	
pg 525	Ishmael	# 3458	H pg 53	***Yishmael***	God will hear	{Ishmael = a wild man	(Gen 16:12)}
pg 431	Hagar	# 1904	H pg 32	***Hagar***	mother of Ishmael – origin and meaning are unknown		
pg 578	Laban	# 3837	H pg 58	***Laban***	Jacob's father-in-law	from #3836 – white	(Gen 29:10)
pg 138	bound	# 6123	H pg 91	***aqad***	bound	*THE Key* Hebrew event	(Gen 22:9)
the binding (from)		# 6123	H pg 91	***Ahkidah***	'binding' of Isaac	on Mt. Moriah	(Gen 22:9)
pg 219	corn	# 1250	H pg 23	***bar***	corn if denotative	gain if conotative	(Gen 42:5)
pg 159	Caleb	# 3612	H pg 55	***Kaleb***	– attack {as a dog}	a great soldier	(Num 14:6)
pg 538	Jehovah-Jireh	# 3070	H pg 46	***Yahweh–yireh***	– LORD will see (– see to it) or provide		(Gen 22:14)

{The verb ***yireh*** is used in the active tense ('see' or 'see to it') – from Abraham's standpoint 'to provide'.}
{Jehovah uses the vowels of ***Adonai*** — (LORD) — with the consonants of ***YHWH***.} Because Hebrews often wanted to avoid pronouncing the ***YHWH*** name of God, some Jewish scribes made marginal notes to the ***Torah*** Scroll so the reader could pronounce ***Adonai*** in place of pronouncing the Tetragrammaton that was in the text. Then, later, ***YHWH*** and ***Adonai*** became mixed as Jehovah, and was subsequently copied into the ***Torah*** text.
[R19] Adventures in Faith: The Life of Abraham\ by M. R. DeHann, MD
[R20] A Walk through the Bible\ by Lesslie Newbigin Ch 2 – Chosen by God - pg 13-21
[R21] Jacob The Fools God Chooses\ by David Roper
[R22] Changing Wanderers to Worshippers\ by Chuck Swindol, PhD (Insights for Living 1-800-772-8888)
[R23] The Life Joseph (radio – April/May 2000)\ by David Jeremiah, PhD; (1-800-947-1993)
[R24] What's in the Bible\ by R. C. Sproul, DrS and Robert Wolgemuth (Ligonier 1-800-435-4343)
[R25] How People Grow\ by Henry Cloude, PhD and John Townsend, PhD (1-800-NEW-LIFE)
[R26] Joseph Beloved–Hated–Exalted\ by F. B. Meyer, BA
[R27] Joseph, The Triumph of Character\ by John G. Butler
[R28] New International Version (1978 'NIV') (radio 05-19-04)\ by Hank Hanagraph of 'CRI' (1-888-7000-CRI)
NIV translated as a 'dynamic equivolent' or 'thought for thought' // KJV and JPS = 'word for word' translation
{NIV may either add clarity to translation or may be misleading – depending upon the translators' perspective.)
[R29] In the Beginning (ARTISAN films movie)\ directed by Kevin Costner (Adam to Moses)
[R30] Great Pharaohs (3 videos)\ by The Learning Channel; (#1) Ramses II – likely Pharaoh during the Exodus
[R31] 3,458 Bible People and Places\ by Thomas Nelson Publishers
[R32] Fascinating Bible Facts, People, Places, Events\ by David Howard, PhD
[R33] God Wrote a Book\ by James McDonald; authenticates the miraculous nature of the Bible

Map 24 – Patriarchs in the Promised Land

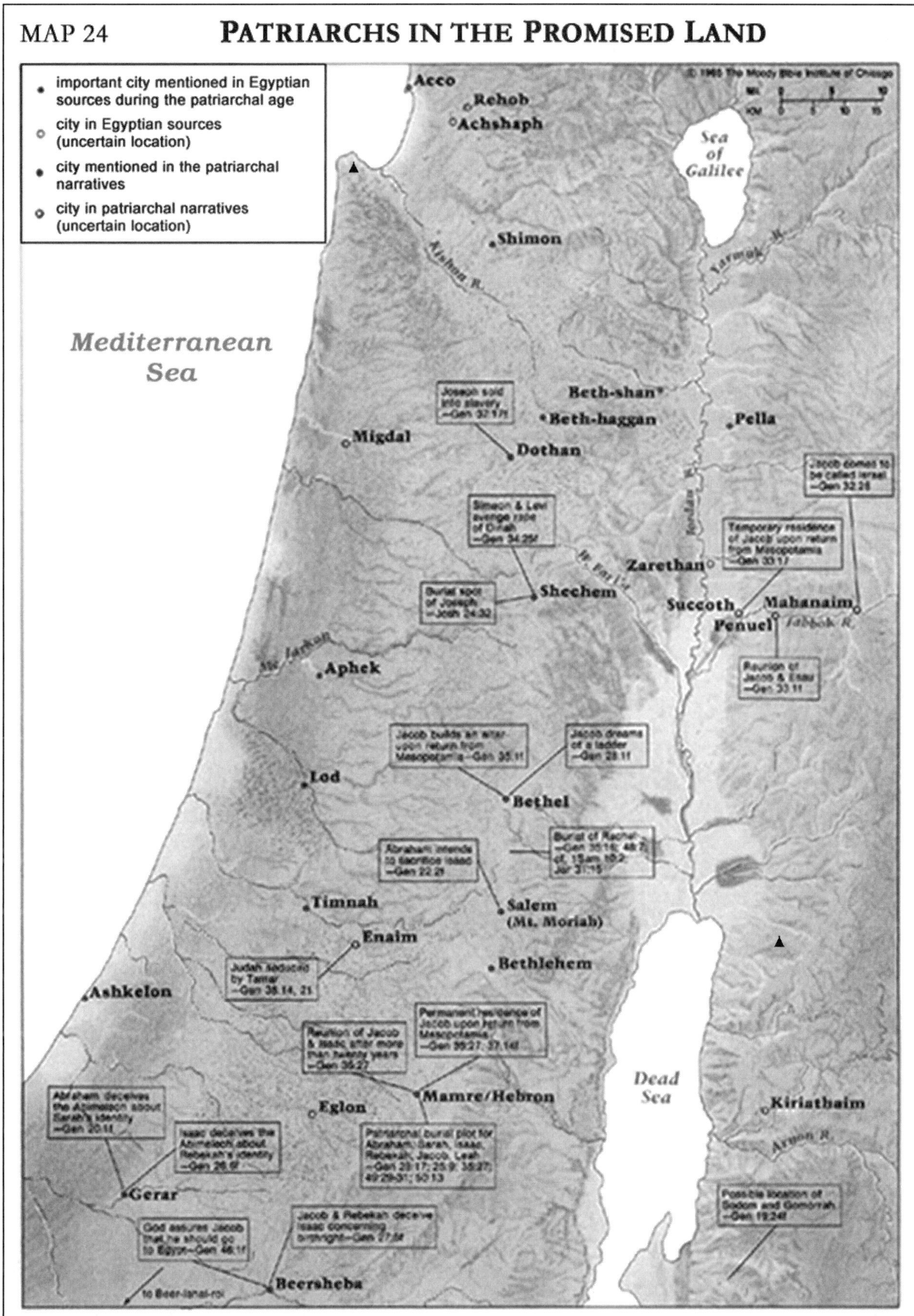

Joseph's Ten Older Brothers

The author suggests that a useful exercise for any ***Torah*** student is to list the examples of love that Joseph demonstrated in his life, and compare this to the examples of improper habits by Joseph's older brothers. Of course, the next and most important activity is to discipline one's own life to maximize the healthy traits of love (Love-Ch 1) and to minimize habits God hates (below). Procedures to develop godly principles and avoid the unwanted character traits are – M and M's – – Memorize and Meditate – upon godly character traits as recommended in *Kingdoms at War*. (Ch 2)

Character traits that the LORD hates include:

A proud look
- an attitude of life that declares its ability to live without the LORD.
- relying upon heritage or boasting of position; rather than seeking personal spiritual growth.
- assumed-righteousness or self-righteousness rather than seeking the LORD's holiness.
- judging oneself to be superior to others.

A lying tongue
- distorting the truth, especially for personal gain.
- not accurately representing the truth, so someone else suffers.

Hands that shed innocent blood
- murder or developing/promoting feelings of anger and hate toward guiltless people.

A heart that devises wicked imaginations
- scheming to do evil rather than looking for ways to do good.
- dwelling upon what's wrong rather than cooperating with what's right.

Feet that are swift to run to mischief
- joining in the rebellion of peers rather than foreseeing evil and fleeting away.
- encouraging others to follow a rebellion.

A false witness that speaketh lies
- when a person's walk is not consistent with his talk.
- gossip: as in discussing grievances with other people who were not part of the original problem, nor are they part of any scenario for a solution.

He that seweth discord amongst brethren
- looking for ways to create doubt, confusion, anger and discord, rather than seeking to create faith, trust and unity.
- murmuring or rebelling against authority.

(As when a few people spoke against Moses and encouraged worship of the golden calf while Moses was up on Mt. Sinai for 40 days, which put the entire Hebrew nation in trouble.)

The '*Echad*' *Torah*

Torah study most often considers the five books of Moses as if they were one (***echad***) book. In ≈550 BC, in Babylonian exile, the ***Torah*** was translated into Aramaic and is called the *Targum*. In ≈250 BC, during Greek occupation of Israel, seventy Hebrew scholars went to Alexandria, Egypt where the ***Tanakh***, including the ***Torah***, was translated into Greek and is known as the *Septuagint*. In the *Septuagint*, the five books of Moses are known as the *Pentateuch*, which means five books. As an aid to clarity, in ***Torah*** study the author often treats the ***Torah*** as a 'penta-unity'. The phrase: 'the whole is greater than the sum of its parts' is certainly applicable to ***Torah*** study, as several aspects of 'one' concept are often discussed in each of Moses' five books. Certainly, any individual book (Genesis, Exodus, Leviticus, Numbers or Deuteronomy) is worthy of being studied on its own. Each book has a unique theme or personality all on its own, apart from the other four ***Torah*** books. Yet, studying the five books a 'whole' allows following the lives of people, or the history of a nation, or the discussion of a concept or the development of a principle, or the application of a principle as it unfolds throughout the ***Torah***. Is the ***Torah*** five individual books, or is the ***Torah*** one united book?

∗ The ***Torah*** is both five books in one unity, and the one ***Torah*** consists of five component books. ∗

Keeping the concept of 'compound unity' in mind during ***Torah*** study will be helpful for all students.
In anatomy, the hand is a compound unity, as the four fingers and thumb function together as 'one'.
In athletics, a triathalon is a compound unity, as swim, bicycle and running races are 'one event'.
In chemistry, at the 'triple point', water exists in three states simultaneously – solid, liquid and gas.
In optics, light is a compound unity, as common 'white' sunlight consists of separate distinct colors.
In music, a chord is a compound unity, where 'three' individual notes are played together as 'one'.

∗ In *Torah* study the concept of 'compound unity' may help to clarify several key issues.

Chapter 4 Emotions
Grace and Trust

After the fall of mankind from the 'Garden of Eden', the LORD recognized His people would be confronted by challenges and difficult circumstances in a world, where not all people desire to do His will or follow His Law. In fact, many people would directly oppose the LORD's will. (Gen 6) God's instructions in the ***Torah*** require His people not to be conformed to the ways of this world; His desire is for them to daily renew in their minds a commitment to do His will. The blessings and benefits of obeying ***Torah*** instructions include living in the world, while not being part of the world; and realizing the emotional balance and stability that are necessary for Mental Health. (Deut 8:1) Ultimately, conforming to the will of the LORD as defined by Moses in the ***Torah*** means being a witness to the people of the world who are lost, so they too may find the LORD's will for their lives.

Moses understood that trust and respect are two basic emotional qualities needed for God's people to enjoy the good health that the LORD desired for them. Conversely, Moses knew fear causes the worry and doubt, which lead to stress and is frequently the root cause of poor health.

Anxiety, worry and stress are best defined as trying to assume responsibility for a relationship, situation or scenario in which case the LORD does not intend that person to take responsibility. [R1]

Moses asked the Hebrews to put their trust in the LORD and follow his statutes. (KJV Deut 5:29)

JPS Deut 5:26 Oh that they [the Hebrews] had such a heart as this always, to fear Me, and keep all My commandments, that it might be well with them, and with their children forever!

When Moses had decisions to make in his life, whether big ones or small ones, he followed a procedure: Moses prayed to God and asked for God's grace. Grace is always a two-way street! **Grace always includes asking God's forgiveness for sin; as well as seeking to do God's will.**

KJV Ex 33:13 Now therefore I pray thee, if I have found grace in thy sight, show me now thy way, that I may know thee, that I may find grace in thy sight: and consider that this nation is thy people.

Moses trusted God and followed His commandments, even during what were very demanding circumstances and events, such as the crisis of having Pharaoh's armies attacking from the rear and having the Red Sea before you and having no place to turn to the left or the right.

JPS Ex 14:13 And Moses said unto the people [Hebrews]:
'Fear ye not, stand still, and see the salvation of the LORD, which He will work for you to-day,
... vs14 The LORD will fight for you, and ye shall hold your peace.'

At this time, God provided a spectacular miracle: the parting of the Red Sea, so the Hebrews could flee the Egyptians and cross to Mt. Sinai on dry ground. The LORD provides miracles for His people today as well. Even though to observers in the world, today's miracles may not be as spectacular as the 10 Plagues on the Egyptians or the parting of the Red Sea, they are no less real and they still are provided by God on the basis of trust, obedience and prayer. Moses called for God's people to trust and rely on God to supply all their needs. For Moses, depending upon God for day-to-day necessities was no different than depending upon Him in crisis situations.

KJV Ex 16:4 Then the LORD said unto Moses, "Behold, I will rain bread from heaven for you: and the people shall go gather a certain rate every day that I may prove them, whether they walk in my law or no."

Fear and the stress that fear causes are not what the LORD wants for His people. Moses encouraged the Hebrews 17 times to 'fear not' and maintain a proper emotional perspective.

JPS Gen 15:1 ...'Fear not, Abram, I am thy shield, thy reward shall be exceeding great.'

NKJV Gen 26:24 ... "I am the God of your father Abraham: do not fear, for I am with you."

NJPS Ex 14:13 ... "Have no fear! Stand by, and witness the deliverance which the LORD will work for you today; for the Egyptians whom you see today you will never see again."

1901 RV Ex 20:20 And Moses said unto the people, Fear not: ...

NASB Num 14:9 Only do not rebel against the LORD; and do not fear the people of the land, ...

RSV Deut 1:21 '... take possession [of the Promised Land] ... ... do not fear or be dismayed.'

KJV Deut 31:6 Be strong and of a good courage, fear not nor be afraid of them [the ungodly nations]: for the LORD thy God, he it is that doth go with thee; he will not fail thee, nor forsake thee.

* Fear is an expensive emotion that will rob people of health and of respect for the LORD.

Bitter Water

For a woman accused of adultery the 'bitter water' test determined her infidelity or innocence.

KJV Num 5:17 And the priest shall take holy water in an earthen vessel; and of the dust that is in the floor of the tabernacle the priest shall take, and put it into the water: ...vs19 And the priest shall charge her by an oath, and say unto the woman, If no man have lain with thee, and if thou hast not gone aside to uncleanliness with another instead of thy husband, be thou free from this bitter water that causeth the curse:

If the woman charged with adultery has committed sin, she already has the feelings of 'guilt'. The LORD would insure that she would respond fittingly to the bitter water challenge either by His miraculous intervention or through the ordinary mind-body interaction — psychoneuroimmunology. Guilty feelings will cause biochemical changes in the body through the psychoneuroimmunology nerve pathway that will weaken the capacity of the immune system to ward off diseases. [R7-8] For a guilty woman, just the thought of being challenged will interfere with the proper function of her immune system. Any harmful microbes that might be in the dirt of the tabernacle floor, which are put in water that a priest tells her to drink, may overpower her under-active immune system and cause an illness. However, should a woman be innocent of any charge, she would be looking forward to demonstrating her innocence; her immune system would be perfectly functioning; and the small numbers of microbes that might be in the dirty bitter water would have no effect on her.

∗ The bitter water challenge may have acted somewhat like a modern lie-detector test.

The LORD knew the consequences of sin, including feelings of guilt, could have a detrimental effect on both mental and physical health. Following the elaborate sacrificial system through the shedding of innocent blood, the Hebrews could know that their sins were covered or atoned for, and they could avoid unhealthy psychoneuroimmunological consequences of guilt that sin causes.

Cain and Abel

Cain and Abel both offered sacrifices to God as part of their worship. Abel offered a sacrifice of faith, with which God was well pleased. Knowing that God was pleased with his offering had to be very uplifting to his Emotional Health. {Apparently, the LORD caused acceptable sacrifices to be 'spontaneously' consumed by fire when placed on the altar; and conversely for an offering that was not accepted by the LORD, it's likely there was no spontaneous fire.} [R35] (II Chronicles 7:1)

When Cain brought his sacrifice to the LORD that was not accepted and not burned, he became very angry. ∗ Thus, Cain's anger toward God caused Cain to be angry with his righteous brother Abel; which led Cain to murder Abel. In this sense, God equates anger with murder. [R33]

JPS Gen 4:3-5 ... Cain brought of the fruit of the ground an offering unto the LORD. vs4 And Abel, he also brought of the firstlings of his flock and of the fat thereof. And the LORD had respect unto Abel and his offering; vs5 but unto Cain and to his offering He had not respect. And Cain was very wroth [angry], and his countenance fell. vs8 ... that Cain rose up against Abel his brother and slew [murdered] him.

As the Hebrews worked as commanded and obeyed the LORD's statutes, then He provided for them. This relationship hasn't changed for today; it is primarily when people do not trust and obey the LORD that life's demanding situations become stressful and lead to health problems.

NIV Deut 8:11 Be careful that you do not forget the LORD your God, failing to observe his commands, his laws and his decrees that I am giving you this day. vs12 Otherwise, when you eat and are satisfied, when you build up fine houses and settle down, vs13 and when your herds and flocks grow large and your silver and gold increase and all you have is multiplied, vs14 then your heart will become proud and you will forget the LORD your God, ... vs18 But remember the LORD your God, for it is he who gives you the ability to produce wealth, ...

This warning from Moses is important today as well. When we live in fine houses, do well in business, accumulate the luxuries of the world, and have sizable bank accounts, then we tend to trust in things rather than to trust in the LORD. When cars break down; or stock prices go down; or houses burn up; or inflation goes up, then security vanishes. This often causes people whom professed trust and faith in the unchanging LORD, to doubt and worry as they see the unstable worldly possessions that they once treasured wither and fad away. Distrust is very damaging to Emotional Health. Emotional Health should always begin with relying upon the LORD's provision.

∗ Trust and obedience are highpoints of walking with the LORD to avoid worry and stress.

Stress

S. I. McMillen, MD in his book *None of These Diseases* wrote that worry and stress are indeed contributing factors to many illnesses. Worry and stress are best defined as trying to assume responsibility for a situation for which God does not intend that person to take responsibility. [R1] In 1948, statistics indicate that two thirds of all patients who went to a physician had symptoms caused or aggravated by mental stress. [R2-3-4] Trusting and obeying the LORD never meant sitting around and waiting for God to dump His provision in one's lap; even the ***manna*** that God provided in the wilderness had to be gathered. Dr. McMillen further illustrates the psychosomatic origin of illness by several case reports. The first involved a young, strong, healthy male, who became fearful about losing his car and losing his girlfriend. This worry caused him to lose his appetite, lose sleep, and lose his strength. Next, a healthy, young married woman found out her husband had been killed. She was so overwhelmed with grief that the next morning her fingers and wrist joints were swollen, stiff and painful. This early onset of arthritis eventually caused the woman to become an invalid. This crippling illness was entirely of an emotional origin that ultimately caused a very real physical disease. Chemical blood tests would have disclosed abnormal toxins from the pituitary, thyroid and adrenal glands as contributing to the illness. [R2A] Dr. McMillen explains that prolonged continued emotional stress (possibly from not trusting in God) can lead to an increase in the size of the stress glands of the body, [i.e. – thyroid and adrenals]. (Autopsies may show one normal-sized adrenal gland and one adrenal gland greatly hypertrophied as a result of stress.) The physical evidence of worn-out adrenal glands that result of stress would likely shorten a person's life, as well as reduce the time that they enjoyed good health. [R2B-3-4]

∗ **Thus, stress can result in tired worn out glands, which can result in tired worn out bodies**.

Hans Selye, MD the world famous researcher on stress, in his book *Stress Without Distress* documented many ways that stress can be unhealthy for the body. Richard Passwater, PhD in his book *Supernutrition* wrote that stress can have very real physiological effects on the body. The demands during the months just prior to April 15 have been documented to raise the cholesterol levels of accountants. [R2-3-4-9-29] The high blood cholesterol levels return to normal after the demands of tax preparation time are over. High LDL cholesterol has been documented to be a risk factor in the developing cardiovascular disease (CVD) like: hypertension, heart attack, high blood pressure, stroke and peripheral arterial disease. [R3A] Very similar physiological reactions also take place for students as they approach their final exams and other people under stress.

∗ **Stress appears to be a leading cause of high LDL cholesterol, which often leads to poor health.**

When people allow these demands to become stressful to the body, not only do cholesterol levels become elevated, but the coronary arteries, which supply blood to the heart, are also affected. These coronary vessels contain a muscular layer that gets its nerve supply from the same sympathetic nervous system that produces adrenaline and causes the body to get geared up for a 'fight or flight' response. In this way, stress causes the coronary vessels to constrict or to 'spasm'. [R4A] This spasm of the coronary vessels in response to stress will restrict the blood flow to the normal heart with no coronary blockage, but can cause arteries that are already restricted to become completely blocked. This stress-induced blockage of the arteries to the heart may result in a heart attack and can be fatal. [R4A] Medical science has recently provided some very exciting documentation for the effects of emotions on health, and especially the biochemistry of the immune system. The immune system is responsible for producing the white blood cells, which are the body's natural defense against disease. Norman Cousins collected the research of other authors and conducted research work at the UCLA School of Medicine on psychoneuroimmunology (PSI) for over 10 years and wrote about the research in his book *Head First the Biology of Hope*. Psychoneuroimmunology is a delicate interaction between brain, endocrine and immune systems of the body. In his book *The Body is the Hero* Ronald Glasser, MD documented that reducing stress and/or increasing beneficial emotions (love, joy, peace, happiness, laughter, etc.) causes increased activity of the immune system. Walter Cannon, MD in his book *The Wisdom of the Body* documented a similar increased activity of the spleen as a result of a positive emotional state. [7-7B]

The ability of the body to ward off and fight infectious organisms is related to the peace of mind and emotional well-being of the individual!

Song and Dance encourages stress relief, as it is impossible to think about two things at once: focusing on scales/notes for song or footwork for dance prevents thinking about stressful events. The most stressful event in the Torah, the Exodus, is immediately followed by song and dance to relieve stress during the song of Moses. Moses prescribed song and dance for relief from stress!

∗ **Stress can devastate Emotional Health, which can return to devastate Physical Health.**

Song and Dance – plus – Laughter

Shortly after the Hebrews crossed the Red Sea (an extremely stressful event), they took time to relieve stress and rejoice unto the LORD with music and dance (Song of Moses). (see pgs 185&204-5)

{ ***Mi Chamocha*** = 'Who is like unto Thee' [in holiness] O LORD amongst the gods?} (Ex 15:11)

KJV Ex 15:1 Then sang Moses and the children of Israel this song (***shiyr***) unto the LORD, and spake, saying, I will sing (***shiyr***) unto the LORD, for he hath triumphed gloriously: the horse and his rider hath he cast into the sea. vs2 The LORD is my strength and song (***zimrath***), and he also has become my salvation. vs11 Who is like unto thee, O LORD, among the gods? who is like unto thee, glorious in holiness, fearful in praises, doing wonders? vs20 And Miriam the prophetess, the sister of Aaron, took a timbrel in her hand; and all the women went out after her with timbrel and dances (***mecholah***). vs21 And Miriam answered them, Sing (***shiyr***) ye to the LORD, ...

Singing and Dancing in ways that are glorifying to God can be a beautiful expression of joy, praise and thanksgiving to God. This author has personally found the activities of singing and/or dancing to traditional Israeli music to be a wonderful expression of worship to the LORD. Unfortunately, singing and dancing can also be done in ways that are distasteful and not honoring to God. Such an incident was associated with idolatrous worship of the golden calf. (Ex 32:19) Today, there is a great variety of music for listening, playing on instruments, singing or dancing. Remember, as always, discretion is wisdom! The choices made will have an influence on your Mental Health and ultimately even affect physical health. [R11] Music with harmonious melodies and words that are glorifying to God can be very uplifting. Music that fails these tests, although seemingly harmless and appropriate for a while, frequently ends up leading a person on a path away from fellowship with God. According to the AMA, six potentially hazardous themes capable of warping certain young minds that permeate the lucrative heavy metal—rap music industry are: drug abuse, alcohol abuse, suicide, violence, satanic worship, racism, and sexual exploitation. [R5]

Robert B. Millman, at New York Hospital–Cornell Medical Center, says:

"There is no question that heavy metal and rap music can have a bad influence on children,"

"Some kids live out their lives according to what these songs say." [R5]

Bill Gothard of *The Institute Life Principles* evaluates that rock and rap music often falls into the category of not honoring the LORD. The author urges the reader to be musically selective and to evaluate how the beat (rhythm), harmony, melody and lyrics might influence Emotional Health. R. C. Sproul, DrS discusses objective standards to evaluate whether music is appropriate or not. Choosing some music may just be personal preference, while occasions: wedding, funeral, ballet or parade may determine the music. Healthy song and dance may be either calming or energizing to the mind and body. The cassette tape *Hear No Evil* helps people to evaluate most music. [R6]

∗ Spiritual music puts people in a proper frame of mind to listen, follow and obey the LORD.

Laughter

Laughter is an important part of Emotional Health. Laughter is well illustrated when the LORD opened the mouth of Balaam's ass, to have Balaam's ass give Balaam advice. (Num 22:28-31)

JPS Num 22:28 And the LORD opened the mouth of the ass, and she said unto Balaam: 'What have I done unto thee, that thou hast smitten me these three times? vs30 And the ass said unto Balaam: 'Am not I thine ass, upon which thou hast ridden all thy life long unto this day? was I ever wont to do so unto thee?' And he [Balaam] said: 'Nay.'

How humorous for a man to talk to his ass. The story of Balaam and his ass may seem mythical; yet when followed by Balaam's sudden demise, it teaches the enduring lesson that Balaam's 'love of money' and his prostitution of his 'gift from God' brought him certain destruction.

Appropriate laughter (as opposed to making fun of other people) is healthy for everyone. Norman Cousins in his book *Anatomy of an Illness* described how he discovered laughter was an analgesic to promote restful sleep, despite great joint pain. Most people will never need laughter to relieve pain or promote sleep, but laughter is very valuable for reducing tension and stress. [R7C] Laughter and vitamin C allowed Mr. Cousins to walk away from crippling ankylosing spondylitis.

Timing is often critical in the usefulness of song, dance and humor to teach a point, encourage learning and promote health. Moses was a master of knowing what to write for the circumstance. In the author's opinion the humor of Mark Twain and Bill Cosby also often teach lessons about life.

Humor often uses the double-meaning of puns, such as < Moses began life as a basket case >.

∗ Healthy Song, Dance and Humor are aspects of Emotional Health that help relieve stress.

Women of the *Torah*

Eve was tempted by Satan to eat the 'forbidden fruit' in the Garden of Eden. Adam must have already taught Eve that 'the fruit' was forbidden. But, when Adam didn't help Eve with discernment, Satan approached Eve with deception. Satan first misquoted the LORD's instructions to Eve. (Gen 3) Eve should have sought her husband Adam and they should have realized that this was rebellion against God. Instead, Eve listened to Satan and she followed his deception and she and Adam ate 'the forbidden fruit', as the LORD commanded them not to. Everyone since is born with an inclination toward sin and rebellion against following the instructions of the LORD. From this time onward, all women were instructed to look to their husbands for strength, wisdom and leadership. (Gen 3:16) **The LORD held both Adam and Eve responsible for the first sin, and they both paid the penalty.**

Sarah followed Abraham and left their home in Ur of the Chaldees to go where she knew not. Ur was an idol-worshipping community. Sarah and Abraham alone had a desire to seek the LORD. Leaving Ur and seeking God in a new land, where they knew no one, took courage, faith and trust. In Egypt, Abraham called Sarah his sister (she was his half-sister) and Sarah trusted his judgment. The LORD promised Sarah a child, but she was barren till after her age of menopause. Sarah was not certain she would bear a child, so she encouraged Abraham that Hagar would bare her child. When her handmaid Hagar bore Ishmael, this immediately caused envy and bitterness in Sarah. After Hagar left, Sarah was restored to fertility and bore Isaac. Despite several understandable lapses, Sarah is credited as demonstrating great trust in her husband and great faith in the LORD. Sarah and Abraham had no role models in trusting the LORD, and all they did was unprecedented.
∗ Should difficult decisions arise today, women may ask: **What Would Sarah Do?** or **W W S D ?**
Rebekah showed good judgment in leaving Nahor to follow a servant to Canaan to marry Isaac. Although Rebekah was a faithful wife to Isaac, she did not learn all the lessons Sarah learned. Rebekah knew Jacob was the more spiritually minded of her two sons. Rebekah wanted the best for Jacob; however, she taught Jacob how to get the blessings from Esau by deceit and fraud.

Rachel was beautiful, but emotionally unstable. Rachel stole Laban's idols when leaving Nahor. Rachel threatened to commit suicide when she didn't have children. Rachel can be contrasted to Sarah, who left Ur and was childless early on, but Sarah had a full vessel and she was content. Rachel, Leah and Laban together deceived Jacob at his wedding. So, Jacob ended up marrying both Rachel and Leah. To the author: Rachel and Leah represent the two sides to every woman. Rachel represents the glamorous woman, who is often idealized concerning romance and love. Leah represents the hard-working wife and mother, who is responsible for caring for the home.

Lot's wife was very likely a glamorous woman, who found her security in the life style of Sodom. (Sarah found her safety and stability in the LORD, and she was content to live in a tent in the hills.) After leaving Sodom, Lot's wife looked back (affectionately), and then she became a pillar of salt. Lot's daughters by incest with Lot both bore sons who opposed the Hebrew descendants of Sarah.

Tamar was widowed of Judah's first son, then Judah's second son died shamefully with her. Later, Tamar was a harlot to Judah, yet Judah declared Tamar was more righteous than himself.

The midwives, Shiphrah and Puah, were ordered by Pharaoh to kill all male Hebrew babies. Shiphrah and Puah defied the order of Pharaoh and sought to do the will of the LORD. Moses and many other male Hebrew babies were saved, and the LORD dealt favorably with the midwives.

Moses' mother, Jochebed, and father, Amram, showed great wisdom, faith and trust in the LORD by putting Moses in an ark of bulrushes and floating him down the Nile. It is very likely that other poor families did this also, hoping that their child would find a more favorable life elsewhere.

Miriam, Moses' sister, was a prophetess and leader of song and dance. Miriam had positions of leadership and responsibility within the congregation. Miriam functioned well in this capacity, until she forgot that Moses was in a higher position of leadership. To Miriam, the LORD spoke in symbols, figures and visions; to Moses, the LORD spoke face to face. When Miriam spoke against Moses for marrying an Ethiopian woman, the LORD rebuked Miriam and she became leprous. Moses prayed for healing for Miriam, and seven days later she was restored to good health.

Zipporah, Moses' wife, was presumably also Cushite. Zipporah didn't want to follow Moses in circumcision for their sons. Zipporah's lack of trust caused the LORD to be angry with Moses. Zipporah finally circumcised her two sons, but she wasn't very happy about it. Zipporah did not always show a submissive spirit to her husband, Moses, that the LORD often praises in women.

The daughters of Zelophehad petitioned for their rights from the Law, and Moses gave them land as an inheritance, since their father had no sons. This is an early example of women's rights.

Rahab heard about the LORD's great works; — she desired to follow Him and to help Joshua. [R22]

∗ The LORD rewarded trust by women in the *Torah,* and some women's lack of trust was very costly.

Boundaries in Relationships

John Townsend, PhD and Henry Cloud, PhD in their book *Boundaries* discuss the dynamics of interpersonal relationships. All relationships that remain stable and beneficial over an extended time period are healthy only because of well established and mutually agreed upon 'boundaries'. In the Garden the LORD immediately established boundaries between Himself, and Adam and Eve that permitted eating of all 'fruit' except 'fruit' from the 'tree of the knowledge of good and evil'. When Adam and Eve ate of the 'forbidden fruit', their relationship with the LORD was broken and this 'fall of humanity" caused all creation to be subject to the 'curse of the LORD'. (Gen 3) Outside the Garden, the LORD established new boundaries by which fallen humanity could be reconciled with the LORD through the shedding innocent blood and offering a sacrifice. Abel had respect unto the LORD's boundaries, but Cain did not respect these boundaries, which led Cain to murder Abel. When Ham did not respect boundaries with Noah, the LORD cursed Ham's son, Canaan. (Gen 9:25) Ham's descendent, Nimrod, was rebellious, did not respect the LORD's boundaries and encouraged others to follow him at the Tower of Babel, which caused the LORD to confuse man's languages. Abraham and Sarah sought to discover the boundaries of the LORD and their lives were blessed. Jacob was terrible at forming boundaries with his brother Esau, and with his father-in-law Laban. Jacob had two wives, two handmaidens and a conniving father-in-law, which immediately caused him boundary problems and contributed to his ten older sons also being terrible with boundaries. Jacob's life was a mess until his conversion experience, when he began to the learn boundaries. Jacob's ten older sons despised Joseph, who often practiced boundaries well. After the Famine, Joseph, as Prime Minister of Egypt, went to great lengths to establish boundaries with his brothers. Moses easily established boundaries with his father-in-law, Jethro; yet his wife, Zipporah, did not always respect healthy boundaries. No mention is made of Moses' relationship with his two sons. Romantic love often 'knows no boundaries' and is 'blind'. Moses loved Zipporah despite her faults. Had Moses established better boundaries before marriage, his marriage may have been healthier. Aaron practiced boundaries well in his role as High Priest, but poorly in forming the 'Golden Calf'. Miriam practiced boundaries well as song/dance leader, yet poorly in challenging Moses' marriage. Korah wasn't content with Moses as leader as he challenged boundaries that the LORD established. Balaam understood the healthy boundaries of the LORD; yet, he violated them for profit and greed. Caleb learned and practiced boundaries, as he was successful with Moses and Joshua as leaders. Slaves have no rights, no healthy boundaries with owners, and emotions are often trampled on.
∗ Relationships without mutually agreed upon boundaries don't last and often result in tragedy.

--- Whoa Unto Us ---

Unfortunately, today much of our entertainment industry seems to provide excuses for people not bringing their lives into conformity with God's standards of conduct. [R2] Comedy, which can be a lighthearted way to look at everyday life occurrences from a new or different perspective, has often declined to ridiculing people who uphold high standards in their lives. The celebrities that this industry creates often provide role models on and off the screen for young and old alike that are socially dysfunctional and in direct opposition to God's standards as stated in the ***Torah*** and the rest of Scripture. Pharaoh Rameses, Ishmael, Esau, Korah, Nimrod and Cain provide examples of people who are so 'busy' trying to accomplish their own means to find 'self-worth' that they fail to put forth the effort needed to develop the character traits that the LORD desires in their lives. Today, unfortunately, there are many people who become workaholics or over-emphasize their recreational and social activities in order to 'feel good' about themselves rather than to put forth the necessary time and effort required to develop these godly personality characteristics in their lives.
∗ Character strength is developed over time with guidance and by making proper choices, just as correctly practicing athletic, aerobic and strength-building activities develops muscular strength. Abraham, Sarah, Isaac, Israel, Joseph, as well as Noah, Moses, Caleb, and Joshua are several people the ***Torah*** who should be looked to as proper role models for all people of all generations. The godly character traits demonstrated in these peoples lives is well documented in the ***Torah***. The fruits of the life that is disciplined and sanctified by ***havdala*** unto God are manifest by the development of these character traits! These character traits are also the greatest means by which God's people can demonstrate the holy righteous character of their LORD to the unbelieving world.

"Truth is often hard if it is not soften by Love.
Love is often soft if it is not strengthened by Truth." [R37]

Truth in Word and Deed

Moses' life was a great example of truth, in which his words and writings were consistent with his behavior. This nearly perfect application of the principles of 'truth' in the life of Moses not only promoted his Mental Health, but also served as a role model for the entire Hebrew nation. Psychologists and Psychiatrists today write about the conflict that develops in the mind when people say one thing and yet do something different. Mental conflicts between ideology and practice can be summed up as 'cognitive dissonance' or a 'false witness'. When someone does that which is against God's laws, they instinctively/intuitively know that it is wrong, which triggers discontented thought patterns in the brain through the psychoneuroimmunological pathway. What an unhappy, unhealthy position people find themselves in when they do that which they know to be wrong and/or do not do that which they know to be right. (How wretched feels the man that does what he would not do; but that which he would not do, he does anyway.) Trusting the LORD always involves making choices according to biblical principles, even when the standards of the world suggest other choices to be acceptable. The mental stress that develops from this double standard often causes the mind to develop psychotic and neurotic mental illnesses. Dr. McMillen states that mental illness is the number one health problem in America today. [R1A] Patterning a person's life after the role-model life of Moses will bring Mental Health today as well.

∗ 'Truth' remains the same: Yesterday, Today and Forever.

Moses warned the Hebrews 13 times in Deuteronomy to remember the situations of the past and the sins of the fathers, so they could avoid repeating the errors (sins) of the past. (Deut 8:18) Obviously, Moses told the Hebrews it is not wrong to have some 'good things' of the world that God intends His people to have. But the key issue is whether God's people are trusting in things or trusting and rejoicing in the LORD God (***Yahweh–yireh***) who provided the good things. These lessons are valuable for God's people today as well. Worry and grief are not intended for believers of God. God instead asks for faith and trust in him as Provider–God. The God who created the heavens and the earth, is same LORD God that knows the heart of each man.

KJV Gen 1:1 In the beginning God created the heaven and the earth.

KJV Gen 6:8 But Noah found favor in the eyes of the LORD.

KJV Gen 15:6 And he [Abraham] believed in the LORD and he counted it to him as righteousness.

It is the LORD who works his divine purpose through people who first trust in Him. Trust is an important step to mental health. The LORD wants men to trust Him – as a child trusts his parents.

KJV Deut 5:16 Honor thy father and mother as the LORD thy God hath commanded thee; that thy days may be prolonged, and that it may go well with thee, in the land which the LORD thy God giveth thee.

Mental Health and peace-of-mind come from practicing emotional discipline, just as physical health comes from the discipline of proper diet and routine exercise. Moses understood that a person's overall health was directly related to his/her state of mind, as is evidenced by the exhortations urging the Hebrews to be joyous and rejoice in the LORD. (Lev 23:40; Deut 12:12; Deut 14:26; Deut 10:11) This healthy exhortation of Moses rings loud and clear today as well.

Rejoice in the LORD Always and Again I Say Rejoice!

JPS Deut 27:7 ... and thou shalt rejoice before the LORD thy God.

JPS Deut 26:11 And thou shalt rejoice in all the good which the LORD thy God hath given. unto thee, and unto thy house, thou, and the Levite, and the stranger that is in the midst of thee.

The *Hebrew Epic* began when Abraham and Sarah left Ur of the Chaldees and culminated when Joshua and Caleb lead the conquest of the 'land promised' to Abraham (≈1,900 BC to ≈1,400 BC). During the *Hebrew Epic* of ≈500 years, the Hebrews experienced the full range of human emotion. Section I: MENTAL HEALTH groups emotional responses from the ***Torah*** and discusses emotions in a manner designed to encourage ***Torah*** students to evaluate emotions throughout the Scripture. ∗ Managing emotions plus prayer will help all ***Torah*** students to grow in the likeness of their LORD.

∗ Rejoicing in the LORD is a great technique to keep emotions in balance and under control.

-------------------------------- References Ch 04 Emotions --------------------------------

[R1] Basic and Advanced Seminars (from the Institute in Life Principles)\ by Bill Gothard; character lessons
[R2] None of These Diseases\ by S. I. McMillen, MD; pg 58 stress
  [R1A] pg 101 toxins from stress [R1B] pg 114 emotional illness – $^{\#}$1 health problem
[R3] None of These Diseases (Revised)\ by McMillen, MD and David Stern, MD; ch 9 – ch 12
[R4] None of These Diseases (Revised and Expanded)\ by McMillen, MD and Stern, MD; pg 184-196 stress
  Part 4 Emotional Wholeness ch 18 – 24 / pg 167-223 // pg 205-210 anger – a dangerous emotion
[R4] The 8 Week Cholesterol Cure\ by Robert E. Kowlowski; pg 109 accountants stress at tax time
  [R4A] pg 108 coronary spasm & heart attack /Ch 8 pg 106-112 Stress /pg 88 Na^{+} and NBP
[R5] American Health (May 91)\ music influences emotions positively or negatively
[R6] 'Hear No Evil' (audio cassette)\ from FireFighters Tape Ministry objective evaluation of music
[R7] Head First the Biology of Hope\ by Norman Cousins; pg 16-18, 36(C), 38-39 psychoneuroimmunology
  [R7B] pg 76 immunology and emotion / pg 36 immunology chart
  [R7C] pg 300 cholesterol and emotional stress / pg 133 laughter relieves stress
[R8] The Chemistry of the Blood\ by M. R. DeHaan, MD/ pg 41-48 bitter water = lie detector test
[R9] Supernutrition\ by Richard Passwater, PhD; pg 96-97 tax time increases stress
  [R9A] pg 74-80 & 96-97 serum cholesterol not related to dietary cholesterol // pg 77 Korean War autopsies
[R10] The Ten Commandments (audio)\ by Laura Schlessinger, PhD and Rabbi Stewart Vogel; commentary
[R11] Time (magazine 12 June 95)\ Violent Reaction; pg 25-35 & A Company Under Fire pg 37-39
[R12] Boundaries\ by John Townsend, PhD and Henry Cloud, PhD relationships require boundaries
[R13] Type A: Behavior and Your Heart\ by Dr. Friedman and Dr. Rosenman; stress damages health
[R14] Anatomy of an Illness\ by Norman Cousins power of placebo – laughter relieves pain
[R15] The Stress of Life\ by Hans Selye, MD adrenal exhaustion from stress
[R16] Stress without Distress\ by Hans Selye, MD remain in harmony with the laws of nature
[R17] The Wisdom of the Body\ by Walter Cannon, MD coined the term – homeostasis [from R16 - pg 69]
[R18] Strong's Concordance \ by James Strong, STD, LLD Who is like unto Thee — ***Mi CHamocha*(*h*)**

pg 1149	who	# 4310	H pg 65	***mi* – *miy* – *me***	Ex 15:11
pg 604	like	# 3644	H pg 56	***chamo* - *kamow***	Ex 15:11
pg 1007	you or Thee	{***cha*(*h*)**}	***chamo* + *cha*(*h*)** as a suffix	=	***CHamocha*(*h*)**
pg 341	fear	# 3372	H pg 52	***yare***	Deut 1:21
pg 955	song	# 7891 / 7892	H pg 115	***shiyr* – *shiyrah***	Ex 15:1
pg 955	song	# 2176	H pg 35	***zimrath***	Ex 15:2
pg 232	dances	# 4246	H pg 64	***mecholah* – *mechowlah***	Ex 15:20
pg 825	Rahab	# 7343	H pg 108	***Rachab***	Josh 2:1
pg 930	sin (miss)	# 2398 / 2403	H pg 38	***chata***	Gen 18:20
pg 516	iniquity (fault)	# 5771	H pg 86	***avon* – *avown***	Ex 34:7
	(moral evil)	# 5766	H pg 86	***evel* – *avel***	Deut 32:4
	false - unjust	# 205	H pg 09	***aven***	Num 32:21
pg 1075	trespass	# 5688	H pg 85	***aboth* – *abowth***	Gen 50:17
	(trespass / sin)	# 817 / 819	H pg 17	***asham***	Lev 6:6
	trespass	# 4604	H pg 69	***ma'al***	Lev 5:15

sin	(# 2398)	to miss the mark – as in archery – trying to hit the target but being off target
iniquity	(# 5766)	may indicate a matter of the heart – wrongful thoughts or motivations
trespass	(# 5688)	may be a purposeful violation of the Law or a willful disobedience of the LORD

[R19] Strong's Guide to Bible Words\ by James Strong, STD, LLD
[R20] The Harlot by the Side of the Road (audio cassettes)\ by Johnathan Kirsch women of the ***Torah***
[R21] All the Women of the Bible\ by Edith Deen; pg 3-69 women of the ***Torah*** (***Miriam* -** 6 yrs older than Moses)
[R22] Women of Faith\ by J. Vernon McGee, PhD redemption and providence through women
[R23] Miriam's Well\ by Alice Bach and Cheryl J. Exum women of the ***Tanakh***
[R24] A Woman God Can Use\ by Alice Matthews Miriam and other women from the ***Torah***
[R25] Women of the Bible\ by Jean E. Syswerda analyzes emotions guiding women of the ***Torah***
[R26] Innocents Abroad\ by Mark Twain; Ch XLIII & XLIV Balaam's Ass, people of the ***Torah*** & ***Eretz*** Israel
[R27] Becoming Strong Again\ by Dr. Greg Jans // [R28] Slouching Toward Gomorrah\ by Robert Borke
[R29] Stress, Diet, and Your Heart\ by Dean Ornish, MD; cassette 1&2 stress, diet and cholesterol
  cassette 4 – stress plus caffeine leads to high cholesterol cassette 7 – high cholesterol and CVD
[R30] The Body is the Hero\ by Ronald Glasser, MD emotional health ⇔ physical health
[R31] Anger Kills\ by Redford Williams, MD and Virginia Williams, RN
[R32] Healing for Damaged Emotions\ by David Seamands (from FoF 04-14-2000)
[R33] This Present Darkness\ by Frank Perette novel – emotions and health
[R34] Winning the War Within & The Glorious Journey \ by Charles Stanley, PhD (In Touch) (1-800-546-0088)
[R35] Genesis 4 Teaching\ by Chuck Missler, PhD Cain and Abel (Koinonia House – 1-800-K-HOUSE-1)
[R36] The Key\ by Nancy Missler (Koinonia House — 1-800-KHOUSE-1)
[R37] Heroes Series (March 2003 radio)\ by Chuck Swindoll, PhD (Insights for Living – 1-800-772-8888 – quote)
[R38] Love Must be Tough\ by James Dobson, PhD live according to the boundaries of love
[R39] Safe People\ by John Townsend, PhD and Henry Cloude, PhD
[R40] Recovering the Beauty of the Arts\ by R. C. Sproul, DrS – music and worship (Ligonier – 1-800-435-4343)

Torah Study

All people respond emotionally to events, and emotions subtly influence all people's actions. One aspect of ***Torah*** study is to look at emotional causes (motive) and effects (action) of people.

Some character in the ***Torah*** or someone elsewhere in the Scripture experienced every human emotional response possible (proper and/or improper). As students progress in ***Torah*** study, they will need to examine their own heart and their own personal emotional responses. The ideal scenario is that a student finds their emotions agreeing with the emotions of the people in the Word who love the LORD and hate sin. Unfortunately, unless the student was trained in these proper emotions from a youth upward, they may find some of their emotions are similar to the emotions of the worldly characters in the ***Torah*** that oppose the instruction of the LORD God.
∗ Emotional growth comes from evaluating emotions, identifying worldly emotions and changing emotions that the ***Torah*** indicates are inappropriate. Changing bad habits is difficult, especially if doing this alone. The LORD knows the iniquities of the older generations will be passed on to the youth until someone calls upon the LORD to help break the habitual worldly emotional patterns. The LORD also knows that people with similar habit patterns will congregate with one another.
∗ Thus, to grow in the likeness of the LORD, the ideal scenario is to congregate with other people who are also growing in the likeness of the LORD. Growing in the LORD is a lifelong process. People insensitive to this growth process may encourage wrong emotions from ***Torah*** students.
∗ People who provoke others to wrath, anger, rage or evil, must be avoided like the plague.
While Lot fellowshipped with the worldly people of Sodom, Abraham avoided this sinful scenario. Lot was a righteous man who didn't transform Sodom. Sodom was devastating to Lot's family. Lot escaped the destruction of Sodom by the skin-of-his-teeth, and by the prayer of Abraham. Noah, guarded his family from sin and people who opposed God, and Noah grew in the LORD. Although it is theoretically possible, as Jonah transformed Nineveh, there are no instances in the ***Torah*** where one godly person enters a sinful society and transforms them to follow the LORD. The ***Torah*** gives an example of how Balaam, a true prophet, was enticed by money to do evil. In the mixed multitude that followed Moses across the Red Sea, a few people that complained may have influenced the entire Hebrew nation to turn from following Moses and following the LORD. A much more ideal scenario is for an ungodly person to fellowship with a group of godly people and desire to be transformed by them, as happened in the book of Joshua with Rahab the harlot. Rahab even married into the Royal Hebrew line, and her distant grandchild was King David.

Joshua, the sixth book of the ***Tanakh,*** is often included with the study of the ***Torah***, and it is often grouped with Genesis, Exodus, Leviticus, Numbers and Deuteronomy as the *Hexateuch.* Many concepts developed by Moses in the ***Torah,*** find their fruition in the book of Joshua. The Gibeonites were one of the people who inhabited Canaan (The Promised Land) that Joshua was told by the LORD to make no covenant with, and to either drive out or kill to the last person. The Gibeonites had other ideas and decided they would rather serve the LORD as slaves, rather than leave Canaan, or fight the Hebrews. The Gibeonites used impersonation to deceive Joshua into thinking they were from a far-away land, and they made a covenant of peace with Joshua. The tactic of imitation, putting up a false front and pretending to have credentials that you don't have is not uncommon throughout history and is still seen today. The Gibeonites did however follow through on their commitment to the LORD and they remained loyal throughout the ***Tanakh***. The Gibeonites used deceit once for spiritual gain, while most often deceit is a person's undoing. This Gibeonite covenant may be considered the first national conversion to the LORD in history. The Gibeonites put away all false gods, burned their idols and gladly performed menial tasks for the Hebrews in the service of the LORD. The Gibeonites are excellent role models for all nationalities.

∗ Moses was famous for his relationship of mutual trust with his father-in-law, Jethro.
∗ Jacob was infamous for his relationship of mutual deceit with his father-in-law, Laban.

A useful ***Torah*** study may be to compare the two father-in-law relationships and to determine dynamics in the lives of Moses and Jethro -plus- Jacob and Laban that fostered these relationships.

Deception, which is the 'work of the Devil', often leads to sin. Have you been deceived lately?
Not trusting in the LORD is the beginning of anyone's rebellion against the authority of the LORD.
Rugged individualistic men often trust in their own abilities, talents and skills to get through life.
Many women desire to trust their husbands for their physical needs and for emotional support.
Children initially learn to trust that their parents will meet all their physical and emotional needs.
Growth through ***Torah*** study requires relying upon 'timeless' principles of health from the ***Torah***.
Wise men, women and children learn to trust the LORD for the ultimate source of Emotional Health.

∗ In ***Torah*** study, the student may find out as much about himself as he finds out about the ***Torah***.

Section II: HYGIENE and SANITATION
Chapter 5 Washings and Cleansings
Tatoos and Cutting the Flesh

The 'Rest of the Story' continues by examining God's concern for the hygiene of His people as they left Egypt, the most advanced society of the world at that time. In 1873 AD, Smith and Ebers discovered and preserved most of the papyri containing Egyptian medical knowledge that may have been 'state-of-the-art' in 1450 BC. [R10] These papyri suggested using such medicinal agents as swine's teeth, putrefied meat, rancid fat and excrement from human beings, dogs and cats for healing human disease. These quote/unquote 'medicinal agents' are now known to be habitats for disease-causing organisms that actually make illnesses worse, not better.* Moses was well schooled in this knowledge of the Egyptians, which was considered state-of-the-art in 1450 BC, yet he did not include any of this misinformation in the text of the ***Torah***. [R2A-3A-4] Undoubtedly the reason none of this Egyptian misinformation is included in the ***Torah*** is that Moses received inspiration for the very words of the text directly from the LORD. (Ex 4:12)

Scientists, who make discoveries in their field, frequently gain insight from proven information of earlier scientists. Scientists following Moses, who have made contributions to sanitation, plague control and personal hygiene, have in no case disproven the scientific accuracy of the ***Torah***. Just the opposite is true. The more researchers learn about these subjects, the more they understand that the writings of Moses represent foundational scientific knowledge. Some scientists, who were considered very knowledgeable in their day, such as Aristotle in 350 BC, wrote about many subjects. However, much of their work has come under examination by later generations and was found to be full of errors. While other people have added to the great truths that Moses wrote in the ***Torah*** ≈3500 years ago, no one has found even one error in the ***Torah***. The instructions of Moses in the ***Torah*** are as accurate today as the day they were written.

Up to the late 1700s, conventional wisdom-treatment in cases of severe infectious illness included draining the blood from a sick person in the hope of eliminating the cause of the illness. Draining blood from someone first requires making a cut in the skin over a blood vessel.

KJV Deut 12:23 The life is in the blood.

By cutting the flesh and draining the blood out of people, physicians frequently, simply bleed their patients to death. When George Washington contracted a severe upper respiratory infection, he was bled at least four separate times. The total amount of blood drained from him has been estimated to be as high as two quarts, which would be nearly half of all his blood. Even for healthy people, losing two quarts of blood would constitute a major health risk, but for someone who was already weakened by an infection, this blood letting undoubted hastened his death. [R5] Today, wise health care practitioners recognize that to cure disease, blood needs to be enriched, nourished, purified and cleansed, but not drained out! 'Cutting the flesh' was a common ritual of the ungodly Canaanites when Joshua lead the Hebrews in the conquest of the Promised Land.

Cutting the flesh (skin piercing) is often unhealthy due to blood loss and chance of infection. Cutting the flesh was a way the priests of Baal called upon their gods for insights. (1Kings 18:28) If the slave of a Hebrew chose to permanently serve the household, he could pierce his earlobe to the door with an awl and become a 'bondservant'. (Lev 25:39) The lower fleshy lobe of the ear is relatively free from blood, and is the healthiest place to pierce the skin and to wear an earring.

Tattoos use needles to permanently inject dyes (inks) into the deepest (3rd) layer of the skin. Tattoo dyes may be toxic to the skin. Tattoos always cause the skin irritation and they may cause skin infections. Tattoos often mark an allegiance to a 'foreign god' and they should be avoided.

KJV Lev 19:28 Ye shall not make any cuttings in your flesh for the dead,
nor print any marks (***qaaqa***) [tattoos] upon you: I am the LORD.

As opposed to tattoos or cuttings, hard physical work that causes sweating helps healthy skin to release toxins. Other Hebrew habits for healthy skin included: 1) washings with Olive oil soap; 2) applications of aloes, such as– Aloe Vera; 3) moderate exposure to sunshine producing a suntan; plus 4) applications of high–mineral mud from the Dead Sea that moisturizes and draws toxins out of the skin. Suntans promote melanin in the skin to convert cholesterol into vitamin D – the sunshine vitamin. Suntans are healthy, especially if obtained at close to 1,300 ft below sea level in the Dead Sea area, where the much denser atmosphere absorbs most UV-b sunlight that may cause an unhealthy sunburn.

*** The Dead Sea with its dense atmosphere and mineral–rich mud is ideal for a health resort.**

Washings

Moses wrote very specific instructions in the ***Torah*** for washing to keep the body clean.

(1) Touching a dead body: (Lev 11:28; Lev 17:15-16; Num 31:19-24)
KJV Num 19:11 He that toucheth the dead body of an man shall be unclean seven days. vs19 .... and on the seventh day he shall purify himself, and wash (***kabac***) his clothes and bathe himself in water and be clean (***taher***) at even.

"For immediately upon death begins a process of corruption which produces compounds not only obnoxious to the senses, but actively poisonous in character; and what is of still more consequence to observe, in the case of all parasitic and infectious diseases, the energy of the infection is specially intensified when the infected person or animal dies. Hence, the careful regulations as to cleansing of those persons or things which had been defiled by the dead; either by water where practical; or where the thing could not be thus thoroughly cleansed, then by burning the article with fire, the most certain of all disinfectants." [R1]

KJV Num 19:6 And the priest shall take cedar wood and hyssop, and scarlet, and cast it into the midst of the burning of the heifer.

Cedar wood, scarlet and hyssop form the basis for an excellent soap. (Num 19 & Lev 14) [R3A]
"It [the soap] was made by burning together in a fire the following: a young cow, cedar wood, hyssop branches, and scarlet wood. The washing solution contained an irritant, cedar-wood oil, that would encourage scrubbing; an antiseptic, hyssop [oregano] oil, that would kill bacteria and fungi; and a scrubbing element, wood fibers, that would dislodge the bacteria." [R3A]

These washings also were repeated several times, and the time between washings would allow drying of the skin and exposure to the sun, which could kill microbes not washed off. [R3A]

(2) Contact with a man's sexual discharge or a woman's menstrual blood: (Lev 15:16-17 & 21-27)
The requirement to keep the skin free of bodily sexual fluids, which could make a person's skin more susceptible to irritation or infection, is facilitated by the commandment to wash.

(3) Contact with any bodily discharges: (Lev 15:2-15)
KJV Lev 15:2 ...When any man hath a running issue out of his flesh, because of his issue he is unclean. vs6 And he that sitteth on any thing whereon he sat that hath the issue shall wash his clothes, and bathe himself in water, and be unclean until the even. vs13 And when he that hath an issue is cleansed of his issue; then he shall number to himself seven days for his cleansing, and wash his clothes, and bathe his flesh in running water, and shall be clean.

The principle of hygienic washings is applied to a person who has a discharge, as in an infection, as well as to his clothes, but also to anyone who comes into contact with his clothes. Bodily secretions that contaminate clothes can later become a source of irritation or infection.

(4) Being infected with a skin disorder, including leprosy (***tsara'at***): (Lev 13:54; Lev 14:9&27)
KJV Lev 14:8 And he that is to be cleansed shall wash his clothes, and shave off all his hair, and wash himself in water, that he may be clean.

The skin/neurological disease of bacterial Leprosy may, in its early stages, be confused with other less severe skin rashes/problems. The principle of washing as a first line of defense against the spread of disease is clearly appropriate, regardless of the severity of the malady.

(5) Touching blood: (Lev 6:27 and Lev 15:23-25 and Lev 16:27-28)
NIV Lev 6:27 if any of the blood is spattered on a garment, then you must wash it in a holy place.

A person's life is in the blood, so long as the blood is circulating in the body. However, when blood is not circulating through the cleansing organs of the body, the blood becomes a perfect breeding ground for unhealthy bacteria. (Ch 9 Blood) Once the blood of man or animal is allowed to contaminate a garment or come into contact with a person, the blood needs to be washed away.

∗ Hyssop (Oregano) formed the basis for a strong anti-microbial soap to cleanse the skin.

Semmelweis, Lister and Pasteur

As simple and easy as washing hands is for cleanliness today, hand washing has in times past been completely ignored and at certain times even ridiculed. Perhaps the saddest example of disregard for the hygienic value of washings occurred in hospitals in Europe in the early 1800s. Many of these hospitals called for physicians to begin their day's work by doing autopsies on the corpses of yesterday's dead. The next duty of these physicians was frequently the maternity ward, where they examined the expecting women and delivered babies with unwashed hands from their duty just before. (These women were expecting the joys motherhood and should not have needed to be expecting infection or death by the hands of the unlearned physicians.) These new mothers frequently suffered tears of the vagina and vaginal bleeding as a result of the delivery of their children, which created an environment that left them very susceptible to disease. In the early 1800's, in the hospitals of Europe many women developed puerperal fever after childbirth. Puerperal fever began at the vagina and the womb, then infected the fallopian tubes and then the blood stream, after which it spread through the entire body. This contamination of new mothers with the germs of yesterday's dead, led to a very high mortality rates amongst these women! In the 1840s, a Jewish physician, Dr. Ignaz Philip Semmelweis noted that women in the same hospitals who were attended by midwives for their birthing and delivery, did not experience this same high rate of fever and death. [R9-10A-14-15] Dr. Semmelweis also reasoned that a cause and effect relationship existed between the blood on the hands of the physicians from the autopsies and the transmission of the disease to the mother during the time of delivery. In one hospital Dr. Semmelweis saw the mortality drop from 57 deaths in April, to one death in each June and July in his obstetrics ward; just by implementing a sanitary hand washing procedure before performing gynecology examinations or delivering babies. Implementation of a hand washing procedure was a beautiful example of application of Mosaic principles (instruction) and should have been applauded by his colleagues. Instead, the unlearned physicians considered hand washing too much of a bother and they had Dr. Semmelweis removed from his position at the hospital. When Semmelweis left the mortality rate went back up again. [R2-3-4-7] In the early practice of medical surgeries the value of washings was similarly ignored. Death by infection after surgery was equally disastrous to childbirth until sanitary washing procedures were developed.

> "From 1867 on, Lister in Scotland had published papers and given lectures showing that just washing hands and instruments could significantly lower the incidence of postoperative wound infections." [R6A]

In the 1870s, Joseph Lister, Louis Pasteur, Robert Koch and others finally convinced the medical community that germs were the cause of many infectious diseases. The unwashed hands of the unlearned physician could spread these disease-causing germs from one patient to another. [R2-3-4] Today, medicine knows that washing in a bowl of water is not as effective for removing germs as washing in running water. Washing in a bowl of stagnant water allows germs from the skin to come back in contact with the skin. These germs will get under the scales of the skin, thus the skin is re-contaminated and is never adequately cleansed of germs. Washing in running water is now the basis of all medical scrubbing before surgery by physicians and patients. (Lev 15:13) [R8] How much pain, misery and death could have been avoided throughout the centuries had the people and the physicians of the world read the ***Torah*** and trusted that following God's instructions would be beneficial for health?

How do we in the 1990s and beyond measure up to obeying God's statutes and hearkening to the voice of the God-physician (***Yahweh–Rapheka***) of Exodus 15:26 for our medical wisdom?

KJV Ex 15:26 And [God] said, If thou wilt diligently hearken to the voice of the LORD thy God and wilt do that which is right in his sight, and wilt give ear to his commandments, and keep all his statutes, I will put none of these diseases upon thee, which I have brought upon the Egyptians; for I am the God (***Yahweh–Rapheka***) that healeth thee.

Do we seek physicians who draw upon the wisdom of God first? In the 1970s, women who had trouble with sleeping and morning sickness during pregnancy turned to a new wonder drug thalidomide, which caused many birth defects. When we have health problems do we first look to the source of all healing for what might be the cause of this problem? Do we look for how our lives might be out of harmony with what the LORD wants for us? Do we and our Physicians seek our solutions in accordance with the proven, age-old principles from Scripture? [R13-15] If we do not keep our medical health in line with the ***Torah***, we may be part of the next medical disaster.

------------------------- References Ch 05 Wash and Cleanse ------------------------

[R1] The Book of Leviticus\ by Samuel Kellogg; pg 292-293 quote - death
[R2] None of These Diseases\ by S. I. McMillen, MD; pg 13-15 various washings
[R2A] pg 9-10 'none of these diseases' & Semmelweis
[R3] None o These Diseases (Revised)\ by McMillen, MD and David Stern, MD; pg 26 -soap quote
[R3A] pg 19-20 'none of these diseases'
[R3B] pg 24-25 Semmelweis
[R4] None of These Diseases (Revised and Expanded)\ by McMillen, MD and Stern, MD; pg 17-26 Semmelweis
The Story of Medicine\ by Inglis A History of Medicine\ by Lehner The Story of Medicine\ by Margotta (historical)
[R5] Head First: The Biology of Hope\ by Norman Cousins; pg 155-156 blood letting
[R6] God and Vitamins\ by Marjorie Holmes; pg 64 *The Body is the Hero* Semmelweis
[R7] The Body is the Hero\ by Ronald Glasser, MD; pg 37-41 Semmelweis
[R8] The Chemistry of the Blood\ by M.R. DeHann, MD; pg 73-74 wash before surgery
[R9] The Cry and the Covenant\ by M. Thompson; Semmelweis died in a mental hospital
[R10] Moses and Preventive Medicine\ Biblio Theca Sacra; vol 147; July-Aug 1990;
by Jay D. Fawver and R. Larry Overstreet; pg 275 Egyptians used donkey feces to treat splinters
[R10A] pg 278-280 Dr. Ignaz Semmelweis began hand-washing
[R11] Killer Microbes All Around (magazine 12 Sept 94)\ in Time; a never-ending battle – man vs microbes
[R12] The Coming Plague\ by Laurie Garrett; history of Plague – past – present – future
[R13] Total Tattoo Book\ by Amy Krakow; pg 8 spiritual dimension //pg 17 Tattoos likely began in Egypt
[R14] What You Don't Know CAN Hurt You\ by Stewart Hughes Dr. Ignaz Semmelweis
[R15] The Joy of Health\ by Zoltan Rona, MD; pg 18 (25+ years later Semmelweis was recognized)
[R16] Outbreak Alert\ by Jason Eberhardt-Phillips, MD; pg 44 – wash – *Cyclospora* infection
[R17] Homeopathic Medicine\ by Lyle W. Morgan; pg 7 used properly may enhance immune function
[R18] Strong's Concordance = Strong's Comprehensive Concordance of the Bible\ by James Strong, STD, LLD

pg 197	clean (pure)	# 2891 (from #2889)	H pg 45	***taher***	Num 19:19
pg 1087	unclean (foul)	# 2930-32	H pg 46	***tame***	Num Ch 19
pg 1106	wash (trample)	# 3526	H pg 54	***kabac***	Num 19:19
pg 1106	wash (water)	# 7364	H pg 108	***rachats***	Lev 14:9
pg 661	marks (gash)	# 7085	H pg 104	***qaaqa***	Lev 19:28
pg 593	leprosy (Grk-*lepra*)	# 6883	H pg 101	***tsara'at* – *tsarara'ath***	Lev Ch 13
pg 593	leprosy	# 3014	G pg 45	*lepra* – scaliness	Mark 1:42
pg 615	LORD (Y-hw-h)	# 3068	H pg 47	***Yahweh* – *Y-HW-H***	Ex 15:26
pg 456	healeth	# 7495	H pg 110	***Rapheka* – *Raphah***	Ex 15:26
pg 795	plague	# 5061	H pg 76	***nega'***	Lev 13:54

[R19] Virus X \ by Frank Ryan, MD; pg 113 Plague from the Latin *plaga*:
a blow, stroke, wound; an affliction, calamity or evil, especially through divine visitation;
a general term for any malignant disease or pestilence with which men or beasts are stricken, especially an epidemic attended by great mortality. (from the Oxford English Dictionary)
"Cholera is a waterborne disease, ... Taken into the body through contaminated water, or food such as shellfish, the germ (*V. cholerae*) attaches to the lining of the human bowel, producing a poison called enterotoxin, which causes the gut to leak fluid. The leak is massive, in excess of a liter per hour. The profuse diarrhea resembles rice water, teeming with germs. This contaminates soil and water supplies, continuing the germ's life cycle of infection to others."
[R20] The Secrets of the Pyramids\ by Peter Tompkins; pg 259 & 262
Moses was trained in wisdom of the Egyptians – which included much 'misinformation'.
[R21] The Book of Leviticus\ by Gordon J. Wenham
[R22] Epidemic\ edited by Rob DeSalle, PhD
[R23] Mapping Epidemics\ by Brent Hoff and Carter Smith III; pg 16-21 Cholera
[R23A] pg 50-51 Leprosy
[R24] Epidemic\ ed by Rob DeSalle, MD; pg 167 many water-borne bacterial diseases
[R25] Or Perish in the Attempt\ by Daniel J. Peck, DO; pg 42 In 1790, Benjamin Rush MD justified blood-letting.
[R26] Epidemics\ by Geoffrey Marks and William K. Beatty
[R27] Virus Hunters of the C.D.C.\ by Joe McCormick, MD, PhD and Susan Fischer-Hoch, MD
[R28] And the Band Played On (movie)\ AIDS + identifying HIV virus + 1) think – 2) know – 3) prove
[R29] Mission Impossible II (movie)\ high tech medicine requires high tech illness/disease
[R30] The First Horseman (audio novel) \ by John Case; 1918 Flu as biological terrorism // Plague (novel//movie)
[R31] The Cure (audio book – tapes 2 to 5)\ by Sonia Levintin; – Jews and plague in medieval 'Dark Ages'
[R32] A Time of Angels (audio book)\ by Karen Hesse; – Jews and the 1918 Flu in New England
[R33] The Journal of the Plague (audio book)\ by Daniel DeFoe; – 1665-6 AD Bubonic Plague in London
(During London's 1665-6 AD Bubonic Plague, Isaac Newton left Cambridge to live on a farm, where he formulated the laws of physics.)
[R34] The Jewish Book of Why (book + audio book read by Eli Wallach)\ by Alfred J. Kolatch; diet, holidays, tradition
[R35] Nostradamus \ by A&E; (Jewish) physician – In 1530, used washings and rose hips (vitamin C) – treated plague.

Chapter 6 Plague and Disease Control
Microbial Control through Sanitation

Moses wrote very specific instructions to the Israelites, requiring them to choose a place away from their dwellings solely for the purpose of isolating and disposing of human waste.

NIV Deut 23:12-13 "Designate a place outside the camp where you can go to relieve yourself.
vs13 As part of your equipment have something [a trowel] to dig with and when you relieve
yourself dig a hole and cover your excrement."

One medical historian wrote that this directive in Deuteronomy 23 is: [R3A]

"certainly a primitive measure, but an effective one, which indicates advances ideas of sanitation."

Fecal matter is a cesspool of toxins, upon which many disease–spreading insects thrive. [R3A-12] Up to the late 1800s, fecal matter was frequently thrown into unpaved, filthy, foul–smelling streets, where flies flourished and spread diseases that killed millions. Outhouses, toilets, sewage treatment plants and septic systems are all based on this Mosaic instruction about confining human waste. Despite the instructions from the ***Torah*** concerning hygiene, which most people in the US take as common knowledge, there are still many places ('third world' countries in which the ***Torah*** is not considered authoritative) that allow unprocessed toilet water to be dumped directly into lakes, rivers and oceans today. [R9A] Many people in these poor countries are sick from bacterial intestinal disease, and they may not have a clue as to what caused their illness, or what to do to stop it.

Donald W. Hewitt, MD in his book *Longer Life: Radiant Health and Dynamic Living* quotes another physician, Dr. Virchow, the father of modern pathology, who stated:

"Moses was the greatest hygienist the world has ever seen." [R1]

Dr. Hewitt also discussed the destructive nature of parasitic and infectious maladies, which has demanded a great amount of attention from modern pathology, appears to have greatly occupied the mind of Moses, and to have dominated all his hygienic rules in the ***Torah***. [R1] **

Greer Williams in his book *The Plague Killers* discusses the hookworm parasite, which gets into the soil by fecal contamination, and is endemic around the globe from 36° N to 30° S latitude. Half the population of the world lives there, and half the people are often infected with hookworm. Hookworm was a huge problem in the US in 'the South' as recently as 1910. Human hookworm requires warm, moist, sandy soil contaminated by infected human feces. Hookworm larvae live in soil, bore through barefoot skin, especially between the toes, get into the bloodstream, live in the intestine and drink blood, causing anemia and bouts of nausea, vomiting, diarrhea or constipation. General malaise, laziness, muscle pain, pot-belly, 'fish-eye' stare and blurred vision are common symptoms, causing much misery and not infrequent death due to secondary infections. Medicine can kill hookworms, but outhouses, which were rare in the 1800s, are the prevention solution. [R20] In 1891, Dr. Charles Stiles began his 20-year effort to cure and prevent hookworm in the South.

Arno Karlan in his book *Man and Microbes* discusses the Typhus epidemic caused by fecal contamination and poor hygiene during WWI that killed 20 million people around the globe. [R24T] Typhus is caused by malnutrition, fecal contamination of water, and *rickettsia* microbes carried by lice on rats, causing skin rash and gangrene in which people literally rot away from the inside, while still alive. Typhoid from fecal (sewage) contaminated water is often associated with Typhus.

Brent Hoff and Carter Smith III in their book *Mapping Diseases* discuss Cholera from fecal contamination of India's Ganges River as a current problem and as initiating global pandemics. [R23]

Today, many societies often do reasonably well in obeying sanitation principles from the ***Torah***.

Despite Jews having not lived in ideal conditions throughout Europe, they bear historical record to the value of the ***Torah*** in preserving health. About one century ago, Professor Hosmer said; [R9]

"Throughout the entire history of Israel, the wisdom of the ancient lawgivers in these respects has been remarkably shown. In times of pestilence the Jews have suffered far less than others; as regards to longevity and general health, they have in every age been noteworthy, and, at the present day, in life-insurance offices, the life of the Jew is said to be worth much more than the life of men of other stock." "Of the facts in the modern world which sustain these statements, Dr. Behrends gives abundant illustration in the article 'Diseases Caught from Butchers Meat' such as the following: 'In Prussia, the mean duration of Jewish life averages 5 years more than that of the general population. In Furth, the average duration of Jewish life is 37, and of Christians 26 years. In Hungary, and exhaustive study of the facts shows that the average duration of life with the Croats is 20.2; of the Germans 26.7; but of the Jews 46.5 years, and that although the Jews generally are poor, and live under much more unfavorable sanitary conditions than their gentile neighbors'."

*** Hebrew history has proven that following Mosaic wisdom yields the fruit of a healthy and long life.**

Bubonic Plague and other Epidemics

In Europe, the Dark Ages of 476 to 1350 AD saw populations grow in the cities, while principles of hygiene, cleanliness and sanitation were not yet well understood and/or not well practiced. Plagues and epidemics in Europe were often more feared than the arrival of an invading army. Timothy Levi Biel in his book *The Black Death* describes Bubonic Plague from 1347 to 1350 AD. This Bubonic Plague began when Mongolians besieging Kaffa on the Black Sea became afflicted. One Mongol general, whose troops were decimated by Bubonic Plague, recognized the contagious nature of plague and catapulted his dead from plague soldiers over a wall of Kaffa before retreating. Black Death was often carried from port to port by the black rat onboard ships. Fleas on a black rat bite a plague-infected rodent, acquire the *Y. pestis* bacillus and then transfer the bacillus to man by biting him. This establishes the rodent–flea–bacillus–man transmission of Bubonic Plague. [R23B] Bubonic Plague or The Plague of the 1300s was the most feared plague of all time, during which ¼ to ½ of Europe or 25 million people – (60 million worldwide) died. People afflicted by Bubonic Plague developed fever, black swollen lymph nodules of the armpits, neck and groin the size of apples that spread over the entire body, frequently followed by lethargy, hallucinations and death. Some people appeared healthy when they awoke, but were dead from Black Death by nightfall. Bubonic Plague of the 14th century is often described as the greatest disaster in human history. When physicians couldn't find answers to stop The Plague, Europe turned to God for the answer. When clergymen required infected individuals to be quarantined, The Plague was stopped. [R2-3-4]

That the environment for all plagues in Europe was hospitable can be traced to the careless hygienic practices of the day. Human waste was thrown into the streets, where it sat and formed a breeding ground for microbes and disease-carrying insects. Cholera, Dysentery and Typhoid were propagated by these practices, which continued through the end of the 18th century. [R2A-3A-4A]

In the 1300s, European Jews, such as the physician Balavignus, must have been meticulous in following Mosaic Law because Jews were largely immune from plagues. Dr. Balavignus recognized that lax sanitary practices could contribute to the spread of disease, so he initiated a community program to improve sanitation in Jewish ghettos. As a consequence of cleanup activities, many rats moved out of Jewish areas and found conditions more to their liking in the 'gentile' sections of town. Since rats were largely responsible for carrying the bacteria that caused Bubonic Plague, fewer rats in the Jewish community translated into only 5% as many deaths from The Plague as their not-so-fortunate gentile neighbors. When the residents of Strasbourg recognized the Jewish death rate was so much less than that of the general population, they too could have searched for the wisdom that is found in the ***Torah***. Instead, a wave of anti-Jewish sentiment developed and the townsfolk began to accuse the Jews, including Dr. Balavignus, of causing The Plague by poisoning the public drinking water from the town wells. So intense was the towns-folks hatred for the Jews, that many Jews were massacred, tortured and persecuted all because the Jews were wise enough to follow levitical principles, when their gentile neighbors didn't follow the levitical law. Dr. Balavignus was even pressured to confess that he and other Jews were responsible for causing Bubonic Plague. [R6] (The environment for Plague during the 1300's may have been worsened by Christian 'witch hunts', since black cats that ate rats were considered part of witchery and were killed along with 'witches'.)

After death a corpse becomes a breeding ground for disease. Moses instructed that a corpse was to be buried the day of death, which would definitely limit the spread of disease. (Deut 21:23)

Arno Karlan in his book *Man and Microbes* discussed that the control of plagues has been an ongoing battle for all human history; and following Mosaic instruction is vital to this effort. [R24]

"In the 1990s, we can see for each disease conquered, another has emerged or reemerged."

Plague and widespread death from infectious disease, especially as encouraged by poor sanitation, seem like issues of the past for people who haven't lived through an epidemic; but Laurie Garrett in her book *The Coming Plague* discusses the great likelihood of future plagues.

Florence Nightingale, John Snow and Charles Stiles cured disease by implementing public health procedures, while Ronald Ross and Walter Reed proved that mosquitoes carried diseases. During the '50 Golden Years' of public health (1854 to 1904), many hygienic principles of the ***Torah*** were re-discovered. Today, Mosaic principles of hygiene are implemented in all modern nations.

'None of these diseases' reflects the cause and effect relationship that ***Yahweh–Rapheka*** – the 'God-that-healtheth' – intended to establish between Himself and His people. (Exodus 15:26) Today, all people of faith should look to the 'LORD God of health' for their well-being and look to follow His instructions in the ***Torah*** as the primary means to maintain their physical health.

∗ Quarantine instructions in the ***Torah*** make Moses the father of public health and bacteriology!

Leprosy (*tsara'at*)

Leprosy (***tsara'at***) as used by Moses in the ***Torah*** could refer to the infectious contagious skin-nerve malady that leaves victims badly mutilated, or to merely a non-infectious skin rash. [R24] ***Tsara'at,*** as Moses used the word, suggests hygienic uncleanness as much as a medical illness. The Greek *Septuagint* translated ***tsara'at*** as *lepra*. In Greek *lepra* is a disfiguring skin disease. Leprosy in English is derived from the Greek *lepra.* [R24] Leprosy in modern times has come to refer exclusively to the infectious bacterial human skin disease that cripples and disfigures its victims. *(This book uses* Leprosy *to refer to the infectious bacterial skin disease; and uses* leprosy *for a non-infectious skin rash.)*

Moses instructed the Levitical Priests to observe the skin and to distinguish non-infectious skin rashes from the moderately contagious Leprosy that has often plagued post-Flood human society.

KJV Lev 13:2 When a man shall have in the skin of his flesh a rising, a scab or bright spot, and it be in the skin of his flesh like the plague (***nega'***) of leprosy (***tsara'at***): ... vs3 And the priest shall look on the plague in the skin of the flesh: and when the hair in the plague is turned white, and the plague in sight be deeper than the skin of his flesh, it is a plague of leprosy (***tsara'at***); and the priest shall look upon him, and pronounce him unclean. vs6 And the priest shall look on him again the seventh day: and, behold, if the plague be somewhat dark, and the plague spread not in the skin, the priest shall pronounce him clean: it is but a scab: and he shall wash his clothes, and be clean. vs7 But if the scab spread much abroad in the skin, after that he hath been seen of the priest for his cleansing, he shall be seen of the priest again: vs8 And if the priest see that, behold the scab spreadeth in the skin, then the priest shall pronounce him unclean: it is a leprosy (***tsara'at***).

The priest may determine that the skin condition is a minor rash or scab, rather than Leprosy. When Moses put his hand under his garment and took it out, his hand became leprous as a sign from the LORD, this was likely just a skin rash, rather than infectious bacterial Leprosy. (Ex 4:6) Miriam questioned Moses and became leprous, which was likely not bacterial Leprosy. (Num 12:10)

Leprous garments and houses may have been fungal, rather human bacterial Leprosy. [R26] Washing clothes, rock walls and skin reduces microbial populations, limiting further outbreaks. Leprous clothes were washed and after washing, if signs persisted, leprous clothes were burned. Leprous houses were to have stone walls scraped clean. Should leprous signs reappear, houses were dismantled, and the stones were taken outside the city and discarded in an unclean place.

KJV Lev 14:37 And he shall look upon the plague (***nega'***), and, behold if the plague be in the walls of the house strakes, greenish or reddish, which in sight are lower than the wall; vs39 And the priest shall come again the seventh day, and shall look, and, behold if the plague is spread in the walls of the house; vs40 Then the priest shall demand that they take away the stones in which the plague is, and they shall cast them into an unclean place without the city; vs43 And if the plague come again in the house, after that he hath taken away the stones, and after he hath scraped the house, and after it is plastered; vs44 Then the priest shall come and look, and, behold if the plague is spread in the house, it is a fretting leprosy (***tsara'at***) in the house: it is unclean. vs45 And he shall break down the walls of the house, the stones of it, and the timber thereof, and all the motor of the house; and shall carry them forth out of the city into an unclean place. vs47 And he that lieth in the house shall wash his clothes; and he that eateth in the house shall wash his clothes. vs49 And he shall take to cleanse the house two birds and cedar wood, and scarlet, and hyssop.

Hyssop, cedar wood, and scarlet are excellent ingredients to make a powerful antiseptic soap. Charcoal, as from burnt cedar wood, contains fibrous elements to absorb toxins and to dislodge microbes from walls, which would make charcoal an excellent additive for soap to cleanse houses.

'Curse of the Pharaoh' disease legends likely resulted from Egyptologists, who entered ancient tombs, but died shortly thereafter from mysteriously illnesses. Curse of the Pharaoh illness was later attributed to leprous mold toxin from water seeping into a tomb creating a dank/damp environment in which mold flourished for centuries on organic pigments used in paints for pictures on tomb walls. Leprous mold toxins in tombs often overwhelmed people with a compromised immune system. [R36] (In Nov 1922, Lord Carnarvon helped discover and enter King Tut's Tomb – he mysteriously died in Apl 1923.)

Sherry Rogers, MD in her book *Tired or Toxic* discusses inadequate nutrition and environmental toxins that result in a weakened immune system and predispose people to acute or chronic illness. Today, people may become ill from leprous mold/fungus found in walls of poorly designed buildings. Dr. Rogers as well as William Crook, MD in his book *The Yeast Connection* discuss Candida yeast overgrowth in people with under active digestive–immune systems that may result in chronic fatigue.

* Toxins from leprous mold may damage health – especially for people with a compromised immune system.

Leprosy and Quarantine

Infectious Leprosy is an old disease that continues to plague some third-world countries today. Symptoms of advanced Leprosy are severe and at times even macabre, yet victims feel little pain.

"Spreading slowly throughout the body, leprosy bacterium damages the nerves and keeps the blood from supplying oxygen and nutrients to the skin; secondary infections descend on dying flesh like birds of prey on carrion. First they raise unsightly calluses and scars; then fingers, toes, and sections of nasal tissues fall away. Hands and feet are twisted into bear-claw shapes; the face becomes broken and twisted; nasal cartilage and vocal cords are damaged, and the voice becomes raspy and honking. As tubercular lesions protrude, the eyebrows become swollen and denuded of hair; the face, the skin, and the limbs take on frightening new aspects; the mouth and nostrils become twisted; the eyes take a on a horrifying stare; and breath and body often give off a disgusting smell." [R13] – pg 26

Damage that advanced Leprosy causes to nerves and skin greatly reduces pain sensitivity, such that a victim may be cut or burned without the benefit of feeling pain to trigger a quick withdrawal. Leprosy is often compared to sin (trespass) by Bible scholars to demonstrate the consequences of sin. Trespass is purposeful sin. Initially committing sin results in feelings of guilt that trigger withdrawal, yet as a trespass is continually practiced an initial feeling of guilt fades and sin becomes normative. The comparison of Leprosy to sin caused society to often look on Leprosy as judgment from God, and treat Lepers as outcasts. Moses expected healing from Leprosy as the offerings indicate. (Lev 14) Washing plus shaving all hair from the body ensures that no harmful bacteria remain on the skin to cause re-infection, as bacteria often inhabit hair follicles. Shaving is common medical hygiene today.

KJV Lev 14:8 And he that is to be cleansed [of ***tsara'at***] shall wash his clothes, and shave off all his hair, and wash himself in water, that he may be clean: and after that he shall come into the camp, ...

Levitical Priests acted like physicians: an unclean diagnosis meant contagious bacterial Leprosy and the isolation of 'quarantine' to prevent an actively contagious Leprosy from spreading to others.

In 1873, Armauer Hansen, MD observed *M. leprae* bacilli that are now known to cause Leprosy. In 1879, Dr. Hansen attempted to transmit Leprosy from a victim to a non-afflicted person when he contaminated a surgical knife with *M. leprae* bacilli from a Leprous tuber and then used the knife to make an incision to a female's conjunctiva. However, the furious woman did not develop a leprous tuber, as Leprosy is extremely difficult to transmit and often has an incubation time of 10 yrs or more. Dr. Hansen helped dispel the myth that Leprosy was inherited or Leprosy was a curse from God. People with malnutrition, poor sanitation and a weak immune system develop Leprosy, since 95% of people worldwide are immune to *M. leprae* bacilli. Leprosy is a human disease with no animal host. Leprosy can only be caught from nasal discharge or skin-to-skin contact with a Leper's open sore. Leprosy eye disease includes unsightly tubers on the eyelids and cornea, reduced blink reflex, reduced corneal sensation and reduced tear production, which can result in blindness from dry eye, corneal ulcers or corneal scars; as well as secondary bacterial infections resulting in red eyes. [R15-16]

KJV Lev 13:46 All the days wherein the [Leprosy] plague shall be in him, he shall be defiled: he is unclean: he shall dwell alone [be isolated in quarantine]: without the camp shall be his habitation.

Quarantine, including rest and *kosher* food, was required by Moses to heal a Leper. (Lev 13:46) Conditions of poor diet and poor sanitation encourage Leprosy and many other plagues–epidemics. The benefit of quarantine to control Leprosy, or other plagues, extends both to victims and society. For the Leper, rest and *kosher* food is the only opportunity of regaining strength, vitality and health. For society, quarantine prevents people with weak immune systems from being exposed to Leprosy.

One medical historian discussed the hygienic insight of Moses in the ***Torah***: [R2A-3C]

"The Laws against leprosy in Leviticus 13 may be regarded as the first model of a sanitary legislation."

Leprosy remains a dreaded disease that has killed or crippled millions throughout the centuries. The 6th and 7th centuries saw Leprosy spread throughout Europe. In the 13th and 14th centuries, Leprosy became endemic in certain areas and especially amongst the malnourished poor. [R2-3-4]

In ≈1950, dapsone, a sulfone drug, was the first successful drug to treat Leprosy, but *M. leprae* bacilli soon developed resistance to dapsone, forcing multiple drug therapy (MDT) since ≈1970. [R7-25] *Microbes that were controlled by antibiotics decades ago have mutated or adapted to more virulent antibiotic-resistant forms that are returning to again cause plagues–epidemics on Earth. [R8-10-13-24] Penicillin, the wonder drug of 1929, is now often worthless due to bacterial resistance and many other antibiotics are now also of limited value to treat bacterial infections, due to bacterial resistance.

∗ Quarantine, *kosher* food and rest was the antidote prescribed by Moses to treat Leprosy.

1918 Flu Pandemic – Purple Death

The last major epidemic was the Spanish Flu of 1918 at the end of The Great War (WW1). Influenza is common and a mild strain of flu emerged from Spain in the winter/spring of 1918, but 'The Spanish Flu' that began in the summer/fall of 1918 was like no other flu before, or since. Symptoms of the 1918 Flu often began like any ordinary flu, with a dull headache, burning eyes and a slight fever. But, bed rest, drinking plenty of liquids, warm blankets and aspirin didn't relieve symptoms. A rest-less sleep often included distorted nightmares and delirium, as the fever climbed. Awaking into semi-consciousness, muscles ached, the head throbbed and the path to death was certain. [R31]

"Your face turns dark brownish purple. You start to cough up blood. Your feet turn black. Finally, as the end nears, you frantically gasp for breath. A blood-tinged saliva bubbles out of your mouth. You die—by drowning, actually—as your lungs fill with a reddish fluid." [R31]

Victims of 'The 1918 Flu' often developed a secondary pneumonia after 4 days of chills/fever.

"... rapidly develop the most viscous type of Pneumonia that has ever been seen. Two hours after admission they have the Mahogany spots over the cheek bones and a few hours later you can begin to see the Cyanosis extending from the ears and spreading all over the face, until it is hard to distinguish the colored man from the white. It is only a matter of a few hours then until death comes and it is simply a struggle for air until they [1918 Flu victims] suffocate." [R31]

"... the lungs were in this [1918 Flu] cadaver – two sacks filled with a thin, bloody, frothy fluid." [R34]

In 1918, 28% of the 80^+ million US populace became ill with the Flu and 2½% of those died, totaling $500,000^+$ American deaths – 'the greatest loss of life in six months of US history'. [R31D]

The 1918 Flu began with US soldiers at Ft. Devens, Mass, but it quickly spread to other military bases.

"Only hours after showing the symptoms of the flu, soldiers were suddenly turning blue and dying." [R30]

Most flues kill only infants, the ill, and the aged, but 21 to 29 year olds were often victims of the 1918 Flu. Initial global estimates of 1918 Flu deaths were 20^+ million, but that many likely died in India alone. [R31D]

The 1918 Flu pandemic circled the Earth in 9 months, killing ≈50 (40^+ to 100) million people in all.

Prior to 1918, flu was unknown in pigs. In 1918, people and pigs transmitted the Flu to one another. [R31J] The 1918 Flu seems to have had an origin closely tied to pigs; and pigs, like humans, were often victims.

In 1976, a US soldier, Dave Lewis, caught a flu, was sick in bed, got up for a 5 mile hike and died shortly after the hike. In 1976, it was feared this flu could become another 'swine flu' global pandemic. Many people were inoculated against a possibly fatal flu, but the warnings were only a false alarm. [30A]

A virus cannot live on its own (outside a host). Viruses wait for a cell that they can enter – flu viruses prefer epithelial cells of the respiratory tract. Once inside a cell, a flu virus forces the cell's biochemistry to reproduce more viruses; later the newly made viruses burst from the infected cell to infect nearby cells.

Viruses, such as a flu virus, often change or mutate. A small yearly change is called a 'drift' and a major (flu) virus change is a 'shift'. [R30] Antibodies defend cells against viruses. Antibodies that kill one years' flu virus often work against a virus 'drift', but not against a virus 'shift'. The immune system makes new antibodies to a 'new or shifted' virus in a week, but the same virus, if seen again, is now 'old' and antibodies are re–made quickly. People who got a 'new' mild 1918 spring flu had antibodies and were often immune to an 'old' 1918 fatal fall Flu. [R31E]

Flu Virus

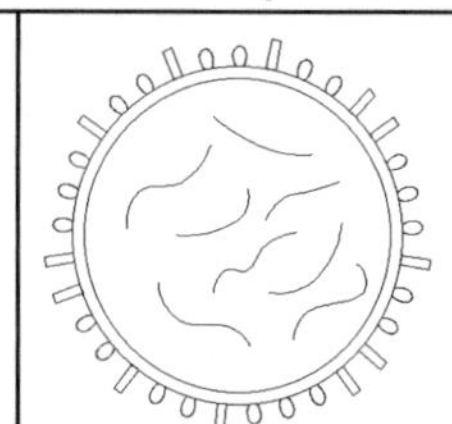

∗ Vaccines stimulate the immune system to produce antibodies, so a 'new' virus is reacted to as if 'old'. Hemagglutinin 'H' proteins protruding from a virus' surface allow a virus to enter a cell and Neuraminidase 'N' proteins enable viruses to exist a cell. The 'H' and 'N' proteins are targets for antibodies to attack. [R31F]

In 1918, soldiers, athletes, police, firemen, nurses and others wore masks to prevent from contracting the Flu, but since a $million^+$ flu viruses fit on a pinhead, the porous gauze made all masks ineffective. [R30]

Vitamin C, discovered in 1928, may help the immune system disable viruses – like the 1918 Flu virus. Anyone, such as soldiers, lacking fresh fruit and vegetables may have been more susceptible to the Flu.

Any severe disease outbreak (Endemic or Epidemic or Pandemic) may be referred to as a 'plague'.

Endemic – localized, routinely found throughout a region (often chronic – for an extended time period)
Epidemic – rapidly spreading over a very large area (often acute – begins quickly – may end suddenly)
Pandemic – widespread over a broad area affecting large percentage of the population (possibly global)

Bubonic Plague = The Plague = Black Death 1918 Flu = The Flu = Purple Death

Malaria is endemic to certain tropical areas and is chronic throughout all recorded post-Flood human history.
The 1918 Flu Epidemic was both pandemic and acute, as it circled the globe in 9 months; but the 1918 Flu has not been heard from since. (In 1976, another bout of The Flu was expected, but it didn't materialize.)
The Ebola hemorrhagic fever was an acute epidemic that stopped very quickly with the help of quarantine.
The AIDS pandemic began insidiously, it is now chronic, it continues to spread rapidly and in some areas of Africa it is endemic, affecting a majority of the population. (Quarantine may not stop AIDS.)

∗ While its origins remain a mystery, immunity to the 1918 Flu pandemic was more precious than gold.

1918 Flu Pandemic – Medical Mystery

The 1918 Flu began mysteriously. – The 1918 Flu ended just as mysteriously; when WW1 ended. How did a common flu virus become so lethal? – Why did 'The 1918 Flu' stop as quickly as it began?

Dr. Pfeiffer identified a bacillus in 1890 flu victims that was also found in many 1918 Flu fatalities. In 1918, physicians theorized: People caught a flu virus and 'Pfeiffer's bacillus' at the same time, causing a secondary pneumonia along with a common flu virus that made the 1918 Flu very lethal. When World War 1 ended on Nov 11, 1918, research on the Flu began. In exchange for having charges against them dropped, some US service men volunteered to find out how people got the Flu. But suddenly, when WW1 ended, nobody caught the 1918 Flu, Pfeiffer's bacillus didn't produce pneumonia in lab animals and no reasonable medical explanation for the 1918 flu was put forth. [R31A]

In 1996, intact 1918 Flu virus was searched for, but not found, in the corpses of 1918 Flu victims who were buried for 75+ years in the permafrost of Alaska and Norway near the Arctic Circle. [R31N]

In March 1918, tons of manure was burned at Ft. Riley Kansas causing a stinking yellow cloud that blackened the sky; soon 500+ soldiers became ill and 48 died, before the healthy left for WW1. (If pig manure ripe with swine flu virus was burned, this may have helped the Flu become widespread.)

Since the 1918 Flu virus was lethal to US hogs in the Midwest, and since people and pigs transmitted the Flu to one another in 1918, early researchers looked for the lethal Flu in hogs. A swine flu has become common in pigs since 1918, but prior to 1918, flu was unknown in pigs. Survivors of the 1918 Flu have antibodies that work against the common flu in swine, and the flu virus that is common in pigs today may also cause human flu, but not flu like the 1918 Flu. [R31E]

In 1997, Jeffrey Taubenberger, MD, PhD of the Armed Forces Institute of Pathology isolated the virus from a preserved 70 year-old piece of lung tissue of a US soldier who died from the 1918 Flu. Dr. Taubenberger's research team also mapped the DNA gene sequence of the 1918 Flu virus. [R22]

Dr. Taubenbeger theorizes: the 1918 Flu may have mutated in pigs to become perfectly lethal in the fall, and then, a further mutation in winter may have caused it to become perfectly harmless. [R31B]

Dr. John Oxford theorizes: the 1918 Flu became global too quickly to have spread just from person to person, and conditions allowing a pandemic must have existed prior to the outbreak. [R31B]

> "The outstanding fact perhaps is the rapidity with which the epidemic spread after it attained the proportions of an epidemic in the first areas affected. The epidemic became nation-wide in the four to five weeks after it appeared in an epidemic stage in the first localities affected. ... the [1918 Flu] disease reached an epidemic state in a number of localities in the central, northern, southern, and western sections [of USA] at about the same time as it did along the northeastern coast." [R31G]

In 1997, a Hong Kong flu yielded many insights into flues. Benign intestinal flu viruses in birds are common. If a bird virus ever jumped species to man, no one would have any antibodies or immunity. Before a bird virus could infect a human it must mutate and become similar to a human flu virus. [R31C]

∗ Virologists Dr. Webster and Dr. Shortridge believe this may have happened in the 1918 Flu.

In China, farmers keep ducks to eat rice crop pests in their rice paddies, and they also keep pigs.

> ∗ "Pigs bridge the gap between birds and humans—both bird flu strains and human flu strains can grow in pigs' bodies. An unfortunate pig that happens to be infected with both a bird and human virus at the same time can become a mixing bowl, with genes from the two types of flu viruses recombining in its cells to form a new hybrid virus that can infect humans but has some genes from the bird flu, genes that make the newly emerging virus more dangerous than any that has been around before. Thus, the stage can be set for a worldwide pandemic." [R31C]

Dr. Webster and Dr. Shortridge theorize: The 1918 Flu began as a duck virus that mutated in a pig and then infected humans, which is why 1918 Flu survivors have antibodies to the swine flu. [R31C]

The article on the 1918 Flu in Science downplayed the duck to pig to man theory, but warned: to prevent a pandemic similar to the 1918 Flu scientists must closely monitor all swine flues. [R22]

The author's theory is: somehow the Flu virus entered pigs, and it may have contaminated US C-rations and pork shipped worldwide, enabling the 'seeds of plague' to be global prior to the Flu being passed between people. Pork eaters may have been the most susceptible to the 1918 Flu. Perhaps pigs were raised differently in 1918 to help supply meat for the war effort. Old US WW1 C-rations that contain pork, if any still exist, may be the best place to find the 1918 Flu virus today.

N.Y. Times science writer Gina Kolata in her book *Flu* wrote her description of the 1918 Flu.

> "They call the plague of 1918 influenza, but it was like no influenza ever seen before. It was more like a biblical prophecy come true, something from Revelations that predicted that first the world was to be struck by war, then famine, and then, with the breaking of the forth seal ... the appearance of a horse, 'deathly pale', and its rider was called Plague, and Hades followed at its heels." [R31K]

∗ The 1918 Flu was the most lethal pandemic in history and it is closely associated with swine flu.

---------------------------- References Ch 6 Plagues ----------------------------

[R1] Longer Life, Radiant Health and Dynamic Living\ by Donald W. Hewitt MD; pg 117 – quote
[R2] None of These Diseases\ by S. I. McMillen, MD; pg 11 Leprosy & Bubonic Plague // R2B] pg 12-13 Cholera
[R3] None of These Diseases (Revised)\ by McMillen, MD and David Stern, MD; pg 21-22 Leprosy & Bubonic P
[R3B] pg 23-24 Cholera // [R3C] pg 22 – Leprocy: (A History of Medicine\ by Arturo Castiglioni; pg 70-71)
[R4] None of These Diseases (Revised and Expanded)\ by McMillen, MD and Stern, MD; pg 12-16 Leprosy
[R4B] pg 27-35 Cholera – sewage – outhouses – Deut 23:12-13// Deut 21:23 bury the dead
[R5] The Black Death - 1361 (Timeline video)\ by PBS 'Bubonic Plague' = 'The Plague' = 'Black Death'
[R6] Principles of Healthy Living\ by World Wide Church of God; pg 14 Jews, sanitation & Bubonic Plague
[R7] The Plague Makers\ by Jeffrey A. Fisher, MD routine use of antibiotics = drug resistance
[R8] The Coming Plague\ by Laurie Garrett; pg 25-27 Mice spread virus in urine to dust to man. (Four Corners)
[R8A] pg 420 Leprosy treated easily with dapsone antibiotic – 1st antibiotic resistance in 1977.
Louis Pasteur - "Discovery Favors the Prepared Mind" // pg 546 – In 1500s, rats 1st came to America on ships.
[R9] The Book of Leviticus\ by Samuel Kellogg; pg 294 quote Jewish health
[R10] You Can Live\ by Lindsey Williams – immunization risks
[R11] Microbial Diseases (20/20 TV program 1994)\ ebb and flow of – man vs microbes
[R12] Germs that Won't Die\ by Marc Lappe', PhD adapted antibiotic resistant microbes
[R13] The Wages of Sin\ by Peter Lewis Allen; pg 26 Leprosy quote
[R14] Plagues and People\ by William H. McNeill Any severe epidemic may be called a plague.
[R15] Ocular Leprosy\ by Schwab, MD; Ostler, MD; Dawson, MD (Clinical Ophthalmology Vol 5 Ch 63); pg 1-7
[R16] Ophthalmic Trials of A. Hansen\ by Michael Marmor, MD (Survey of Ophthalmology Vol 47 #3 My-Jn2002); pg 275-287
[R17] The Eye in Systemic Disease\ by Gold, MD & Winegeist, MD (Ch 64 Leprosy\ by T. J. Ffytche, MD pg 193-196)
[R18] Strong's Concordance\ by James Strong, STD, LLD
pg 593 Leprosy (Grk-*lepra*) # 6883 H pg 101 ***tsara'at*** – ***tsara'ath*** Lev 13:2
pg 615 LORD # 3068 H pg 47 ***Yahweh*** – ***Y-hw-h*** Ex 15:26
pg 456 which 'healeth' thee # 7495 H pg 110 ***Raphah*** – ***Rapheka*** Ex 15:26
[R19] Outbreak Alert\ by Jason Eberhart-Phillips, MD; pg 92 Hepatitis C /pg 169 – 1918 Flu
[R20] The Plague Killers\ by Greer Williams; pg 3-17 Hookworm from fecal contamination of soil
[R20] pg 16 thymol and Epsom Salts as a cure // pg 17 outhouses for prevention
[R20A] pg 101 malaria plasmodium protozoan of Anopheles mosquito causes human Malaria
[R20B] pg 191-192 mosquitoes living in public water supply often cause Yellow Fever
pg 189 Malaria and Yellow Fever epidemics stop with first frost – Smallpox and Measles continue despite frosts
[R21] Viruses, Plagues, and History\ by Michael B. A. Oldstone; pg 9 drawing of Influenza virus
[R22] Virology (Science: vol 275 - 21 March 97)\ by Elizabeth Pennisi; pg 1739 Taubenberger –1918 Flu virus
[R23] Mapping Epidemics\ by Brent Hoff & Carter Smith III; pg 16-21 Cholera // [R23A] pg 50-51 Leprosy
[R23B] pg 68 Rats carry *Y. pestis* in fleas of fur //Latin *plaga* – to strike out violently with divine intent
pg 70 Jews blamed/killed – C. Priests died tending sick – allowed P. Reformation // pg 104-107 Plague Chronology
[R24] Man and Microbes\ by Arno Karlan; pg 4 – quote emerging disease
[R24T] pg 3&143 Typhus in WWI // pg 113-119 Typhus = malnutrition & filth = victims rot to death
[R24H] pg 82-85 Hansen's Disease = Leprosy (***tsara'at***)) // pg 83 *lepra* in Greek *Septuagint*
[R25] Leprosy\(VineNetwork)–(Internet); pg 3 – 95% of people immune to *M. leprae* bacilli & (American Leprosy Mission)
[R26] Leprosy in the Bible-part III\ in Catholic Encyclopedia from Diseases in the Bible\ by Bennett (1887)
[R27] X-Rated Animal Imports\ by Marty Stouffer – Rats brought diseases to US on ships (1700-1800s) – killed many
[R28] A Field Guide to Germs\ by Wayne Biddle; pg 36-43 Cholera
[R29] The Gift of Pain\ by Paul Brand, MD and Phillip Yancy; Leprosy and the lack of pain
[R30] Purple Death\ by David Getz; pg 33-37 define virus [R30A] pg 49-55 1976 Swine Flu – Lewis' death
[R30B] pg 46-47 viruses often change = drift or shift [R30C] pg 15 quote soldiers death
[R31] Flu\ by Gina Kolata; pg 4-5 – 1st quote symptoms // pg 14-15 – 2nd quote – death
[R31A] pg 64-69 Pfeiffer bacillus [R31D] pg 7 & 285-6 death statistics
[R31B] ch 7 pg 187-218 Taubenberger // pg 304 mutation theory
[R31C] pg 222-224 Webster and Shortridge & 1918 Flu = duck to pig to man – 3rd quote
[R31E] pg 66-67 & 223 1918 – 1st swine flu // antibodies to 1918 Flu = swine flu antibodies
[R31F] pg 118-119 H and N proteins on flu virus - stimulate antibodies to attack virus
[R31G] pg 290-291 & 61-62q global to quickly to be spread just from person to person – 4th quote
[R31H] ch 8 pg 219-241 Hong Kong flu // [R31J] pg 80 - 1918 Flu - pig to man to pig
[R31K] pg 4-5 – 5th quote Plague from *Revelations* // [R31N] Ch 9 pg 243-280 victims in permafrost
[R32] The Plague of the Spanish Lady\ by Richard Collier – The 1918 Flu pandemic
[R33] Influenza 1918 (TV – video) \ by PBS 600,000 US deaths // 21-29 yr olds // burning of manure
[R34] America's Forgotten Pandemic\ by Dr. Alfred Crosby; pg 8 quote – 1918 Flu victim's lungs
[R35] The Hot Zone\ by Richard Preston Ebola virus – very high mortality – caregivers frequent victims
[R36] Howard Carter and the 'Curse of the Mummy' – www.unmuseum.org/mummy.htm – aspergillus mold
[R37] The Forgotten Plague\ by Frank Ryan, MD //and Tuberculosis in America (video)\ by PBS
[R38] War on Disease\ pg 4-31 & (both National Geographic Feb 2002) AIDS Turns 20\ pg 32-43
[R39] Secrets of the Dead – Killer Flu (06-23-04)\ by NOVA-PBS (1918 Flu – bird virus origin? – 1916 Etaple France?)
[R40] Secrets of the Dead – Black Death (09-02-03)\ by NOVA (Bubonic Plague + Pneumonic Plague = Black Death)

Chronology of Plague – plus – The Author's Commentary

≈ 2400 BC	1st Malaria begins in China
400 BC	1st Leprosy in China and India
48 BC	1st Smallpox in China
165-180 AD	Smallpox and Measles in Rome
395-410 AD	Malaria is common in Rome
542-543 AD	1st Bubonic Plague in Mediterranean
535-536 AD	Smallpox in Japan
1343 AD	Dysentery in English troops
1347-1351	Bubonic Plague – Black Death
1400-1500s	Leprosy was endemic in Europe
1489-1494	Typhus in Spain -1st Syphilis in France
1525-1527	Smallpox in Incas – 200,000 dead
1576	Diphtheria in Paris
1617-1619	Smallpox kills Massachusetts Indians
1643	Typhus in England
1665-1666	'Great Plague' kills 20% in London
1710	1st Influenza in Russia
1720	Plague kills 33% in Marseilles
1721-1722	Smallpox in Boston
— 1798 AD	Edward Jenner -1st Smallpox vaccine
1803	Yellow Fever in French army in Haiti
1812-1813	Typhus-Dysentery stops Napoleon
1815	Tuberculosis (TB) plague in England
1817-1823	1st Cholera epidemic from India
1826-1828	Dengue Fever in Georgia
1826-1837	2nd Cholera pandemic in India
1853	Yellow Fever in New Orleans
1853-1856	Diphtheria in England - pandemic
1854	Cholera – Dysentery in Turkey
— 1854 AD	Florence Nightingale stops diseases
— 1854 AD	J. Snow stops Cholera in England
1863-1866	3rd Cholera pandemic from India
— 1873 AD	A. Hansen isolates Leprosy bacteria
— 1876 AD	R. Koch isolates Anthrax bacteria
1881-1896	5th Cholera pandemic from India
— 1882 AD	Koch isolates Tuberculosis bacteria
— 1884 AD	Louis Pasteur – 1st Rabies vaccine
— 1891 AD	Stiles – outhouses stop hookworm
— 1897 AD	R. Ross – Malaria from mosquitoes
1890-1900	3rd Plague epidemic from China
— 1904 AD	Reed –Yellow Fever from mosquitoes
1916	1st Polio outbreak in USA
1918	Flu pandemic – Purple Death – WW1
— 1929 AD	Fleming discovers penicillin
1930s	TB, the modern plague, declines
1950	1st Dengue hemorrhagic fever (HF)
1950-1953	Hantaan HF in Korea kills US soldiers
— 1955 AD	Jonas Salk – 1st Polio vaccine in US
1957-1958	Asian Flu pandemic from China
1975 AD	1st Lyme Disease in USA
1976 AD	1st Ebola HF in Sudan
1976 AD	1st Legionnaire's disease
— 1977 AD	Smallpox – global eradication
1980	1st AIDS – HIV infection in USA
1981-1985	Dengue HF from Latin Am. to USA
1986	1st Mad Cow Disease in England
1989	1st Hepatitis C (non A-non B) in USA
1993	1st Four Corners Hantavirus in USA
1993	1st deadly *E. coli* in burgers in USA
2003	1st SARS in late winter in China

– ≈1450 BC Moses directed '10 Plagues' in Egypt
– Plagues have played a major role in world history. Which nation won a war was often determined by the health of its soldiers rather than superior weaponry.
– India, China and southeast Asia are often a breeding ground for diseases that become global pandemics.
– Malaria was the 1st recorded disease after the Flood. Malaria remains one of the biggest killers in human history.
– Leprosy was endemic in the malnourished of SE Asia.
– 1096 to 1219 – Crusades from Europe to the Holy Land.
– Black Death began in SE Asia and spread to Europe via the 'Silk Road' used by traders. – {1250 Marco Polo}
– ≈1200-1800 – Inquisition – Jews & heretics condemned
– 1350 – the worst Bubonic Plague epidemic in Europe.
– 1340-1440 - 100 Years War devastated Britain & France
– 1430 Joan of Arc lead France to victory over Britain
— 1459 Protestant Reformation followed 100 Years War

– Leprosy maimed many before killing them, is linked to poor nutrition, and was considered a curse from God.
– 1500s European s brought diseases to the New World.
– The Incas, Mayans and Aztecs had no resistance.
– Native people throughout the 'New World', including Hawaiians, were often nearly annihilated by plagues.
– In 1763, British army intentionally distributed blankets contaminated with Smallpox to the Potomac Indians. This biological warfare killed many Indians in the tribe.
– In 1804, Napoleon's troops were decimated in Haiti.
– In 1812, Napoleon's troops were decimated in Russia.
– 1840s Semmelweis began hygienic hand washing.

– 1854 Florence Nightingale practiced public health in accordance with Mosaic principles that halted diseases (i.e.-Cholera) plaguing British soldiers fighting in Turkey.
– Cholera in London from contaminated drinking well John Snow closed the well and stopped the Cholera.
– India, with its large population and complete lack of Mosaic insight, continues as a source for epidemics.
– 1867 Mark Twain developed Cholera in Syria, fortunately he recovered and continued his journey to the Holy Land.
– 1904 Walter Reed stopped Yellow Fever by drying up swamps during the building of the Panama Canal.
– Nightingale, Snow, Koch, Pasteur, Stiles, Ross, Reed strove to research–control–prevent infectious disease.
— 1854 to 1904 were '50 Golden Years' of public health

– In 1940s, infectious disease declines with antibiotics.
– The author theorizes: The 1918 Flu virus may have contaminated US military C-rations that contained pork as part of its rapid global distribution, and when WW1 was over, most people stopped eating their C-rations.
— Servicemen were frequent fatalities of the 1918 Flu.
– 1918 Flu, Ebola & HIV may be newly adapted viruses.
– *E. coli* became deadly after mutating to antibiotics.
– Mad Cow Disease has no treatment – is 100% fatal.
– Experts predict: – more new epidemics will occur.
– and old epidemics will reoccur.
– Mosaic public health principles are still the first line of defense to prevent and/or control all infectious disease.
– SARS could become the next global epidemic

Map 11 – Mountains and Rivers of Palestine

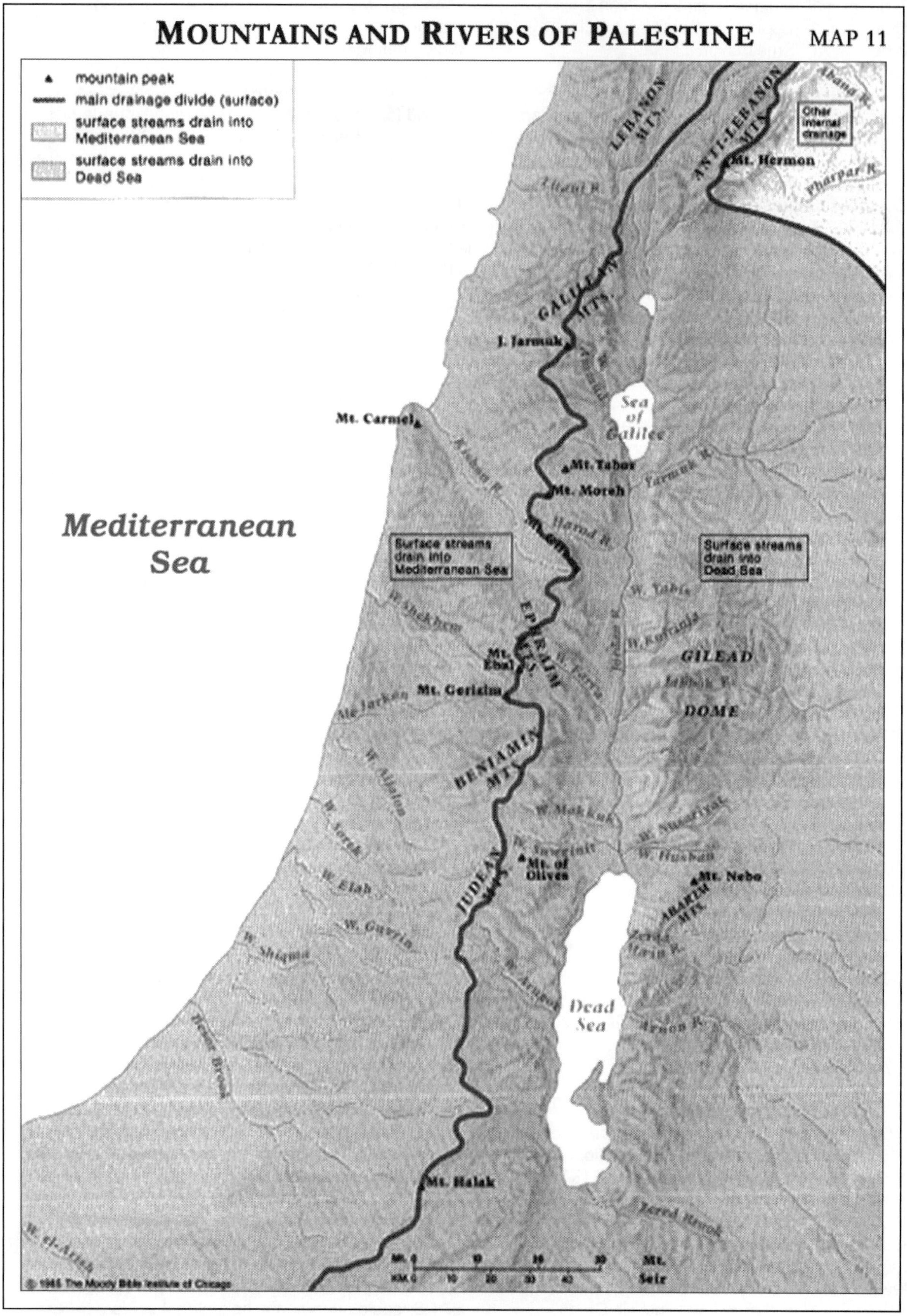

Section III: AGRICULTURE and the LAND
Chapter 7 Perfect Plants
Selective Breeding

The 'Rest of the Story' continues by examining the instructions that God gave to Moses, so the Hebrews could be good stewards of the Promised Land that they were soon to possess (conquer). The Promised Land's highly varied climate and topography is suitable for agriculture and farming.

JPS Deut 1:8 [Moses spoke to the Israelites]: 'Behold, I have set the [Promised] land before you: go in and possess the land which the LORD swore unto your fathers, to Abraham, to Isaac, and to Jacob, to give them and to their seed after them.'

Today, we are familiar with the knowledge that selective breeding of plants and animals is important to maintain the strongest and healthiest plants and animals. Breeding the healthiest males and female with one another produces the strongest herds. Cattle produce better beef and more milk this way, and sheep produce better wool. Apparently, Jacob understood some of these principles when he contracted with Laban for the speckled and spotted animals. (Gen 30) [R3] With crops, selective seeds from strong pure strains produce better fruit, vegetables, and grains. To grow pure non-hybrid strains, farmers must avoid cross-pollination with other similar plants. Watermelons grown too close to squash and citron will yield melons that have a citron-like taste. Similarly, planting a pure strain of corn near a different strain will yield corn of mixed tastes. [R1]

KJV Lev 19:19 Thou shalt not let thy cattle gender with diverse kinds (***myin***): thou shalt not sow thy field with mingled seed (***zera'***).

KJV Deut 22:9 Thou shalt not sow thy vineyard with diverse seeds (***zera'***), lest the fruit of thy seed which thou hast sown and the fruit of thy vineyard be defiled.

Today, scientists try to tamper with God's intended varieties that are also called 'land races', to produce crops (and livestock) for greater yield or more resistance to disease. These resultant new varieties often seem to be an improvement over land-race varieties, but there are often unwanted traits among these new varieties that detract from their overall vitality. These resultant new strains of seeds may not absorb nutrients from the soil as well as the land-race seeds, producing crops that are less nutritious and plants that are less resistant to disease. [R14-15]

Now, the farmer or rancher, who trusted the scientist for his newly designed variety, must trust the same scientist to keep these plants healthy and producing a high yield. This usually requires the use of artificial fertilizers for proper plant growth and the use of insecticides to control insect pests. Unfortunately, pesticides kill more than insects, and harmful residues toxic to health frequently remain in foods people eat, as discussed in Sections 4 and 5 of this book. [R6-8-10]

Hybrid plant technology began in the late 1950s as a means of increasing food production for 'Third World' countries, by breeding and distributing 'high-yield' varieties, principally cereal grains. Plant breeders utilized genetic material containing dwarfing genes, which encouraged the shifting of biomass from stems and leaves into grain. In other words, the 'new improved' varieties produced fewer leaves and more harvestable grain. The technology developed during WWII to produce bombs requiring nitrogen chemicals made possible the production of high technology phosphorous-nitrogen-potassium (P-N-K) fertilizers after the war. The new (hybrid-plant) varieties turned out to be very fertilizer responsive: they were capable of taking the added (synthetic) nutrients in fertilizers and translating them into greater yields. Hybrid-seeds with P-N-K fertilizers produced increases up to 50%. [R7C] But, while food production increased on 'green revolution' lands, hunger persisted. From the beginning, the hybrid-seeds did not grow as well for the poor farmers as for the richer ones. Achieving high yields required fertilizer and irrigation. Fertilizer and irrigation nourished weeds as well as crops, requiring new herbicides (chemicals to kill weeds). Crop pests found the genetic uniformity within crops made new varieties appetizing (vulnerable), which created the need for new high-technology insecticides (chemicals to kill crop pests) as well. The would-be beneficiaries of the 'green revolution' hybrid technology, the poor and starving, found that food produced by the fancy imported technologies was often too expensive to buy. [R7]

**"The [new high-technology] fertilizers made the new varieties [of hybrid plants] possible.
The new [hybrid] varieties made the [high-technology P-N-K] fertilizers necessary."** [R7A]

Today, often the companies that are among the leading producers of fertilizers, herbicides and pesticides are also among the largest hybrid plant breeders and hybrid seed distributors. [R7B]

∗ High-tech hybrid seeds and P-N-K fertilizers go hand-in-hand – as do computers and software.

Land Races – the Right Stuff

Since man left the Garden of Eden, he has been tilling the ground and sewing the seed to produce crops that provide food to eat. Many plants have required 'domestication' from wild varieties to produce the crops that man has relied upon for food over many centuries. [R27]

KJV Gen 3:23 Therefore the LORD sent him [mankind] forth from the garden of Eden,.
to till the ground from whence he was taken.

Many traditional plant varieties, called 'land races', likely developed shortly after the Flood in response to newly formed ecosystems. Today, plant breeders manipulate germ plasm (the place within the seed in which the genetic code responsible for determining the characteristics of each plant are kept), to produce a few 'improved' varieties. As these new and 'improved' varieties are being developed and planted for the purpose of higher yields, they are replacing the sustainable 'land race' varieties. Although these new hybrid varieties do seem to yield more crops, they have done so at the expense of reducing the growing of 'land race' variety crops. Since the vigor and genetic diversity of the 'land race' varieties help provide insurance against pest blights for the future of our food supply, it has become essential to rediscover and protect these old strains. [R4]

In the 1960s, scientists developed new 'miracle' seeds by carefully crossbreeding germ plasm to increase food production — mostly rice and wheat — in poor nations. As more and more hybrid varieties were grown, the natural 'land race' varieties became extremely scarce, sometimes to the point of extinction. John Fagan, PhD in his tape *Genetic Engineering* discusses that: [4A-5-6-8-14-15]

"Crops from hybrids often contain less protein and poorer quality protein than land races."

Garrison Wilkes, Professor of Biology at the University of Massachusetts, and a leading authority on genetic erosion (the loss of bio-diversity from 'land race' plants), states: [R4A]

∗ "The extinction of local 'land races' by the introduction of improved varieties is analogous to removing stones from the foundation to repair the roof."

A huge problem with new 'miracle' crops is that they are all genetically identical. Genetic uniformity in crops increases yield, but it makes each plant <u>identically vulnerable</u> to insect blight. Genetic crop uniformity may insure a desirable response to fertilizers from new hybrid seed, but:

∗ A single field or a whole nation's production of a food crop that is grown from genetically uniform seeds, will produce uniform plants that are all identically susceptible to crop pestilence. [R7D]

"In a field of land races a pest might gobble up one plant but find the next one different enough to be distasteful. In a field of modern varieties, if the first tasted good, they were all going to taste good." [R7D]

One hybrid crop danger is: <u>a single crop pest has the potential to devastate the entire crop</u>. This scary scenario became reality several years ago for much wheat grown on the Great Plains. Today, attempts are being made to safeguard hybrid crops from such ultimate devastation. [R4]

Dan Barry says, if foods that have never existed in nature find their way into the food supply:

"All of us will become guinea pigs in a colossal biological experiment." [R13]

Fortunately, today there are several international research groups collecting these land race varieties worldwide as a means of preserving the genetic bio-diversity that the LORD intended. Today, there are also many regional 'seed-saving' groups that offer non-hybrid, land race seeds for local commercial farmers and backyard gardeners. People, who grow these plants, whether commercially or for private use, help maintain the bio-diversity that is necessary for the preservation of 'land race' varieties, which is vital to the continued production of the foods we eat.

God stated 10 times in Genesis 1 that each creation should reproduce 'after its own kind'.

KJV Gen 1:11 And God said, Let the earth bring forth grass, the herb yielding seed, and the fruit yielding fruit after his kind (***myin***), whose seed is in itself, upon the earth: and it was so.

Farmers who grow hybrid varieties of crops recognize one of the problems with seeds from these new varieties, is that they are often sterile, or the fruit or vegetable that results from the hybrid seed is not always like the parent plant from which it came. This is in direct contrast to the statement from the LORD, that each kind (***myin***) of his variety should faithfully reproduce itself. [R15]

∗ Crops from seeds of hybrid varieties often produce no yield or a poor, inconsistent yield.

Genetic engineering, gene splicing, and genetically modified food (GMO) are techniques that might seem to promise great benefits, but are certain to have unwanted consequences. [R15-22]

Hybrid foods like brocci-flower or canola oil from rape-seed should be discouraged.

∗ Wise farmers need to grow land race variety crops, to ensure the 'survival of the species'.

Pesticides and Herbicides – the Wrong Stuff

On June 28, 1972, United States Senator Alan Cranston of California stated; [R1]

"Environmentally speaking, I believe that the organic farming method is superior to modern farming methods. The organic method is based on respect for the soil – respect which views the soil as a long-term resource – and requires considerable care of the soil. It repudiates the need for pesticides and artificial fertilizers, relying instead on the additions of organic matter and natural mineral fertilizers to replenish the soil and on the use of predator insects to control harmful plant pests." [R1]

When crops are grown in accordance with the principles of 'sustainable agriculture', that Moses wrote about in the ***Torah***, there is never a need for the pesticides, herbicides, fungicides and harsh chemical P-N-K fertilizers that farmers use today. This 'chemical rescue agriculture' kills the natural life properties of the soil, and also leaves the crops nutrient-poor and laden with chemical-toxins.

Pulitzer Prize winning author William Longgood in his book *The Poisons in Your Food* warns that many of the pesticides used for growing fruits are chemical cousins to nerve poisons called 'organo-phosphates' (developed for chemical warfare). [R6-8B] While the acute effects of these poisons are well established and documented — nausea, vomiting, abdominal pains, gastritis, coughing, etc.; the signs of chronic, long-term exposure to small amounts of these poisons are not as easy to document or diagnose; but may include hyper-sensitive skin, headaches, numbness and tingling sensations, twitching of muscles from nerve involvement or depression. [R8D] The AMA council on pharmacy and chemistry issued a warning about the use of insecticides, indicating that it is not reasonable to expect that humans can avoid injury if they are exposed year after year to a toxic agent in concentrations that kill insects in a few hours. The AMA states;

"The resultant injury may be cumulative or delayed or simulate a chronic disease of other origin, thereby making identification and statistical comparison difficult or impossible." [R8C]

Medical Researcher and Nobel Prize winner Dr. Otto Warburg warns that: [R8A]

"any poison that interferes with the respiration (normal routine function) of cells causes irreparable damage and inevitably leads to deterioration in the form of degenerative disease including cancer. ... a poison need not be stored cumulative in the body to have a cumulative effect on the health; the effect of each dose adds to that of the previous one."

Marc Lappe', PhD in his book *Chemical Deception* also warns about nerve-gas pesticides. Many pesticides, like DDT (now banned in the USA), cannot be washed off foods. [R8B]

'The Public Health Service has said that it is virtually impossible to find a meal that is not laced with some insect poison. They will penetrate the skins of fruits, vegetables and grains and concentrate in the fat of animals we eat.' [R8B]

Unfortunately, only 0.1% to 2% of pesticides released by spray ever reach the targeted pest. Pesticides often end up in air, water, soil, and food and kill beneficial organisms and people. [R27]

In 1989, many apples were found tainted with a pesticide, alar which caused wide spread problems for people who ate these apples. Despite the public awareness of this problem, the residues of pesticides found on foods in California actually increased from 1987 to 1988. [R11]

In the Garden of Eden, the LORD God commanded man to rule over the land and be stewards of the land. (Gen 2:15) After leaving the Ark, God told Noah how the new post-flood Earth climate would affect agriculture and Noah received the same instruction for stewardship of the Earth. (Gen 9:1-7) Unfortunately, this need for stewardship of the land has often been overlooked or misunderstood by farmers, businessmen and politicians throughout the centuries.

Moses states that God will withhold rain for disobeying His commandments. Farmers and non-farmers are always fearful of what may lie ahead in a severe drought. Even with modern scientific knowledge, only God is the Weatherman and He alone controls the life-giving rain.

KJV Gen 8:22 While the earth remaineth, seedtime and harvest, and cold and heat, and summer and winter, and day and night shall not ceases.

KJV Lev 26:4 Then will I [the LORD] give you rain in due season, and the land shall yield her increase, and the trees of the field shall yield their fruit.

Today, society must re-examine management priorities of the resources God has given us. Acres USA Conferences have supported farmers in pursuit of sustainable agriculture for years.

Farmers who practice sustainable agriculture recommend, to grow the strongest crops: begin with rich, hearty soil and grow land race varieties to end up with nutritionally rich crops. [R12-23]

*** <u>Feed the Soil</u>, let the soil feed the plants, and let nutrient-rich plants feed animals/people.**

---------------------------- References Ch 07 Perfect Plants ----------------------------

[R1] Organically Grown Foods\ by Rodale Press; pg 34 Senator Alan Cranston
[R2] The Chemistry of the Blood\ by M. R. DeHaan, MD; pg 77 avoid diverse seeds
[R3] Genesis and the Big Bang\ by Gerald Schroeder, PhD; pg 143 Jacob and sheep breeding
]R4] World's Food Supply at Risk\ in National Geographic; April 1991;
[R4] pg 77 traditional land race varieties of crops are domesticated from wild varieties
[R4A] pg 83 new high-yield crops are uniformly vulnerable to pests
[R5] Enduring Seeds\ by Gary Nabham; the health value of heirloom and non-hybrid seeds
[R6] Food Healing for Man\ by Bernard Jensen, DC; pg 336 hybrids often lose nutritional value
]R7] Shattering: Food, Politics and the Loss of Genetic Diversity\ by Cary Fowler & Pat Mooney
[R7] pg 57-58 loss of 'race races' - replaced by hybrid varieties
[R7A] pg 60 quote nitrogen fertilizer relationship with hybrid seeds
[R7B] pg 125&128 companies often produce both fertilizers and hybrid seeds
R7C] pg 71 hybrid seeds increased yields
[R7D] pg 46-47 pests may find hybrid crops uniformly attractive
[R8] Poisons in Your Food\ by William Longgood (Pulitzer Prize); pg 55 chronic pesticide poisoning
[R9] Chemical Deception\ by Marc Lappe', PhD; warns of toxic pesticide residues in food
[R10] The Organic Revolution (Audubon magazine-Mar/Apl 99)\ by Joel Bourne; pg 64-82
pg 64 organic revolution pg 71 bugging out
pg 74 lessons from the Land Institute pg 80 greener cleaner
[R11] Feed the Soil (audio tape 1999 Acres USA Conference)\ by Neil Kinsey; 'Albrect System' of soil fertility
[R12] Soil Food Web (Internet site)\ by Elaine Ingham, PhD www.soilfoodweb.com/phpweb/ – soil health
[R13] Brave New Food (American Health – Jan/Feb 94)\ by David Schardt; pg 60-63 danger in GMO food
[R14] The True Cost of the Failed Agricultural System\ by Arden Anderson, DO, PhD
(audio tape 1999 Acres USA Conference) – genetically engineered food is always nutritionally inferior
[R15] Genetic Engineering – Tampering with the Blueprint of Life (audio 99AcUSA)\ by John Fagan, PhD; GMO food
[R16] The New Garden #407 – 8 Organic Principles (video)\ by The New Garden – PO Box 2267 – San Antonio, Texas 78298

***** Between 50% to 80% of all micronutrients from plant crops are lost due to processing, freezing, transporting, storage, cooking, spraying and chemical additives.**

[R17] An Acres USA Primer\ by Charles Walters, Jr. – www.acresusa.com – (1-800-355-5313)
[R18] Strong's Concordance\ by James Strong, STD, LLD

pg 796	plant	# 7880	H pg 115	***siyach***	Gen 2:5
pg 1074	tree(s)	# 6086	H pg 90	***ets***	Gen 1:11
pg 1099	vineyard(s)	# 3754	H pg 57	***kerem***	Gen 9:20
pg 562	kind(s)	# 4327	H pg 65	***myin***	Gen 1:11 & Lev 19:19
pg 896	seed(s)	# 2233	H pg 36	***zera'***	Lev19:19 & Deut 22:9

[R19] Vegetables (Strategies for Sustainable Agriculture)\ by Rodale Press
manure and compost adds to the total topsoil - green manures or cover crops fix nitrogen out of air
- takes land out of production for one season, but makes land more productive
- weed control is a huge problem for an organic farmer, but timing and balance is the key
- pesticides kill crop pests, but always kill beneficial native predatory insects as well
- best to introduce/support foreign predatory killer insects - principles of Integrated Pest Management (IPM)
[R20] Rotational Grazing; (Strategies for Sustainable Agriculture)\ by Rodale Press
ruminants eat grass (8 in - 4 in) - grasses are 25% protein - don't need high protein from grain (corn)
aids the land - clover (green manure) fix nitrogen - healthy soil microbes - adds manure to soil w/o work
- don't feed corn - grow with no or few pesticides - less tractor time needed - don't confine cows
[R21] The Joy of Health\ by Zoltan Rona, MD; pg 60 loss of nutrients in current crops
[R22] Genetically Engineered Food\ by Ronnie Cummings and Ben Lilliston
[R23] Mental and Elemental Nutrients\ by Carl Pfeiffer, PhD, MD; pg 108 Green Revolution - 1960s
[R24] Environmental Science\ by G. Tyler Miller, Jr.; pg 301-402 pesticides
[R25] Global 2000 (cassette tape)\ by Barry Smith; potential agricultural collapse
[R26] Seed Savers Exchange – Seeds of Time & Horse Creek Seed Sanctuary – sell land race seeds
[R27] Guns, Germs and Steel (book or audio)\ by Jared Diamond; Tape2 Many prominent and useful food-producing plants of today began as wild varieties that were 'domesticated' to become food crops.
[R28] Travels in the Genetically Modified Zone\ by Mark L. Winston
[R29] Fateful Harvest\ by Duff Wilson – toxic waste ends up in fertilizer – ends up in crops
[R30] Why Our Food is Making Us Sick: and What We Can Do About It \ by Nicols Fox
[R31] Genetically Engineered Food: Changing the Nature of Nature\ by Martin Teitel, PhD and Kimberly Wilson
[R32] Man on Earth\ by John Reader (from Salmon of Doubt\ by D. Adams) Bali, Indonesia /pg 67-72 rice – old vs new
[R33] Sacred Balance #2 – PBS 1-800-543-3764 /Penta-water /PCBs Bali – water & agriculture
[R34] BBC Radio (10-16-03) – GMO crops may alter insect populations living in GMO crop fields.

*** note- Between 50% to 80% of all nutrients from plants may be lost from processing, freezing, transporting, storage, cooking, spraying and chemical additives.** [R16]

Chapter 8 Sabbath Rest for the Land
Fallow the Land – Save the Soil

God instructed Moses that the Hebrews should plant the field for six years but on the seventh or Sabbath (***Shabbat***) year, no crops were to be grown. During the Sabbath year, clean animals would wander or graze on the land and deposit their manure, which would then enrich the soil.

KJV Lev 25:2-5 & 21 ... When you come into the land which I give you, then shall the land keep a sabbath unto the LORD. vs3 Six years thou shalt sow thy field and six years thou shalt prune thy vineyard, and gather the fruit thereof; vs4 But in the seventh year shall be a sabbath of rest unto the land, a sabbath for the LORD: thou shalt neither sow thy field, nor prune thy vineyard. vs5 That which growest on its own accord of thy harvest thou shalt not reap, neither gather the grapes of thy vine undressed: for it is a year of rest unto the LORD. vs21 Then I will command my blessing upon in the sixth year and it [the land] will bring forth fruit for three years.

Crops that might grow on their own were plowed under on this Sabbath year. By plowing under what might grow this Sabbath year, the nutrients of the crops are returned back to the soil. Today, to enrich the soil, 'green manures' or 'cover crops' are grown just to be plowed under. [R4]

'Green manures' or cover crops feed micro-organisms and help the soil continue to be fertile. [R10]

The relationship between nutrients in the soil resulting in nutrients in the crops is very clear.

"For many years our agricultural chemists and agronomists have been stressing the fact that our soil is steadily being depleted of its trace elements by the combination of excessive cropping and leaching through broken sod. This loss of minerals from our soil is now being reflected in trace-element-deficient food on our dinner tables." [R7]

"Experiments conducted by the Agriculture Department of the Federal Government and many of our states have led to the prescription of mineral supplements to be added to the soil with the usual P.N.P. (Phosphorus-Nitrogen-Potassium) [i.e. – P-N-K] fertilizers and lime. Stress, however, has been on the replacement of these elements that are essential to plant growth, and no effort has been made to replace trace elements which, although not essential for plant growth, are essential to human health." [R7]

∗ If the nutrients aren't in the soil, nutrients won't be in the plants and nutrients won't be in the crops.

Joel Wallach, DVM, ND and Ma Lan, MD in their book *Rare Earths Forbidden Cures* discuss the use of P-N-K fertilizers and the loss of soil fertility that results in nutrient deficient crops.

"Our Earth is anemic!!!! A potentially apocalyptic mixture of mining, deforestation, farming, irrigation and acid rain has shifted, eroded or leached our life-giving and life-sustaining raw materials from our formerly mineral-rich land." [R10A]

University of West Virginia researchers Dr. Rabindar Singh and Dr. Robert Keefer found that the use of agricultural fertilizers does alter the nutrients in the soil and in the resultant crops.

"The changes occur in the amounts of trace elements contained in grains and leaves. The most important trace elements [minerals] from a nutritional point are iron, manganese, copper and zinc ... extremely important in human diet. ... One of the most interesting results of the studies on sweet corn is that the more phosphorus applied to the soils, the less zinc is found in the grains. Results of this nature suggest that one should examine carefully the long term effect of heavy fertilization rates from the standpoint of human health." [R9]

Farmers today have abandoned God's wisdom of the Sabbath rest and grow crops on the land without the required rest. The apparent gain of more profit is quickly negated as the soils become worn out. Tired soils require the use of harsh rescue Phosphorus-Nitrogen-Potassium (P-N-K) fertilizers to grow a crop. [R4-9B-11] Crops grown on mineral-depleted soils and with harsh P-N-K fertilizers are not as nutritious as crops grown organically. P-N-K fertilizers produce luxurious plants, but this is the result of over-stimulating plant roots. P-N-K fertilized plants use their energy to produce size rather than to extract the essential trace minerals from the soil. [R9A]

All soils may need mineral fertilizers. Sustainable-agriculture organic farmers treat the soil as a resource, so soil bacteria, worms and cover crops can convert inorganic minerals into organic matter that crops need. Soil bacteria that are necessary for this critical conversion of inorganic material to organic nutrients are often destroyed or crippled by harsh, chemical, P-N-K fertilizers.

Crop plants literally 'mine' minerals from the soil, so animals or humans can obtain essential minerals by eating the crops or eating the animals that were fed on the mineral-rich crops. [R10B]

The Hebrews were to trust that the LORD would supply abundantly on the sixth year so they would not go hungry by letting the land lay fallow during the seventh or Sabbath year.

∗ A Sabbath rest of the land is a principle of sustainable agriculture that will improve soil quality.

Sabbath and Jubilee Rests – Pest Control

The Sabbath rest of the land encourages natural pest control. Farmers must always be concerned about what insect blight might be lurking ahead, ready to wipe out a crop. Many insects that infest crops, such as the corn borer, the tomato worm, or the Colorado beetle have a one-year life cycle. After their eggs remain dormant all winter, the larvae hatch in the spring as full-grown insects, ready to feed on the crop for which they are adapted. Alas, if there is no crop, the insects have nothing to feed on and they all die shortly after being hatched. This breaks the life cycle of the insect because there are no adults left to lay eggs at the end of the season, and no larvae to infest next year's crop. [R2] Other pest insects have life cycles covering several years and at least one insect pest has a seventeen-year life cycle. The Year of Jubilee rest requires that after seven Sabbath rests, an additional year of rest be given to the land. [R2A] Thus, the land is to be rested every 7th (Sabbatical) year for 49 years and then rested again on the 50th (Jubilee) year. To be effective for pest control 'fallowing the land' must be practiced faithfully by all farmers within a region so a crop pest could not just migrate to a neighbors field to find suitable crops to eat.

KJV Lev 25:11 A jubilee shall that fiftieth year be unto you; ye shall not sow neither reap that which groweth of itself in it, nor gather the grapes in it of thy vine undressed [wild vine].

Breeding patterns of multiple year life cycle insect pests would be interrupted by a Jubilee rest to the land. [R2A] Few farmers practice a Sabbath year of rest or an additional Jubilee rest, so very little data exists to confirm the pest control value to agriculture from these rests for the land.

Some farmers rotate crops during alternate years on one parcel of land. This practice often provides some pest control value, and is certainly a step in the right direction toward a Sabbath rest of the land. Rotating certain crops and planting cover crops that are plowed under help soils to retain more organic nutrients, as some crops encourage healthy biochemical changes to soils. The Sabbath rest principle for the land is sown into the very fabric of the soil, and is as vital to the continued production of healthy crops as is the rain the LORD provides in due season.

KJV Lev 26:4 Then I [God] will give you rain in due season, and the land shall yield her increase, and the trees of the field shall yield her fruit.

∗ The Sabbath year rest provides a natural, healthy opportunity for crop pest control.

The Israelites were unfaithful to keep the Sabbath of the land for 490 years. During the first 490 years that Israel ruled the land, they did not once obey God's command to rest the land.

KJV Lev 26:14 But if you will not harken unto me and will not do all these commandments ... vs33 And I will scatter you among the heathen and will draw out a sword after you: and your land shall be desolate and your cities waste. vs34 Then shall the land enjoy her sabbaths, as long as it lieth desolate and ye be in your enemies' land; even then shall the land rest and enjoy her sabbaths.

As the LORD had warned, the LORD removed the Hebrews from ***Eretz*** Israel and scattered them abroad during the Babylonian and Persian captivity for exactly 70 years.

KJV II Ch 36:21 Until the land enjoyed her sabbaths: for as long as she lay desolate she kept her sabbaths, to fulfill three score and ten [60+10=70] years.

The Persian king Cyrus issued his decree ending the Jews' 70 years of captivity. (Ezra 1:1-3) The Hebrew's captivity in Babylon/Persia lasted exactly one year for each year the Sabbath rest was unkept to the land and unkept to the LORD. Hebrew years are calculated on a 360 day year. The 70 years Desolation of Jerusalem captivity in Babylon and Persia fulfilled prophecy, lasted from 606 to 537 BC, and showed that the LORD is serious about following His commandments! [26]

These principles for land management and sanitation/hygiene (Section 2) in the ***Torah*** are complete instructions to care for ***Eretz*** Israel that are also applicable for the care of other lands.

KJV Lev 25:10 And you shall hallow the fiftieth year, and proclaim liberty throughout all the land unto all the inhabitants thereof: it shall be a jubilee unto you ....

The French recognized the Year of Jubilee symbolism was Liberty, which meant: Freedom to pursue the healthy life that the LORD intended. In 1886 AD, the French inscribed Leviticus 25:10 on the Statue of Liberty on Ellis Island, New York, which they delivered to the USA as a great gift.

∗ Rejoice in the Jubilee of the LORD and find wonder in the majesty of His Commandments.

Stewardship of the Land

In the Garden of Eden, the LORD told man to rule over and to be stewards of the land (***eretz***). After leaving the Ark, God told Noah how Earth's new post-Flood climate would affect agriculture and Noah received the same instruction as Adam for stewardship of the Earth. (Gen 9:1-7)

KJV Gen 2:15 ...and put him [man] in the Garden of Eden to tend it and keep it.

NIV Gen 1:28 God blessed them and said to them, "Be fruitful and increase in number; fill the earth and subdue it. Rule over the fish of the sea and the birds of the air and over every living creature that moves on the ground."

A practical example of the stewardship required by Genesis is demonstrated in Deuteronomy.

NIV Deut 22:6 If you come across a bird's nest beside the road, either in a tree or on the ground and the mother is sitting on the young or on the eggs, do not take the mother with the young. vs7 You may take the young, but be sure to let the mother go, so that it may go well with you and you may have a long life.

The consequences of poor stewardship of the land are discussed by Farley Mowat in his book *Sea of Slaughter* and Rachael Carson in her book *Silent Spring*. Poor stewardship of the land is exemplified by the Eskimo Curlew bird that used to migrate back and forth between the pampas plains of South America and the great plains of North America. The Curlew arrived in North America just in time to devour the Rocky Mountain grasshopper and other corn crop pests. In the 1870s, Curlews were slaughtered to extinction for food, profit and sport and God's natural means of pest control was lost forever. To save crops, farmland now became an experimental laboratory for pesticides such as DDT, lead arsenates and others that kill a lot more than insects. When men are not good stewards of the land, the results are always disastrous. [R4-5-8]

As Moses provided instructions so the land (***eretz***) would not become physically defiled, he also warned against spiritual defilement of the land. Moses knew that physical defilement of the land and spiritual defilement of the land were often linked. (Lev 18-19 – Num 35:34 – Deut 24)

KJV Lev 19:29 Do not prostitute thy daughter to cause her to be a whore: lest the land (***eretz***) fall to whoredom and the land fall to wickedness.

KJV Ex 23:32-33 Thou shalt not make covenant with them [the inhabitants of the land] nor with their gods. They shall not dwell on the land (***eretz***) lest they make the sin against me: for if thou serve their gods it will surely be a snare unto thee.

The LORD treasures the Promised Land and He wishes to have this land spiritually undefiled. The LORD's people are commanded not to follow the idolatrous ways of other peoples, but are to hearken diligently to His voice. A physically and spiritually undefiled land (***eretz***) are necessary for perfect health of the land to be maintained. So the Hebrews could live the life that the LORD intended for them, the LORD put His commandment in their hearts. (Deut 30:14) The LORD promised blessings for obedience, and He promised peril for disobedience. (Deut 30:15-18) The LORD gave His people free choice of life and blessing; or death and cursing. (Deut 30:19)

JPS Deut 6:3 —— a land (***eretz***) flowing with milk and honey.

NKJV Deut 30:16 "I [Moses] command you today to love the LORD your God, to walk in His ways and to keep His commandments, His statutes, and His judgments, that you may live and multiply; and the LORD your God will bless you in the land (***eretz***) which you go to possess."

In 1990, the California Department of Agriculture sprayed 16 square miles of El Cajon with the insecticide malathion three times in one month. The reason for concern was three Mexican fruit flies found in this region that might threaten fruit crops. [R13] This is not good land stewardship.

The Sabbath and Jubilee rests of the land are only the beginning of stewardship. Integrated Pest Management (IPM) includes fallowing the land one year in seven, crop rotation and cover crops. Ultimately the health of the soil is critical for sustainable agriculture without toxic rescue chemicals such as: herbicides, pesticides, fungicides and harsh chemical P-N-K type fertilizers. Elaine Ingham, PhD on her web site discusses measuring the quantity and quality of life in the soil. Acres USA Conferences have helped farmers to farm according to the principles of sustainable agriculture for many years. Unfortunately, the stewardship of the land has often been overlooked and/or abused by farmers, businessmen, landowners and politicians throughout the centuries.

'Sustainable agriculture' requires widespread support to be effective as good stewardship.

---------------------------- References Ch 8 Sabbath Rest ------------------------------

[R1] Environmental Science\ by G. Tyler Miller, Jr.; pg 402-406 alternative pest control
[R2] The Chemistry of the Blood\ by M.R. DeHaan, MD; pg 78 Sabbath rest = pest control
[R3] Silent Spring\ by Rachael Carson; pesticides kill more than pests - accumulate in predators
[R4] Organically Grown Foods\ Rodale Press; pg 54 green manures = cover crops = feed the soil
[R5] Sea of Slaughter\ by Farley Mowat; eskimo curlew and other birds eat/control crop pests
[R6] Organic Plant Protection\ ed by Roger B. Yepsen, Jr.; pest control w/o pesticide chemicals
[R7] Food and Nutrition\ by Rodale Press; pg 304 quotes – P-N-K fertilizers and no trace minerals
[R8] The True Cost of the Failed Agricultural System\ by Arden Anderson, DO, PhD (Acres USA 99)
[R9] God and Vitamins\ by Marjorie Holms; pg 266 – more trace minerals in organically grown food
[R9A] pg 268-269 – soil fertility = vitamins and minerals in crops
[R9B] pg ch 14 - 257-273 – The Magic Minerals and Organic Foods
[R10] Rare Earths: Forbidden Cures\ by Joel Wallach, DVM, ND; ch 3 pg 37-52 Our Anemic Earth
[R10A] pg 37 quotes - formerly mineral-rich farm land (USA) are no longer mineral-rich - Dr. Airola
[R10B] pg 40 crops: concentrate nutrients from the soil - leave the soil depleted - require soil renewal
[R11] The Airola Diet and Cookbook\ by Paavo Airola, ND, PhD; from [R10] Rare Earths; pg 37
"Those who now advocate eating natural foods as the only source of vitamins and minerals live in a dream world of yesterday. What was yesterday's law is today's folly. It doesn't matter how well you balance your meals, or if you're a meat eater, vegetarian, or a raw-foodist, you still run the risk of malnutrition if you try to get all your vitamins and minerals exclusively from the [nutrient-deficient] foods you eat."
[R12] The Soil Food Web (Internet)\ by Elaine Ingham, PhD; feed soil ⇒ healthy crops w^3.soilfoodweb.com
[R13] San Diego–El Cajon (summer 1990) – county-wide malathion spray to kill 3 Mexican fruit flies
[R14] Green Manures (Internet)\ by FAIRS – (Florida Agriculture Interdisciplinary Research Station) – cover crops & soil
[R15] The Joy of Health\ by Zoltan Rona, MD; pg 60 nutrients in soil & food
[R16] New Garden #407 – 8 Organic Principles (video)\ by (New Garden – PO Box 2267 – San Antonio, Texas 78298)
[R17] An Acres USA Primer\ by Charles Walters, Jr. – www.acresusa.com – (1-800-355-5313)
[R18] Strong's Concordance\ by James Strong, STD, LLD

pg 855	Sabbath	# 7676	H pg 112	***shabbat***	Lev 25:2
pg 552	Jubilee	# 3104	H pg 48	***yobel***	Lev 25:10
pg 581	land - earth	# 776	H pg 17	***eretz***	Lev 19 - Deut 6:3

[R19] Vegetables: Strategies for Sustainable Agriculture (video)\ by Rodale Press
manure – compost adds to total topsoil - green manures or cover crops fix nitrogen out of air
- takes land out of production for one season, but makes land more productive
- weed control is a huge problem for an organic farmer, but timing and balance is the key
- pesticides always kill all beneficial native predatory insects – alternative - introducing foreign predatory killer insects that are not native - principles of Integrated Pest Management
[R20] Rotational Grazing: Strategies for Sustainable Agriculture (video)\ by Rodale Press
grasses eaten 8 in to 4 in - grasses are 25% protein - don't need high protein from grain (corn)
aids the land - clover that fix nitrogen - healthy soil microbes - more manure to soil w/o work
- don't feed animals corn - need less pesticides - less tractor time needed - don't confine cows
[R21]Handbook of Natural Insect and Disease Control\ by Rodale Press (Rodale Garden Books)
pg 365 — Tilling the ground kills plant pathogens — Rotating crops may kills pathogens
(Legumes 'fix' nitrogen from the soil, which makes them useful as cover crops and in crop rotation.)
[R22] Organic Gardening Under Glass\ by George (Doc) Abraham and Katy Abraham
[R23] Food for Everyone\ by Jacob Mittleider and Andrew N. Nelson, PhD
[R24] Organic Plant Protection\ by Rodale Press
[R25] Mental and Elemental Nutrients\ by Carl Pfeiffer, PhD, MD; pg 23-24 - nutrient deficient soil
[R26] The Rise of Babylon and the Persian Gulf Crisis\ by Hal Lindsey, PhD & Chuck Missler, PhD;
pg 8-10 & 26 {BC = BCE dates & AD = CE dates & based on 360 days/year} (1-800-KOUSE-1)
[R27] 100 Scientists Who Shaped World History\ by John Hudson Tiner; pg 32 Linnaeus – herbal medicine
pg 74 George Washington Carver – peanuts & soybeans as cover crops to revitalize soils in the 'South' US.

Incidentally, plowing with an ox and an ass together is awkward for the animals and results in great difficulty for the farmer to plow a straight furrow that is necessary for efficient farming. For a farmer to attempt to plow a field yoking an ox and an ass together is almost comical.

KJV Deut 22:10 Thou shalt not plow with an ox and an ass [NKJV - donkey] together.

This verse discusses the physical awkwardness of plowing with an ox, a clean beast, and an ass, an unclean beast, together; and the verse may also have a spiritual message as well.

*** People who have mastered the principles of health from the *Torah* shall inherit the Earth.**

Section IV: KOSHER (Clean) MEAT
Chapter 09 Meat Fat
Fat Chemistry

Almost all the fats in food are in the form of triglycerides, which are individual fatty acids (fats) linked together on a backbone of a molecule of glycerol. [R1] The types of individual fatty acids that are attached to this carrier molecule of glycerol are responsible for determining the physical properties of the fats (triglycerides). [R2A] The properties of individual fatty acids also determine the biochemical and physiological effects of the fats on the body. When triglycerides in foods (fat) are eaten, digestion breaks the triglycerides down into individual fatty acids and glycerol. [R2A] Fatty acids are composed of two parts: a chain of Carbon molecules of variable length; and at one end a carboxylic acid group, where the fatty acid is attached to the molecule of glycerol. [R2C] All fatty acids (FAs) have even numbers of Carbons, with 4 the shortest and 28 the longest chain. The chain of Carbon atoms is what differs from one fatty acid to another and causes the unique properties of each fatty acid. Each Carbon atom in a fatty acid (FA) chain must bond with four other atoms around itself. Carbons that are not in an end position have two bonds occupied by other Carbons and two more bonds that can either be filled by Hydrogen atoms or can be filled by a second 'double bond' to an adjacent Carbon. If all Carbons are attached to one another by single bonds, the FA is called 'saturated' with Hydrogen. If there are one or more 'double bonds' between Carbons, the fatty acid is called 'unsaturated' (UFA). If there is only one double bond between adjacent Carbon atoms, the fatty acid is called 'monounsaturated' (UFA). If there is more than one double bond in the Carbon chain, the fatty acid is called 'polyunsaturated' (UFA). [R2D] 'Hydrocarbon' is the term for the endless combinations of Hydrogen and Carbon along with Oxygen and Nitrogen that are used to make the 'organic' molecules necessary for life, of which fats are a necessary part. Many saturated fatty acids (SFAs) can be converted to unsaturated fatty acids (UFAs) within the body by enzymes that remove Hydrogens from adjacent Carbons, resulting in a double bond between these two Carbons. These enzymes may also shorten (reduce) the number of Carbons in the chain. [R2J] Certain polyunsaturated fatty acids (UFAs) that are necessary for life <u>cannot</u> be manufactured within the body. These fatty acids must be obtained by the foods people eat and are termed 'essential fatty acids' (EFAs). [R2F] EFAs are very important for health and some EFAs are found in most categories of foods. (Ch 22 Eggs - Oils) All saturated fatty acids (SFAs) are straight chains. In nature, all UFAs (one or more double bond between adjacent Carbons) are in 'cis' configuration, resulting in their bent 3-D molecular shape. If UFAs are 'partially hydrogenated', the Carbon chain is straight and is in 'trans' configuration.

* UFAs in foods are always found in 'cis' configuration, which is the only way they are healthy.

* **The biological value of a UFA to health is determined by its unique 3-D molecular shape.**

The main uses of FAs in the body are: for the structure of the membranes (walls) of all cells; or to be converted to glucose and used for energy; or to form reservoirs of body fat under the skin and surrounding the internal organs; or as components of required chemicals, such as hormones. The most critical tissue needs for EFAs are in cell walls and to manufacture body chemicals. [R2B]

Most FAs from animals are saturated (SFAs). Most SFAs in meat fat have a long-chain length (12^{+} Carbons), while many SFAs in dairy products have a short-chain length (4 to 10 Carbons). The longer the length of the Carbon chain of SFAs, the poorer is their solubility in water or blood. Long chain length SFAs, because of their inability to mix well in a water medium like blood, are likely to clump together forming aggregates or clots and are frequently described as 'sticky'. [R2B] Long-length SFAs are more difficult to metabolize (burn) for energy than the shorter chain SFAs.

UFAs are liquid at room temperature, and SFAs, such as butter, are solid. If Hydrogen is added to a UFA, then a double bond between Carbons is filled with Hydrogens, making the UFA 'partially hydrogenated'. Partially hydrogenated fats, such as margarine, are often solid, and the fats are always in 'trans' configuration. Trans-FAs are sticky in blood, just like long chain SFAs.

** **Tight compacting of SFAs and trans FAs is what makes them solid at room temperature.**

SFAs withstand heat better than UFAs, but the heat of deep-frying is destructive to all fats. Deep-frying any UFA produces trans fats, other toxic byproducts and destructive free radicals.

Cholesterol is only an animal product, it is not a true fat, but it is often found with animal fat. Cholesterol is a nutrient needed by every cell in the body. Cholesterol is not soluble in blood, and must be transported as a soluble complex. The liver makes cholesterol but the liver cannot break down cholesterol. Medication to hinder the liver's production of cholesterol may damage the liver.

* **Fats can be either <u>healthful</u> or <u>harmful</u> to life depending upon their structure and biochemistry.**

Meat Fat

Moses told the Hebrews not to eat any fat, also called 'suet', from animal meats. (Lev 7:25)

JPS Lev 3:17 It shall be a perpetual statute throughout your generations in all your dwellings, that ye eat neither fat nor blood.

Most fatty acids in meat fats are long chain SFAs, and meat fat contains few, if any, EFAs. All animals convert extra calories from carbohydrates, fats or proteins into storage as fat. SFAs are most efficient for storage because they are straight molecules that can be packed tighter in a smaller volume than UFAs. [R14] Non-essential long chain SFAs are often stored as adipose tissue to cushion internal organs. Long chain SFAs are more difficult to burn for fuel than the short chain SFAs found in milk. Long chain SFAs from meat fat can be used in only limited amounts in cell walls before damaging the efficiency of cell walls. Cell walls allow nutrients to enter and toxins to leave the cell. [R2B] Long chain SFAs have very limited usefulness for health.

Rex Russell, MD in his book *What the Bible Says About Healthy Living* discusses that the fat just under all animals skin is called 'suet' or cover fat, and has a much higher concentration of undesirable, long chain SFAs than the small amount of fat that may be 'marbled' within meat. [R12]

Francis Moore Lappe' in her book *Diet for a Small Planet* wrote that 150 years ago buffalo eating only grasses were much leaner than any commercially raised meat from cattle today. [R15]

Animal fat usually contains much cholesterol. Cholesterol is needed by every cell for health. Cholesterol that the body cannot transport efficiently (i.e.- LDL cholesterol) may turn from being a nutrient to a detriment and may be deposited on the walls of arteries as plaques. Plaques along with SFA deposits can narrow the volume of blood that the artery can carry and cause the artery walls to thicken and lose their elasticity (hardening of the arteries). These conditions also lead to cardiovascular disease (CVD), such as high blood pressure, stroke and heart attack. [R2-3-14]

The best evidence concerning the development of chronic degenerative diseases concludes: while SFA plaques and cholesterol deposits are part of the disease process, foods containing cholesterol and SFAs by themselves may not be responsible for causing CVD disease. The true cause of chronic degenerative diseases (CVD) appears to be the lack of all the micronutrients necessary to metabolize, process, distribute and utilize SFAs and cholesterol before they are oxidized in the bloodstream as plaque! [R2E-33-34-6-14-28] All meat fat contains high amounts of long-chain SFAs and cholesterol and few micro-nutrients. * Cholesterol and SFAs alone do not appear to be the cause of CVD; rather, the lack of all the micro-nutrients in sufficient quantities for the body to properly utilize and transport cholesterol and SFAs appears to cause much CVD.

*** Meat fat contains few, if any, essential micro-nutrients (vitamins, minerals, essential fatty acids).**

Udo Erasmus, PhD states this quite clearly in his book *Fats and Oils*. [R2H]

"To the nutritionists, the cholesterol 'problem' is secondary to disruptions in the biochemistry of life."

All fats store fat-soluble toxins. Agricultural toxins and chemicals that may be stored in meat fat include pesticides, herbicides, fungicides, as well as growth hormones and antibiotics. [R16-17] Pesticides are close cousins to chemical warfare nerve gas. Pesticides stay on plants, and are stored in meat fat, especially in suet adipose tissue of animals that eat pesticide-laden plants. Antibiotics are useful to treat infections, but should not be used as a routine part of animal feed. Antibiotics can harm the normal healthy bacterial flora of the animal and/or the human who eats the meat of the animal. Growth hormones fed to animals will get the animal to market faster, but may also have an adverse effect on the animal and people that eat the hormones in meat fat.

*** Toxins from all animals are stored in meat fat. If you eat meat, eat only very lean meat.**

In the phrase the 'fat of the land', the word 'fat' is used as an adjective in a metaphorical and descriptive sense, rather than as a noun to refer to any specific fat, such as meat fat. (Gen 45:18)

Paul Dudley White, MD, the heart specialist who treated President Eisenhower while he was in the White House, once quoted Leviticus 7:23. Dr. White asserted; [R4]

"It is conceivable that a few years from now we medical men may repeat to the citizens of the United States of America the advice that Moses was asked by God to present to the children of Israel 3,000 years ago." [R4]

KJV Lev 7:23 You shall eat no manner of fat, of ox, or of sheep, or of goat.

Dr. White's words of wisdom have come true today, as nutritionists such as Monte Kline, PhD, Rex Russell, MD and Ted Broer, PhD discuss avoiding meat fat as a dietary principle from the ***Torah***.

*** Meat fat, especially suet, always contains unwanted long-chain SFAs and unwanted toxins.**

------------------------------ References Ch 09 Meat Fats ------------------------------

[R1] Nutritional Almanac\ (1979 Ed) pg 112 diagram artery clogged by plaque
[R2] Fats and Oils\ by Udo Erasmus, PhD: pg 45 triglyceride defined
[R2A] [R2C] pg 3 & 45-47 & 212-216 triglyceride discussion and fats in meats
[R2B] [R2G] [R2J] pg 21 &162-163 SFAs [R2D] pg 29-33 UFAs
[R2E] [R2L] pg 312 deficiency theory – quote [R2F] pg 34-35 &163-165 EFAs – LA & LNA
[R2H] pg 193 CVD quote - deficiency like an orchestra
[R2K] pg 34-35* & 216 essential FAs - EFAs
[R2M] pg 59 and 56 cholesterol and lecithin stick models
[R2N] pg 96-106 trans-fats
[R2O] pg 30-32 & 163-164 Olive oil and mono-UFAs
[R3] Fats that Heal Fats that Kill\ by Udo Erasmus, PhD; pg 68-69 fats and cholesterol quote
[R3B] pg 23 &29-31 fats in butter Buyteric FA
[R4] Principles of Healthful Living\ (Worldwide Church of God); pg13 quote Dr. White
[R5] Are the Dietary Laws Scientific?\ by Harold Hemenway avoid meat fat
[R6] The Book of Vitamin Therapy\ by Dr. Harold Rosenberg; pg 232 meat fats
[R7] Clean and Unclean Foods\ by Gordon Tessler, PhD; pg 20 avoid meat fat
[R8] Good Fat Bad Fat\ by William P. Castelli, MD and Glen C. Griffin, MD; pg 52 trans-fatty acids
[R9] Your Health Under Siege\ by Jeffrey Bland, PhD; pg 20, 94, 75 trans-fat elevates blood cholesterol
[R10] Swearing off the Miracle (Vegetarian Times Feb 94)
[R11] God's Key to Health and Happiness\ by Elmer Josephson; pg 112-117 avoid meat fat
[R12] What the Bible Says About Healthy Living\ by Rex Russell, MD; pg 136&146 suet or cover fat
[R12A] pg 139 processed vegetable 'white oil'
[R12B] pg 128-130 margarine and trans-fatty acids
[R12C] pg 129 cover fat a repository for toxins
[R13] The Pritikin Diet\ by Nathan Pritikin – advocated very low fat diet – {the author's opinion – likely too little fat}
[R14] Essential Fatty Acids in Health and Disease\ by Edward Siguel, MD, PhD
[R14] pg 163-164 storage of calories as SFAs
[R15] Diet for a Small Planet\ by Francis Moore Lappe': pg 4-5 lean Buffalo meat
[R16] Germs that Won't Die\ by Marc Lappe', PhD antibiotics routinly feed to animals ⇒ antibiotic resistant bacteria
[R17] Poisons in Your Food\ by William Longgood
[R18] Strong's Concordance\ by James Strong, STD, LLD { ***chalav*** – as 'milk' – (Ch 14 pg 125)}

pg 335	fat	# 2459	H pg 39	***cheleb***	Lev 3:3
pg 335	fat	# 6309	H pg 93	***peder – peduth***	Lev 1:8 & Lev 8:20
pg 131	blood	# 1818	H pg 31	***dam***	Lev 3:17
pg 846	right	# 3787	H pg 58	***kawsher***	Esther 8:5

{Hebrew is at times very economical with nouns as #2459 (CHet-Lamed-Bet) may mean 'fat' – ***cheleb*** or 'milk' – ***chalav*** depending upon the context. This book uses ***cheleb*** for meat fat and ***chalav*** for milk.}
[R19] The Zone\ by Barry Sears, PhD; pg 120-127 good fat vs bad fat //pg 141-147 cholesterol
[R20] Nutrition and Your Body\ by Benjamin Colimore, MA & Sarah Stewart Colimore, LPT
[R21] Medicinal Fatty Acids in Inflammation\ by Joel M. Kremer, MD
[R22] Counsel on Diet and Health\ by Ellen G. White eat no meat; including no meat fat
[R23] Omega 3 Miracle\ by Garry Gordon, MD; nutrition (*w*3 oils) and the biochemistry of health
[R24] Help Yourself to Better Health Manual and Body, Mind and Health\ by Monte Kline, PhD (1-800-255-4246)
[R25] Proof Positive\ by Neil Nedley, MD/ pg 67 SFAs raise cholesterol twice as fast as UFAs lower it
[R25A] pg 56-57 & 91-94 diagrams of artery clogged by plaque
[R26] Controlling Cholesterol\ by Kenneth Cooper, MD – improved diet and exercise help reduce cholesterol
[R27] Antioxidant Revolution\ by Kenneth Cooper, MD; pg 12-13 CVD & foam cells
[R28] The 28-Day Antioxidant Diet Program\ by Steven Masley, MD; pg 50-62 fats
[R28B] pg 52 cholesterol – LDL vs HDL //[R28C] pg 61 arterial plaque from LDL
[R29] Nutrition Against Disease\ by Roger Williams, PhD; Ch 5; pg 75 Cholesterol is not the villain.
[R30] Good Cholesterol Bad Cholesterol\ by Eli Roth, MD and Sandra Streicher Lamkin, RN
Lecithin is a special case of triglyceride with a molecule of choline attached to one end of the glycerol. The highest quality lecithin has an EFA in the middle position. Lecithin's configuration allows it to emulsify many fats (FAs) and keep FAs suspended in a water medium, such as blood.
[R31] Omega 3 Oils\ by Donald Rudin, MD and Clara Felix; *w*3 fish oils – heart health – degenerative disease
[R32] Lifeclinic (website) & pharmaceutical inserts – risk of liver damage from (statin) meds to lower cholesterol
[R33] Supernutrition\ by Richard Passwater, PhD; pg 71-103 plaque and CVD
[R34] New Supernutrition\ by Richard Passwater, PhD; pg 136 & 166 plaque and CVD
[R35] The New Whole Foods Encyclopedia\ by Rebecca Wood; pg 54 Canola oil is bad news
[R36] The 8 Week Cholesterol Cure\ by Robert Kowlowski \\ [R37] Diet for a New America\ by John Robbins
(videos) – show long ropes of cholesterol–SFA plagues in arteries being removed by surgeons
[R38] Antioxidant Revolution (audio)\ by Ken Cooper, MD – risky pair – low HDL cholesterol – high Triglycerides (fat)
[R39] Living in Devine Health (audio cassettes)\ by Ted Broer, PhD and Sharon Broer www.TedBroer.com
[R40] Maximum Energy\ by Ted Broer, PhD – eat no fat & no blood & no unclean meat (1-800-592-4325)

Chart 09 Good Fat / Bad Fat

Fats are chains of Carbon atoms with Hydrogen atoms attached to the Carbons. Fatty acids are chains of Carbon and Hydrogen atoms with a molecule of carboxylic acid at one end. Fatty acids are usually connected to a molecule of glycerol at the carboxylic acid end to form a triglyceride. Triglycerides are the way the blood carries fatty acids and is the way 95% of fat is found in food. Fatty acids always have an even number of Carbons and vary in length from 4 to 28 Carbons. The length of the Carbon chain and the way the Carbons and Hydrogens are attached to one-another determines the physical properties and biological value or usefulness of the fatty acids. Carbon has 4 positions to attach or bond to other atoms. Hydrogen only bonds with 1 other atom. Carbon and Hydrogen combine to form many complex, varied molecules called 'hydrocarbons'. Carbon and Hydrogen along with Oxygen and Nitrogen are basic to all 'organic' or life molecules. Combinations of Carbon, Hydrogen, Oxygen and Nitrogen into molecules are basic to all organic chemistry, like combinations of the notes: do - re - mi - fa - so - la - ti - do are basic to all music.

—C— Carbon bonds to 4 atoms	N— Nitrogen bonds to 3 atoms
H— Hydrogen bonds to 1 atom	Ammonia - NH_3 - is very toxic to health.
—O— Oxygen bonds to 2 atoms	

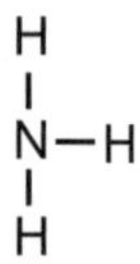

Methane, a gas, is the simplest hydrocarbon. Methane is not a fat.

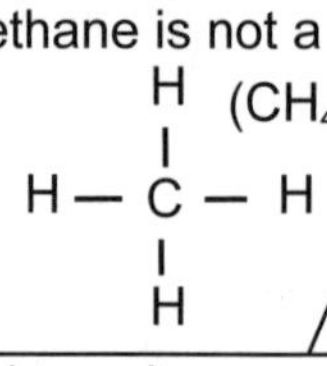

(CH_4)

($C_4H_8O_2$)

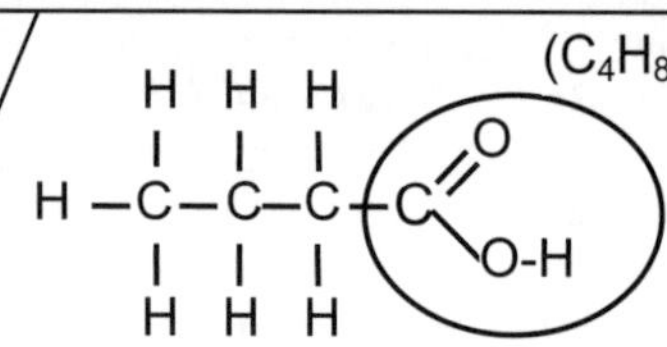

All Fatty Acids, such as Butyric FA, have a Carboxylic Acid end group.

Methane is CH_4. Nutritionists use shorthand to write names of fats. Butyric fatty acid is $C_4H_8O_2$. Fatty acids always end as a group of: Carbon with a double bond to Oxygen and a single bond to Oxygen that is also bonded to Hydrogen (Hydroxyl). This end group is called 'carboxylic acid'. Bonds between Carbons in Fatty Acids (FAs) are always bent, but for convenience they may be drawn straight as above - and often FAs are drawn without all Hydrogens or Carbons in place.

Fatty Acid = Carbon Chain + Carboxylic Acid

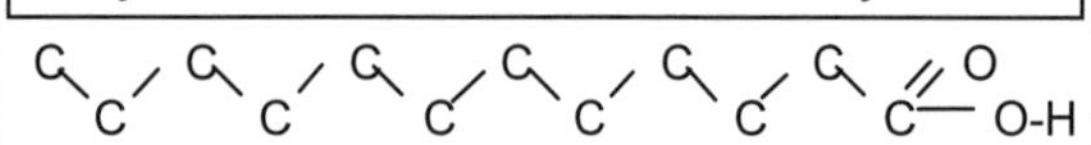

Chemical formula of Lauric SFA [12:0]

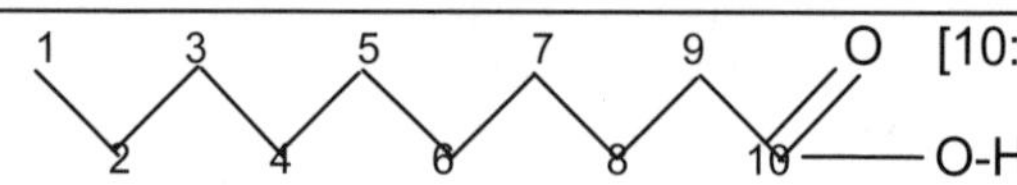

[10:0]

Stick model of Capric SFA using the *w* (omega) system for numbering Carbons in Fatty Acids

If all the middle Carbons in the Fatty Acid chain are bonded to two Hydrogens and two other Carbons the Fatty Acid is called 'saturated' with Hydrogens. When there is only one double bond between two adjacent Carbons the Fatty Acid is called 'monounsaturated' with Hydrogens. When there is more than one double bond between Carbons the Fatty Acid is called 'polyunsaturated'. Body enzymes can create double bonds in Saturated Fatty Acids and convert some Saturated Fatty Acids (SFAs) into Unsaturated Fatty Acids (UFAs). Some UFAs can not be created from SFAs by human enzymes. Two UFAs that can not be created by human enzymes are called 'Essential Fatty Acids'. Essential Fatty Acids (EFAs) have two or three double bonds in their Carbon chain. These EFAs are called 'Linoleic Acid' (LA) and 'Linolenic Acid' (LNA).

Glycerol

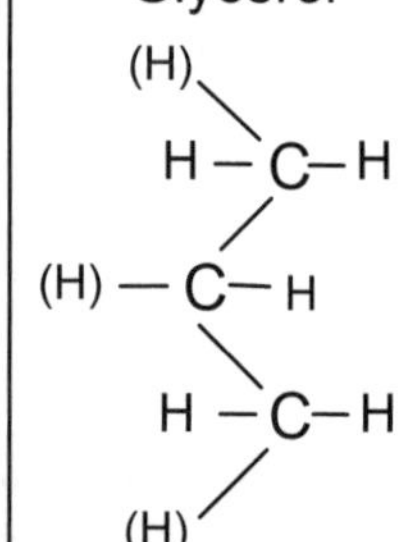

Meat fat contains many long chain SFAs, much cholesterol but very few precious EFAs. "Cholesterol is unique in that our body can make it but, once made, cannot break it down. The removal of cholesterol is increased by dietary fiber. If fiber is absent, up to 94% of the cholesterol and bile salts are reabsorbed and recycled. This is one of the reasons why low-fiber diets increase blood cholesterol levels." [R3] "Proponents of orthomolecular nutrition suggest that the 'cholesterol' problem is really caused by dietary deficiencies of micronutrient vitamins and minerals required to properly metabolize cholesterol in our body. ... diets that are moderately high in cholesterol, which also include sufficient quantities of all vitamin and mineral micronutrients, keep blood cholesterol levels normal and prevent atherosclerosis. [R3]

The fat-soluble vitamins are A, D, E, F and K. Vitamin D is more like a hormone than a vitamin. Vitamin D is primarily formed from cholesterol interacting with tanning sunshine (UV-a) via melanin in the skin. Meat fat, especially suet (i.e.– cover fat), often contains few or no fat-soluble vitamins.

Essential Fatty Acids and Cholesterol

[18:2*w*6] =18 Carbons -2 double bonds -Carbon #6 has the 1st double bond

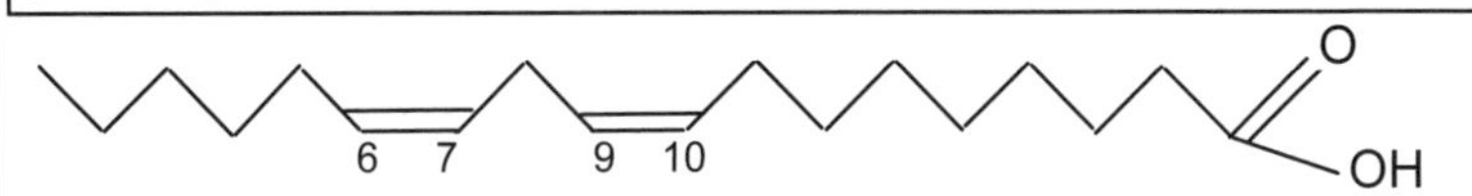

stick model of essential Linoleic Fatty Acid (LA) [18:2*w*6]

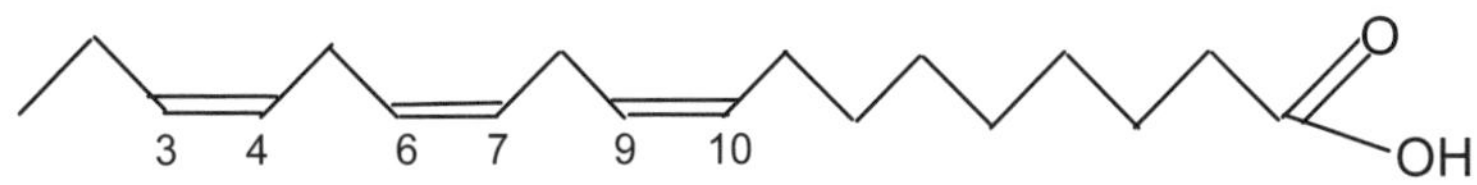

stick model of essential Linolenic Fatty Acid (LNA) [18:3*w*3]

Triglyceride

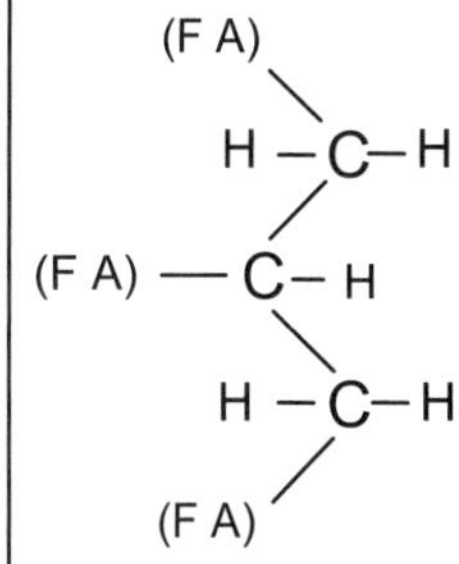

Cholesterol
27 Carbons

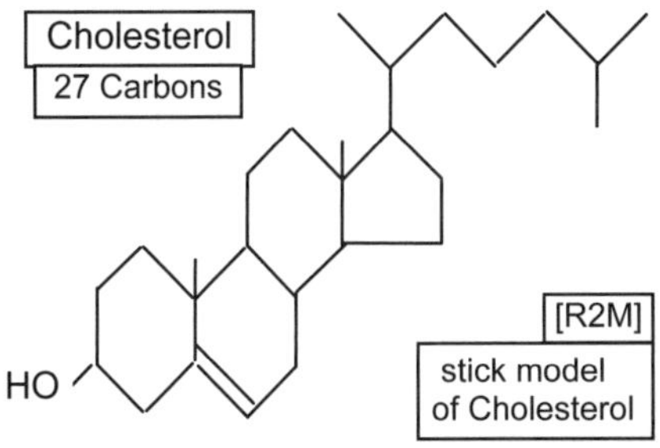

[R2M]

stick model of Cholesterol

Healthy cell walls are vital for normal function of all cells. Fats are an integral part of all cell walls. UFAs keep walls loose and fluid. SFAs keep membranes hard and rigid. All cell walls (membranes) need both UFAs and SFAs in the proper balance. Cholesterol helps keep cell walls healthy and functioning properly by adding to rigidity if walls are too fluid or by adding to fluidity if walls are too rigid. Cell walls allow respiration as nutrients enter and wastes leave. Cell walls also act as a barrier against harmful microbes. Nearly 80% of all body cholesterol is produced in the liver.

Steven Masley, MD discusses the pneumonic **L**ethal for LDL cholesterol (**L**ow-Density-Lipid) and **H**ealthy for **H**DL cholesterol (High-Density-Lipid {Lipoprotein}). HDL-cholesterol is safely transported through arteries. Cholesterol in an LDL-complex is often subject to oxidative damage when it is transported back to the liver. Antioxidants like Vitamin E, EFAs, Vitamin C, carotenoids and flavonoids make up the LDL-cholesterol complex, but if too many oxidants are encountered the antioxidants are exhausted. An LDL-cholesterol complex damaged by oxidants is engulfed by a white blood cell. If this happens, the white blood cell containing the oxidized LDL-complex dies and forms artery clogging plaque. Think of the cholesterol as if it were a VIP being transported to town by stagecoach, a small safety escort being the antioxidants and the well-armed assassins as being oxidants. If the escort is well enough armed, the VIP will get to town safely. If the VIPs are not well protected, the stage, the VIPs, and the escort will all die in a big heap in the roadway. Later, scavengers may come to clean up the mess. In this scenario, the scavengers might be the rescue antioxidants from micronutrient rich food sent to clean up the plaque deposits in arteries. Antioxidant cleanup is critical before more VIPs need to travel on the same clogged road. [R28]

Oxygen is an oxidant used to burn sugars, fats and even proteins for energy. Oxidation in the proper place is a necessary part of healthy biochemistry, but unwanted oxidation is extremely damaging to all tissues. Burning wood in a fireplace is a form of oxidation, but if the fire gets out of the fireplace, tables, chairs, rugs, beds and even the whole house can be quickly burned up.

Barry Sears, PhD in his book *The Zone* discusses that high LDL-cholesterol is a symptom of underlying metabolic dysfunction and a poorly balanced diet, but not from dietary cholesterol. [R19]

Cream has 10% short-chain SFAs (4 to 6 Carbons). Butyric SFA is 4 Carbons long and is named for its content in butter. Short-chain SFAs have many healthy qualities, including being easy to burn for fuel. Butyric SFA helps feed friendly bacteria in the colon. Medium-chain SFAs (8 to 12 Carbons) are easy to digest, are as easy to burn for energy as short-chain SFAs, are not stored in the body as fat, and may be beneficial in diets of people with liver or digestive disorders. Butter contains many short-chain and medium-chain SFAs between 4 and 14 Carbons in length. Caprylic SFA (8 Carbons) inhibits the growth of yeasts, like *candida albicans*, in the intestines. Many athletes include short and medium-chain SFAs in their diets for energy before workouts. Butter contains some long-chain SFAs that are required in healthy cell walls for stiffness. [R8B] Cream in milk has been highly prized since Abel was a keeper of the flocks. Churned, cultured cream becomes butter. Butter, cream and fat in milk are easiest to digest before pasteurization and homogenization. SFAs in milk fat, cream and butter are less likely to suffer free-radical oxidative damage from the high heat of cooking, especially frying, than UFAs in vegetable oils.

∗ Raw fresh butter and milk are desirable for healthy SFAs, cholesterol and other nutrients.

Unsaturated Fatty Acids

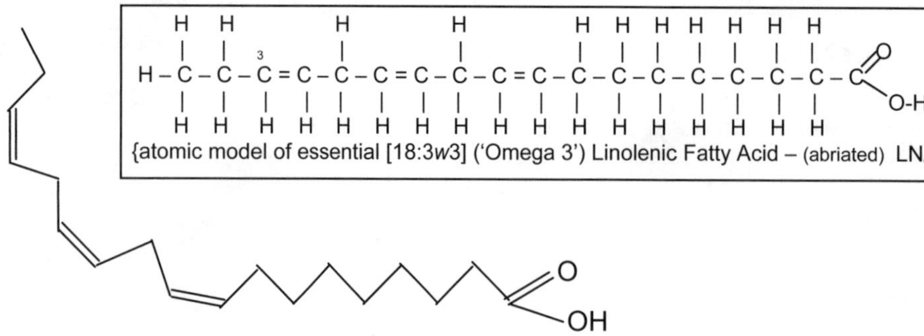

{atomic model of essential [18:3*w*3] ('Omega 3') Linolenic Fatty Acid – (abriated) LNA}

{spatial (3-D) model of [18:3*w*3] all-cis essential Linolenic Acid}

Omega 3 (*w*3) FAs are found in fish liver oil. Omega 3 FAs are converted in the body to superior quality synovial fluids that lubricate between bones in joint spaces.

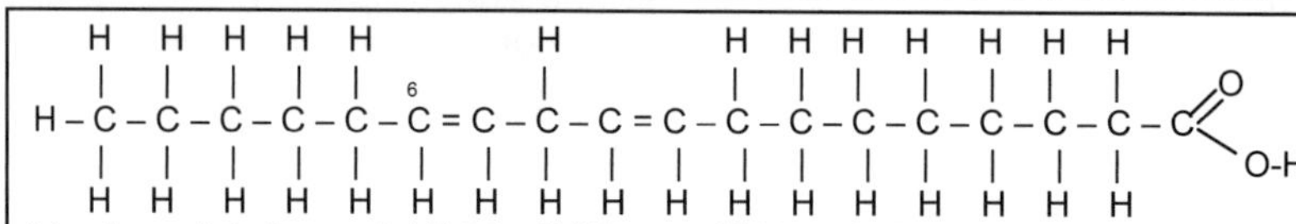

{atomic model of essential [18:2*w6*] ('Omega 6') Linoleic Fatty Acid – (abriated) LA}

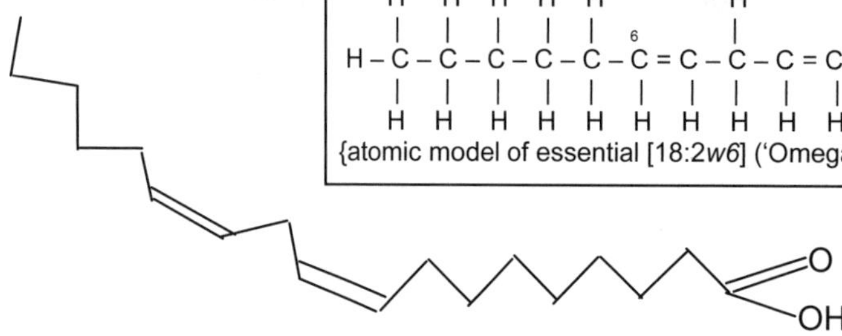

{spatial (3-D) model of [18:2*w*6] all-cis essential Linoleic Fatty Acid}

Health requires twice as much *w*3 EFA as *w*6 EFA. [*w*3 LNA X 2 = *w*6 LA]

A Carboxylic Acid end group may be written as COOH and also as CO_2H.

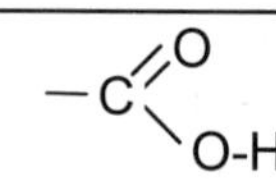

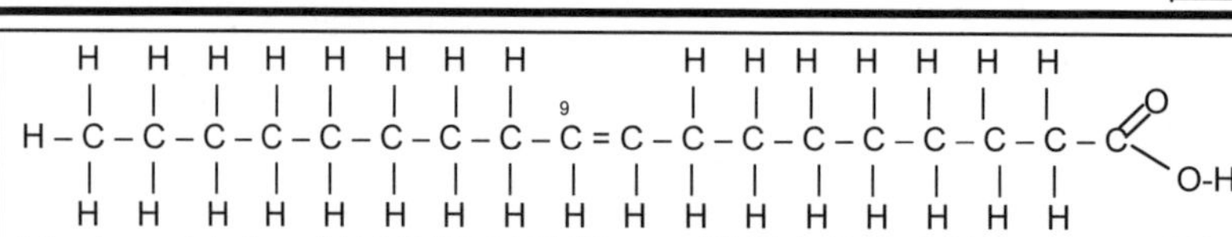

{atomic model of useful UFA [18:1*w9*] ('Omega 9') Oleic Fatty Acid – (abriated) OA}

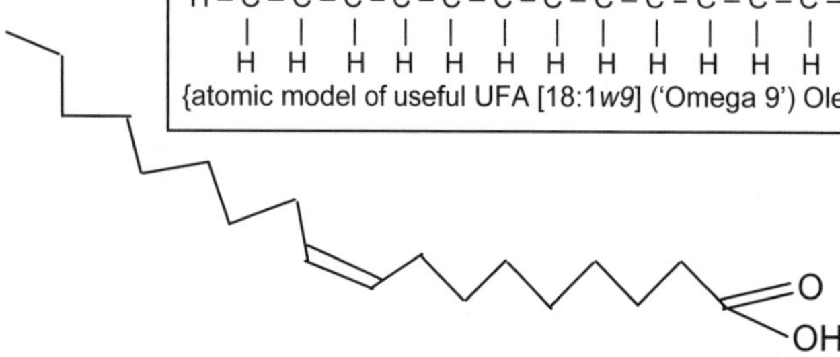

spatial model of [18:1*w*9] (cis) monounsaturated Oleic Fatty Acid

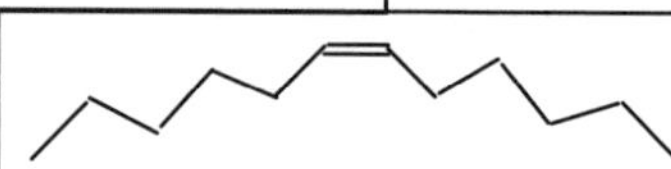

Cis-fats, as found in nature, have Hydrogens at the double-bond on the same side & are always bent. The bent shape of UFAs produces many essential properties of UFAs.

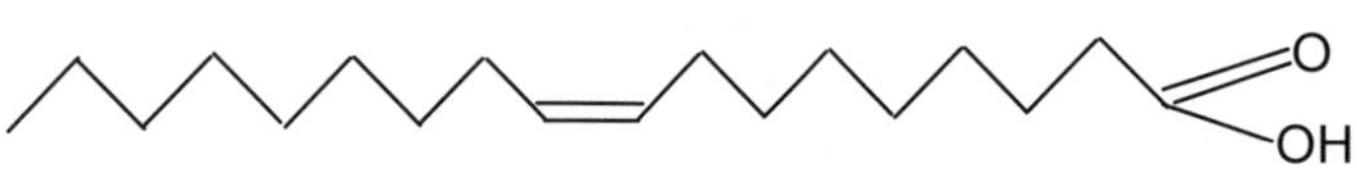

spatial model of non-useful [18:1*t* 9] (trans) Fatty Acid

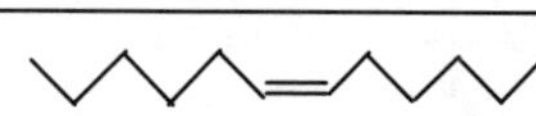

Trans-fats, as in partially hydrogenated fat, have Hydrogens at the double-bond on the opposite sides & all are straight molecules.

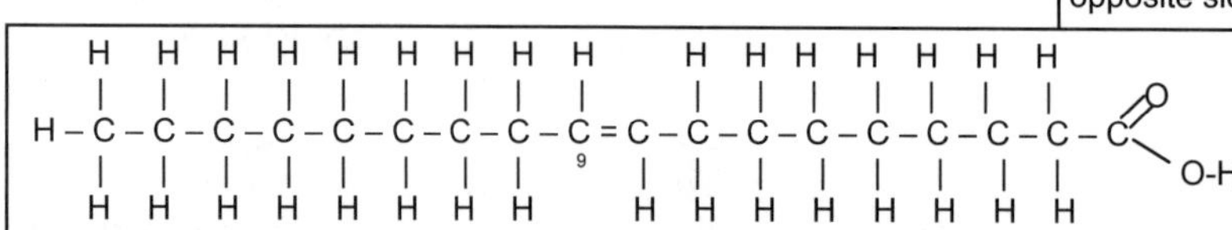

{atomic model of non-useful, straight, disruptive 'trans FA' – never found in nature }

partial hydrogenation of UFAs produces straight 'trans FAs' that are 'sticky' like long-chain SFAs

Using 'Trans FAs' in cell membranes and other essential cellular biochemistry may be analogous to using the wrong make and the wrong model carburetor parts to repair the engine your automobile; components would not be put together as designed, nor fit as designed, nor function as designed.

Trans FAs that are incorporated into a cell and used in biochemistry, may slowly degrade cellular efficiency.

Saturated Fatty Acids – Lecithin – Protein – Urea

spatial model of [18:0] saturated Stearic Fatty Acid

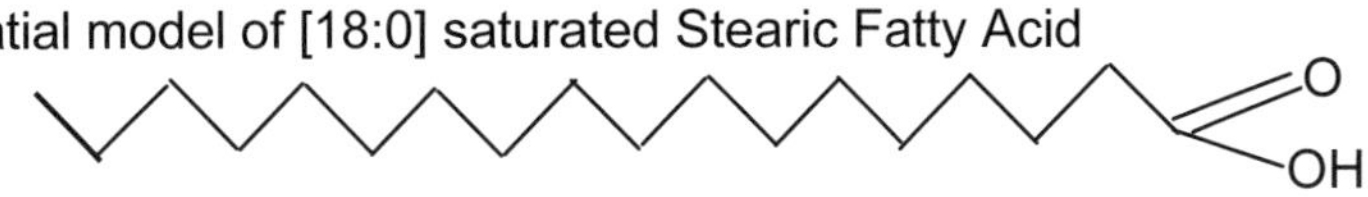

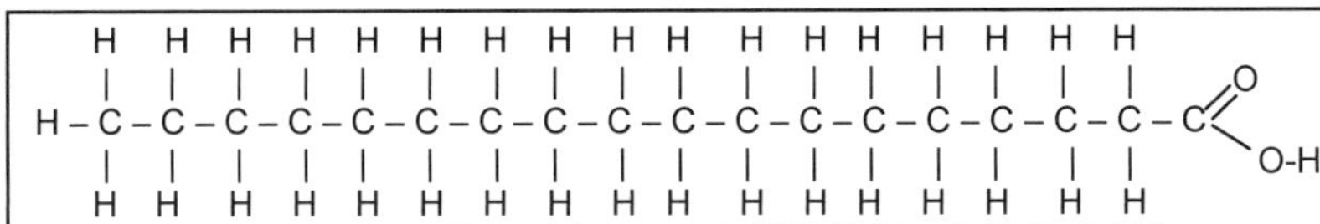

{atomic model of 'long-chain', straight, saturated [18:0] Stearic Fatty Acid }

'Long-chain' Stearic SFA has 18 Carbons. Long-chain SFAs have 12+ Carbons and are of limited value to build the functional cell walls that are essential to life. Too many long SFAs and all trans-FAs are sticky in blood. [R2N]

spatial model of [4:0] saturated Butyric FA

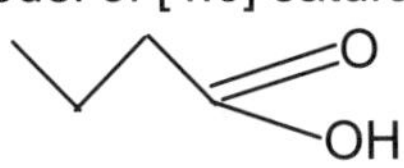

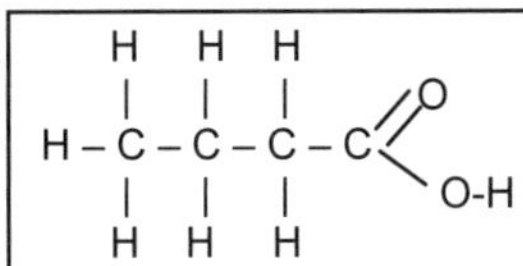

'Short-chain' Butyric SFA is common in dairy products Butter–Cream.

{atomic model of saturated [4:0] Butyric FA }

Short-chain SFAs 4 to 10 Carbons are liquid at body temperature 37°C. Long-chain SFAs 12 to 24 Carbons are solid at body temperature 98.6°F.

spatial model of [8:0] saturated Caprylic FA

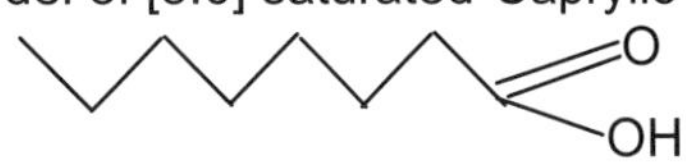

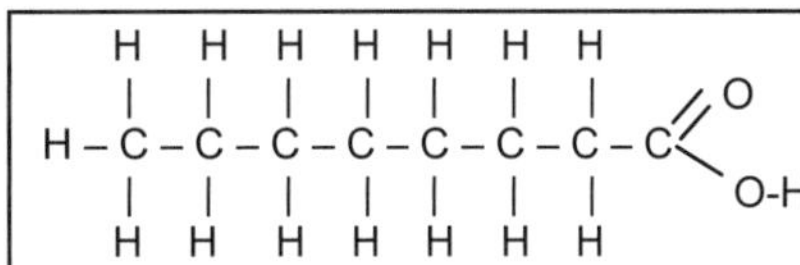

{atomic model of saturated [8:0] Caprylic FA }

Lecithin – a backbone of Glycerol &
– H_3PO_4 plus Choline on one end
– an unsaturated FA in the middle
– a saturated FA on the other end

Phosphoric Acid (H_3PO_4) is attached to Glycerol – and is attached to Choline.

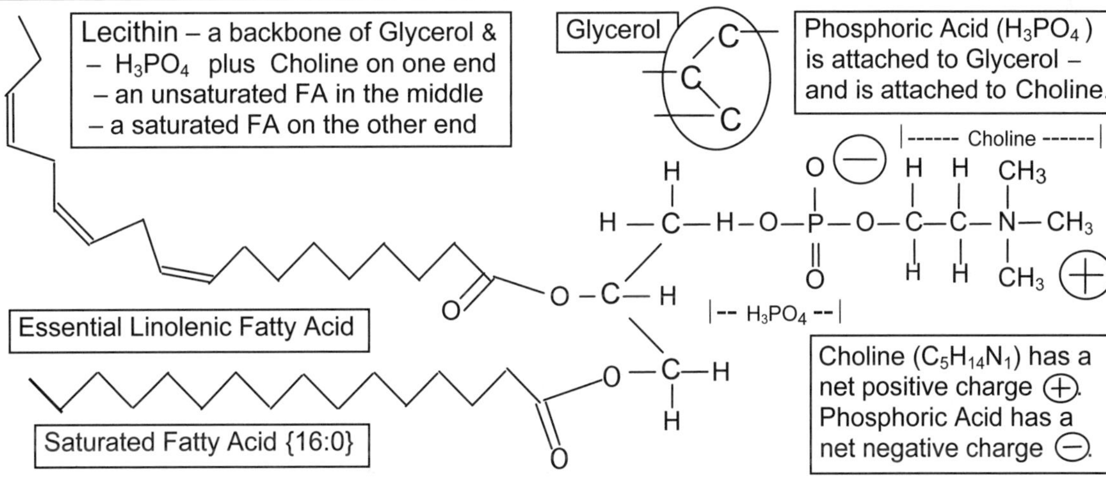

Choline ($C_5H_{14}N_1$) has a net positive charge ⊕. Phosphoric Acid has a net negative charge ⊖.

The highest quality Lecithin has an essential FA, such as Linolenic (LNL) in the middle position. The fatty acid end of Lecithin is soluble in fats, but the choline end of Lecithin is soluble in H_2O. Lecithin will also help other fats (SFAs) that aren't soluble in water, to be soluble in water (H_2O). Whoever said 'fats and water don't mix' didn't know about Lecithin. Lecithin is the fat equalizer. Lecithin is an important, complex molecule found in greatest abundance in milk, eggs and soy.

Water (H_2O) is polarized with a negative end ⊖ and a positive end ⊕.

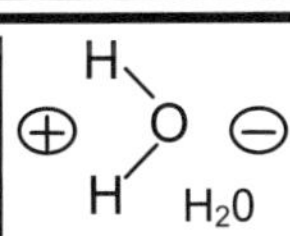

Carbon Dioxide is (CO_2) O=C=O. CO_2 is a gas.

Oxygen is found as (O_2) O=O. O_2 is a gas.

Methane (CH_4) & Ammonia (NH_3) are both gases.

Proteins are made of Amino Acids (AAs) – complex chains (rings) of Carbon, Hydrogen, Oxygen and Nitrogen.

AA – Phenylalanine

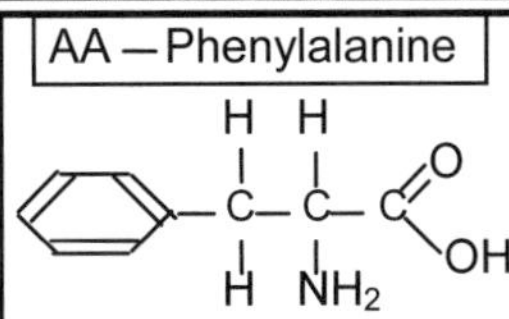

Tryptophan

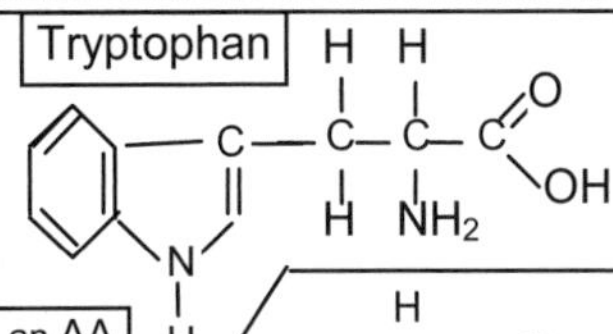

an AA

Urea – CN_2H_4O

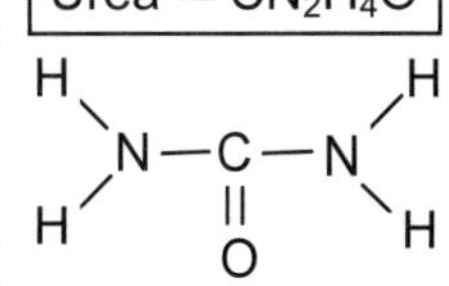

Protein is degraded to ammonia that is eliminated by the kidneys.

6-Carbon Benzene rings

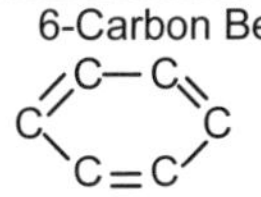

also contain unshown Hydrogens.

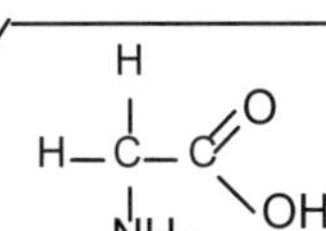

Glycine is the simplest AA.

Urea = 2 HN_3 + CO_2
Urea is 2 Ammonia plus Carbon Dioxide.

Chapter 10 Blood

Moses commanded the Hebrews not to eat any blood. (Lev 1:15, Lev 7:26 and Deut 15:2)

KJV Deut 12:23 Only be sure that thou eat not the blood: for the blood is the life; and thou mayest not eat the life with the flesh.

Cutting an animal's throat and allowing the heart to pump the blood out of the arteries is the 'kosher' method of butchering. Kosher means clean, fit or proper. Kosher butchering produces meat free from blood, which allows meats to keep longer before spoiling, and produces meats with very few impurities. Jewish butchers have practiced this healthy kosher procedure for centuries.

Blood contains some elements of food (proteins, fats or carbohydrates), but blood also carries many waste byproducts of metabolism for detoxification and elimination by the liver and kidneys. Ammonia and CO_2 are common waste byproducts of metabolism. [R2] These waste products are cleansed from the blood by the kidneys as urea. [R3] If people eat an animal's blood, they get some blood-borne wastes, and their kidneys must now work to eliminate these wastes. [R2-3]

If an animal is in poor health, disease-causing organisms or toxins from the microbes would also be found in the blood. Microbes and toxins could be transferred to people by eating blood. God further protected the Hebrews from contracting illnesses due to eating meat from diseased animals (zooanosis), by ordering that no meat can be eaten of any beast that is not freshly killed. Blood can not be purged from the muscle of an already dead (and possibly unhealthy) clean animal.

NIV Lev 22:8 "... he must not eat anything found dead or torn (***terephah***) by wild animals ..."

If the circumstances of an animal's death are not known, the butcher may not know whether a disease may have contributed to the animal's death and it can't be eaten.** When an animal dies with blood still in it, the corpse will soon decay and the meat becomes unclean or unhealthy.

> "For immediately upon death begins a process of corruption which produces compounds not only obnoxious to the senses, but actively poisonous in character; and what is of still more consequence to observe, in the case of all parasitic and infectious diseases, the energy of the infection is specially intensified when the infected person or animal dies." [R4]

Today, cattle may be electrically stunned and hung by the hind feet, before the throat is cut and the heart pumps the blood out of the muscle meat as the cow dies. This is kosher butchering.

An animal's blood also carries the life-regulating chemicals called hormones. Hormones stimulate the glands of the body to perform their normal activities, including sexual activity. Hormones are essential to healthy function for the animal that made the hormone. If eaten in blood, life-supporting animal hormones may become life-altering and life-damaging for humans. Today, livestock are routinely fed synthetic hormones to cause them to grow faster and get to the market faster. Elmer Josephson discussed how both animal and synthetic hormones in blood, if eaten as part of meat, may contribute to abnormal human sexual desires and activity today. [R1]

In some places, snake blood is drained into wine and is drunk as an aphrodisiac. [R11]

Today, farm animals are also routinely injected with antibiotics to 'prevent' contagious illness or to keep otherwise unhealthy animals alive long enough to get to market. [R7] Marc Lappe', PhD in his book *Germs That Won't Die* discusses that routine use of antibiotics for livestock provides an excellent environment for microbes to 'mutate' and become resistant to these antibiotics. [R8B] Antibiotic-resistant microbes, such as *E. coli*, may be found in an animal's blood or fat, where they may cause life-threatening human disease. Microbes that develop antibiotic-resistance in livestock may inadvertently contaminate other food, such as fresh fruit juice, causing further human illness.

> "... antibiotics are to livestock production what the assembly line was to the auto industry: without it, production would stay at the level of the home industry: ... [R8] The most dramatic results came with the advent of intensive rearing practices in which animals were raised in even more confined quarters. There the risk of epidemics or chronic infections normally cut back on gains made by increased efficiency of production, until antibiotics came along. Antibiotics seemed to make it possible to raise more animals in less space, using less feed, and over a shorter period than through the use of conventional methods." [R8A]

Laurie Garrett in her book *The Coming Plague* discusses that eating blood, fat or meat may introduce unwanted antibiotics and unwanted mutant antibiotic-resistant bacteria into humans. The recent outbreak of *E. coli* from ground hamburger beef may be traced to this practice. [R7]

Pesticides, herbicides, fungicides and harsh chemical fertilizers that are used in agriculture, may remain on crops and are found concentrated in animal fat and may also be found in blood.

*** Blood is always an unwanted contaminate of healthy lean kosher meat from clean animals.**

Mad Cow Disease

** Even meat from clean animals may be unhealthy to eat if the animal is improperly raised. In 1986, the development of 'Mad Cow Disease' in Britain and later in Europe can be traced to improperly enriching the diet of dairy/beef cows with offal: the remains of dead 'downer' animals.

"Offal often includes brain, spinal cord, spleen, eyes, intestines and other organs." [R19]

Ruminant animals aren't designed to eat any animal matter in their feed! Downer animals are animals that die before slaughtering from undiagnosed diseases. Enriching the diets of grazing animals with downer animals offers the opportunity for a disease that caused the downer animal to die to be amplified and recycled back into the food chain. A small family of fatal neurological diseases, called transmissible spongiform encephalopathies [TSE], have recently been discovered. *Mad Cow Disease is a recent TSE in humans caused by eating cattle fed downer-enriched feed.

"An alternative source of protein supplement in Britain and many other countries, including the United States, is meat-and-bone meal from the knacker's yard: the ground, cooked and dried remains of dead animals, including downer cattle and sheep dead of undiagnosed disease. Cattle (and sheep, pigs, and chickens) are thus made cannibals in the interest of cheaper milk and meat." [R14] {'Downer' animals are dead from disease.}

Said Dr. Richard Marsh about the family of TSE, 100% fatal, neurological diseases:

"If spontaneous cases of prion [a TSE] disease can occur in humans, they likely also occur in animals. Normally not naturally transmitted, these spontaneous incidents [of animal TSE] can still pose a danger by the unnatural act of cannibalism as seen in kuru [a TSE] in humans, or by the intervention of man and the feeding of [downer] animal protein to ruminants." [R14A]

'Prion', a renegade protein, is the TSE disease agent that is 100% fatal in the brain of man and animal. Mad Cow, Kuru and CJD are all TSE diseases. Kuru was the first recognized TSE, occurring in cannibals of New Guinea. In 1976, Carlton Gajdusek, MD received a Nobel Prize in Medicine for his work on Kuru. {CJD (Creutzfeldt-Jakob) is a very rare, 100% fatal human TSE disease.}

"The British disaster makes it grimly evident that the high-tech cannibalism of recycling animal protein risks spreading lethal disease. The practice continues in the United States for the same reason that it continues in Britain even as the death count rises: because the meat industry and its allies in government assess the risk differently from the scientists and physicians who know most about the transmissible spongiform encephalopathies [TSE]." [R14B]

Scientists, Physicians and ***Torah*** scholars who know the LORD's instructions should stand together to stop downer and offal feed for cattle. In Britain, Mad Cow Disease became common when the percentage of downer/offal feed for cattle was significantly increased to save feed cost. In many countries, cattle continue to be fed a low, hopefully safe amount of downer and offal feed. In 1997, US legislation was finally passed to restrict the use of downer/offal in cattle feed. [R19]

NIV Lev 22:8 He must not eat anything found dead or torn (***terephah***) by wild animals, and so become unclean through it. I am the LORD.

After first becoming aware that force-feeding downer bone/meat meal to dairy/beef cattle caused the fatal Mad Cow Disease in humans, the practice continued in Britain until the enormity of the problem was recognized and 140+ people died. Britain could have responded quickly and immediately stopped the use of downer animals as feed and saved many human lives and most of their cattle. Eventually, after many more dairy/beef cattle acquired Mad Cow Disease and after 140+ people died, Britain and Europe finally recognized how widespread Mad Cow Disease was. Now they were forced to destroy most of their dairy/beef cattle, causing many people to turn to unclean meat, from horse, as a replacement for the beef they no longer considered safe. Cooking kills many blood-borne disease-causing microbes, but cooking does not inhibit/kill (TSE) prions.

Mad Cow Disease is an epidemic that never had to be, if cattle were fed a vegetable-matter only diet.

The LORD's purpose for the dietary laws is to distinguish between meat (animal, fish or fowl) that is clean and healthy to eat from meat that is unclean and unhealthy to eat. The dietary laws require avoiding fat and blood, as well as meat from even clean animals that die on their own.

KJV Lev 11:46 ... for this is the law of the beasts, and of the fowl, and every living creature that moveth in the waters, and of every creature that creepeth upon the earth:
vs47 To make a difference between the clean and the unclean, and between the beast that may be eaten and the beast that may not be eaten.

The Mosaic dietary Laws discuss concepts in human health that are as old as the earliest written books, and at the same time, are as modern as today's newspapers or magazines.

---------------------------------- References Ch 10 Blood ----------------------------------

[R1] God's Key to Health and Happiness\ by Elmer Josephson;
pg 111 animal hormones in blood may encourage perverse sex
[R2] Nutrition and Your Body\ by Benjamin Colimore, MA and Sarah Stewart Colimore, LPT;
pg 167-168 albumen in blood collects waste products for excretion by the kidneys
[R3] Textbook of Physiology\ by Arthur Guyton, MD; pg 933 $CO_2 + 2NH_3$ = urea
[R4] The Book of Leviticus\ by Samuel Kellogg; pg 292-293 eat no blood
[R5] Are the Dietary Laws Scientific?\ by Harold Hemenway eat no blood
[R6] The Poisons In Your Food; by William Longgood\ (Ch VI) pg 109-126 carcinogens in food
[R6A] pg 116 co-carcinogens [R6B] (Ch VII) pg 129-164 Test-tube Meats = carcinogenic toxicity
[R7] The Coming Plague\ by Laurie Garrett; pg 424-428 antibiotics in livestock
[R8] Germs that Won't Die\ by Marc Lappe', PhD; Ch 10 - pg 123-149 antibiotics at the feedlot
[R8] pg 14 quote 1st – ½ //[R8A] pg 126-127 quote 2nd – ½ //[R8B] pg 133-135 mutant *E. coli*
[R9] Guess What Came to Dinner\ by Ann Louise Gittleman; Ch 3 pg 37-56 - various parasites
[R9A] pg 49 quote symptoms of trichinosis
[R9B] pg 64-66 microwaving meat, especially pork, doesn't kill all parasites
[R10] The Chemistry of the Blood\ by M. R. DeHann, MD; Ch 1 – pg 13-40
[R11] Ripley's Believe it or Not\ hosted by Jack Palance; snake blood drank as an aphrodisiac
[R12] What the Bible Says About Healthy Living\ by Rex Russell, MD
[R13] Food in History\ by Reay Tannahill; pg 55-56 *kashrut* - no blood
[R14] Deadly Feasts\ by Richard Rhodes; pg 174-175 quote downer animals
[R14A] pg 228 quote Dr. Richard Marsh - Mad Cow disease
[R14B] pg 232 quote failed warning s //[R14C] pg 135-136 Carlton Gajdusek, MD Oct 14, 1976 Nobel Prize
[R15] Man and Microbes\ by Arno Karlen; (1995 Putnam Sons) [R15A] pg 199; Mad-Cow Disease
[R15B] pg 8-38-143-144-145 (swine flu) / book - Pale Horse, Pale Rider
[R16] Mad Cow Disease\ by Dr. Richard Lacey and The Dines Letter (March/April 2001) – Mad Cow Disease
[R17] Washington State 12-26-2003 Seattle P.I. – US Cow found with Mad Cow Disease – 143 died in Britian
[R18] Strong's Concordance\ by James Strong, STD, LLD {***diaspora*** = dispersion – as in seeds}

pg 197	clean (pure)	# 2891 (# 2889)	H pg 45	***tahor – tahowr***	Num 19:19
pg 1087	unclean (foul)	# 2930-32	H pg 46	***tame***	Num Ch 19
pg 335	fat	# 2459	H pg 39	***cheleb***	Lev 3:3
pg 131	blood	# 1818	H pg 31	***dam***	Lev 3:17
pg 936	slaughter	# 7821 (from #7819)	H pg 114	***shehitah – shechiytah***	Hosea 5:2
pg 846	right	# 3787	H pg 58	***kasher – kawsher***	Esther 8:5

{***Kawsher*** is transliterated to *kashrut*, *kashruth* or kosher. ***Kawsher*** is translated: right – clean, fit or proper.}
[R19] Mapping Epidemics\ by Brent Hoff and Carter Smith III; pg 54-55 Mad Cow Disease
[R20] Mad Cow USA\ by Sheldon Rampton and John Stauber
[R21] Oprah Winfrey (1996 TV program)\ discussed Mad Cow Disease
[R22] Diet for a New America\ by John Robbins overcrowding animals – antibiotics in feed – poorer protein
[R23] The Serpent and the Rainbow (DVD-movie #15)\ by Wes Craven – Human blood is drunk in voodo.
[R24] What Would Jesus Eat?\ by Don Colbert, MD;pg 55-58 Mad Cow Disase and pg 58-61 ***shehitah*** (noun)
Rabbis state that the LORD gave Moses an 'Oral ***Torah***' – the ***Mishnah*** – on Mt. Sinai along with the ***Torah***. In 70 AD, the destruction of the Jerusalem Temple began the ***Diaspora***. In ≈75 AD, in Yavneh, Israel, Jews of the ***Sanhedrin*** began to write down the ***Mishnah***. In ≈220 AD, in Sepphoris, Israel, the ***Mishnsh*** was finished. In ≈250 AD, Rabbinical scholars in Babylon and Palestine began the ***Gemarah*** commentary on the ***Mishnah***. In ≈400 AD, work on the Palestinian (i.e.– Jerusalem) ***Gemarah*** ceased. In ≈550 AD, the Babylon ***Gemarah*** was completed and it was added to the ***Mishnah*** to the finish the ***Talmud***. ***Shehitah*** slaughtering as described in the ***Mishnah*** requires using a to-and-fro cut with a long sharp knife to quickly severe the trachea, esophagus, two vagus nerves, both carotid arteries and the jugular vein. ***Shehitah*** slaughtering is minimally painful to the clean animal (herbivore) and produces the maximum blood loss from the animal by the still pumping heart.
[R25] Kashruth \ by Rabbi Yacov Lipschutz (Brooklyn, NY – Mesorah Pub., 1988) – reference ***shehitah*** in [R24] {see pg 112}
[R26] Outbreak Alert\ by Jason Eberhardt-Phillips; pg 113-120 Mad Cow Disease //pg 194 antibiotics in feed
[R27] Living in Divine Health (audio)\ by Ted Broer, PhD; T2-s2 *broma* – I Tim 4 /T5-s2 Peter's Vision – Acts 10

Prions and resultant TSE disease may be possible in meat from any clean or unclean animal that is force fed ground-up offal (i.e. – from a downer animal) as bone meal or meat meal. — from 1996 to 2002 ≈100+ Mad Cow Disease fatalities in Europe –

Meat(s) may be used in a narrow (denotative) sense to refer only to flesh from animals; or in a broader, general (connotative) sense to group flesh from animals, fish and/or fowl together. {pg 25}
The context in which meat(s) is used in this book will make its proper meaning easily understood.
Kine, Hefer or Bullock are used denotatively in the ***Torah*** (KJV) to refer only to bovine animals.
Cattle is used connotatively in the ***Torah*** (KJV) to group all clean ruminant animals together. {pg 98}

The LORD dictated important health information to Moses. What a shame that throughout history, and even today, medical science has not regarded the instructions in the ***Torah*** authoritatively.

Chapter 11 Meat
Unclean Pig

All grazing animals that both chew the cud and part the hoof are clean and healthy for meat. The digestive system of these clean ruminants has four stomachs that pass cud (partially digested grass or leafy plant matter) back and forth, allowing bacteria in the stomachs to digest the cellulose. A ruminant's digestion system is virtually a protein factory, changing low quality plant protein into high quality muscle protein. [R1] Animals that do not both part the hoof and chew the cud are unclean and aren't fit for food. Unclean animals are often predator/scavengers. Noah also knew the clean/unclean distinction before he entered the Ark. (Gen 7:2) Adam used the general (connotative) terms: 'cattle' for all the clean farm animals and 'beasts' for all the unclean wild animals. (Gen 2:20)

JPS Lev 11:3 Whatsoever parteth the hoof, and is wholly cloven-footed (***sheca***), and cheweth the cud (***gerah***), among the beasts, that may ye eat.

JPS Lev 11: 4 Nevertheless these shall ye not eat of them that only chew the cud, or of them that only part the hoof: the camel, because he cheweth the cud but parteth not the hoof, he is unclean unto you. vs6 And the hare, because she cheweth the cud but parteth not the hoof, she is unclean unto you. vs7 And the swine, because he parteth the hoof, and is cloven-footed, but cheweth not the cud, he is unclean unto you. vs5 And the rock-badger, because he cheweth the cud but parteth not the hoof, he is unclean unto you.

Understanding the physiology of pig and other unclean animals explains why the LORD made this distinction for the health of His people. Pig is always susceptible to infestation with the trichina worm, which can cause the disease trichinosis for people who eat the flesh of the pig. Trichina, the 'worm that never dies', is one of eighteen parasites that routinely live in pig. [R3B]

Laird Goldsborough, MD wrote about the dangers of trichinosis from eating pork:

> "In the pork which we Americans eat, there too often lurk myriads (countless numbers) of baffling and sinister parasites. They are minute spiral worms which scientists call *Trichinella spirals*. A single serving of infected pork – even a single mouthful – can kill or cripple or condemn the victim to a lifetime of aches and pains. (Regulations as of 1976.)" [R3A - R4]

For the disabling and potentially deadly tichinae parasite, there is no wonder drug, nor cure. Flagel, the first anti-parasitic drug, was developed in the 1930s, but it not a cure-all for trichinosis. Prevention is the best choice for health, and prevention is found in obedience to the ***Torah***.

Dr. Goldsborough's warning continues in an excerpt from Readers Digest (Mar 1950). [R3A-4]

> "In the flesh of a pig, the trichinae are often so minute and so nearly transparent, that to find them, even with a microscope is a task for expert scientific inspectors ... Remember this: when you see stamped on a pork product the words, 'U.S. Government Inspected and Passed', those words do not mean that any official inspection whatever has been made as to whether this pork has trichinosis or not. It has merely passed the routine inspection given meat in general."

Senator Thomas Desmond, chairman of the New York Trichinosis Commission stated: [R3B]

> "Physicians have confused trichinosis with some fifty ailments ranging from typhoid fever to acute alcoholism. That pain in your arm or leg may be arthritis or rheumatism, but it may be trichinosis; that pain in your back may mean gall bladder involvement, but it may mean trichinosis." [R3B]

Pig keeps an environment inside its body that is undoubtedly part of the reason a pig is such a hospitable host for a huge variety of parasites, including trichinae. London's eminent scientist, Sir James Paget, who discovered the trichinae parasite in pork in 1835, wrote: [R3B]

> "Fancy the body of a single pig supporting more separately existing creatures [parasites] than the [entire human] population of the world." [R3B]
>
> "Contrary to popular belief, even well-cooked pork harbors viable *trichinella* worms and a tapeworm that may infiltrate human brain and muscle tissue." [R19-14A]

Pig is the glutton of all gluttons who will eat any animal flesh. The idiom for a gluttonous person is to 'pig out' or 'pork out'. Hog or Swine, from whom this idiom comes, is well deserving of this reputation, as dead, decaying, maggot-ridden, putrefied, animal flesh is a delicacy for a pig. Swine, if left alone with excess food, may continue to eat until they eat themselves to death. [R16] Hogs raised in a farm lot with horses and cows, will eat these animal's refuse, feces and urine. [R3] Pigs have been seen to chew cancerous growths off other animals. [R3] A scavengers physiology allows them to survive or even thrive when eating animal matter that is unfit for any other animal. Swine are scavengers on land; just as are crustaceans in the sea; and as vultures are in the air.

∗ Hog, Razorback or Swine, a Pig on the dinner plate by any other name is still called pork.

Trichinosis

Ann Louise Gittleman discusses trichinosis in her book *Guess What Came to Dinner*. [R14]

"Just about any symptom known to man can be caused by the various stages of trichinosis infection, which can masquerade as at least fifty more familiar diseases ranging from flu to generalized and specific aches and pains. These tiny [trichinae] roundworms can become enclosed in a cyst inside the muscles of bear, walrus, or pig. If pork is eaten and not thoroughly cooked, the cysts are dissolved by the host's digestive juices, and the worms mature and travel into the muscles, where they become encased. Eventually, the worms can burrow themselves into the larynx, chest, diaphragm, abdomen, jaws, and upper arms. Then they calcify, causing severe muscle soreness and fever. The symptoms of trichinosis change according to the progress the trichinella makes through the body. During the first week of infection, acute diarrhea, nausea, vomiting, and colic occur as the larvae penetrate the first part of the small intestine. Then, when the larvae migrate to muscle tissue, about two to four weeks after the infected meat was eaten, the most classic symptom, severe muscle pain, is experienced. When the larvae finally encyst themselves in muscle fiber, extreme dehydration and toxic edema can be caused. Edema of the lip, face, or eyelids, difficulty in breathing or speaking, chewing problems, enlarged lymph glands, meningitis, and encephalitis can take place. Brain damage, pneumonia, pleurisy, and nephritis are further complications of the disease." [R14]

Hans-Heinrich Reckeweg, MD, compared the physical characteristics of pork to other meats. Dr. Reckeweg found that pork is inferior in quality due to the toxins and fat it always contains.

"Pork should be regarded as an important homotoxin (human poison) which initiates activation of the body's defense mechanisms. [R2] Pork contains much intra-cellular fat or particles of fat inside the cell themselves, while in other animals, the fat is found almost exclusively outside these cells in the connective tissues, in the form of fat cells." [R2A]

Other problems can arise from consuming the sulfur-rich substances (mucopolysaccharides) of the connective tissues of pork, which have a specific mucous character. Mucopolysaccharides in pork allow the butcher to produce sausage meat that can be spread. Mucopolysaccharides, when eaten by people, can cause a mucous swelling of the connective tissue, which then results in water retention. Storage of mucopolysaccharides from pork by human tissues can result in a number of health issues including rheumatism, arthritis and damage to inter-vertebral discs. [R2A] There are certain skin-irritating effects from the histamine content in pork, which often initiate an inflammation. According to Professor Shope, an important factor in the toxic effect of pork is the influenza virus that remains infectious in a pig's lungs. As pork is used in sausage, hot dogs, liverwurst, luncheon meats, etc. the pig viruses may be transmitted to the consumer in pork. [R2B]

Today, the probability of infestation of pork products by trichinella and other parasites can be greatly reduced by not permitting pigs to eat raw flesh [R9]; but this restricted diet does nothing to eliminate the toxins that always accumulate in pig tissues or the viruses that thrive in the lungs. The tissues (meat) of pig remain toxic even if pigs are fed an otherwise healthy vegetarian diet. Pigs have very poorly developed organs of elimination, including the absence of sweat glands. [R7] Other animals, including humans, have well developed sweat glands, often called a 'third kidney'. People sweat away pounds of water through the skin; and with water goes unwanted wastes and toxins. (toxins + bacteria = body odor) ∗ **Pig retains many wastes and toxins as part of the flesh.** Sweating also helps to cool animals when the sweat evaporates from the skin. Pigs compensate for not sweating by wallowing in the mud to get moisture on their skin; and this muddy water later evaporates for cooling. Pig always maintains an unclean physiology both internally and externally.

"Viewed overall the pig is a very sick animal having few muscles and small bones, but with an abundance of mucous and fatty connective tissue, suffering from fatty degeneration of the cardiac muscle and liver." [R2C]

Anything a swine eats is very quickly digested and after about four hours may become part of the pig's flesh. All pork products contain contaminants from the food that the pig may have eaten. Pig is very profitable to raise, as everything the pig eats soon becomes fatty meat on the hoof. A slaughterer in Minnesota discussed that when butchering a pig, nothing goes to waste: [R3]

"… pork chops, ham, bacon; the intestines for sausages, hot dogs and wieners; head cheese from the head, pickle the feet, brains, liver, the hide for bacon rind and salt pork; etc." [R3]

Other common pork products include baloney or bologna from intestines and meat scraps, liverwurst from liver, sausage from meat, pork fat and lungs, as well as pepperoni and pastrami.

∗ No matter how you slice it, eating pork always presents a risk of developing trichinosis.

The Trichinosis Masquerade

The reported incidence of trichinosis in recent years gives the impression that the trichinosis epidemic is on the decline in the United States; however, this idea may be a misrepresentation of the true scenario. Certainly, the incidence of death from trichinosis is on the decline recently, but many trichinosis cases are of a milder variety and are not correctly diagnosed as trichinosis. Trichinosis, like any other disease, must be correctly diagnosed before meaningful statistics concerning its true incidence can be tabulated. Trichinosis often presents symptoms similar to general gastric distress, with an upset stomach or nausea, possibly diarrhea or cramps, a slight fever and headache. A bismuth remedy like bismuth carbonate might be commonly prescribed, along with bed rest and fluids. Many people could consider these initial symptoms as no big deal. If symptoms abate, the cause of the gastritis is then unimportant and a diagnosis is unnecessary. If symptoms persist, a heart disorder or an inflamed aorta or cirrhosis of the liver is considered. More advanced symptoms of trichinosis may include severe itching all over, eyelid edema that may swell the lids shut, a faded or failing voice, and seething pain in the chest and abdomen that may spread to the arms and legs. Since trichinae eventually lodge in muscle tissue, muscle ache is a classic symptom of trichinosis, and the muscle of choice for trichinae is often the diaphragm. Chest pain and pain on breathing are classic symptoms of trichinosis that could be symptoms of many ailments, such as heart attack or appendicitis. White Blood Cells fight all chronic infections. When trichinosis symptoms are advanced, blood chemistry will show elevated White Blood Cells. Trichinae enter human intestines via digestion of infected meat and penetrate intestinal walls to enter the bloodstream, and seek to lodge in muscles, where they classically cause muscle pain. Rob DeSalle, PhD in his book *Epidemic* wrote of a man who died of trichinosis from eating pork. A biopsy revealed tissue teeming with trichinae, which led the pathologist to estimate 12 million trichinae parasites infested his body; while an infestation of 5 million is generally lethal. [R23]

> "The worm is staggeringly prolific, and it has been known to remain alive, though quiescent, in the body of a surviving victim for more than thirty-one years. In general, the number of trichinae that succeed in reaching the muscle determines the severity of an attack. As such parasitic organisms go, adult trichinae are relatively large, the male averaging one-twentieth of an inch in length and the females about twice that. The [trichinae] larvae are less statuesque." [R23]

Pathologists have found as many as twelve hundred trichinae encysted in one gram of tissue.

> "Numerous animals, ranging in size from the mole to the hippopotamus, are hospitable to the trichinae but it has a strong predilection for swine and man. ...Few acute afflictions are more painful than trichinosis, or more prolonged and debilitating. Its victims are occasionally protracted for many months, and relapses after apparent recoveries are not uncommon. Its mortality is disconcertingly variable. It is usually around six percent, but in some outbreaks nearly a third of those stricken have died, and recovery of a patient from a full-scale attack is almost unheard of. Nobody is, or can be rendered, immune to trichinosis. Also, there is no specific cure. ...any therapeutic agent potent enough to kill a multitude of embedded trichinae would probably kill the patient too. ...Some authorities, in fact, regard the Mosaic proscription of pork as the pioneering step in the development of preventative medicine. [R23A] Trichinosis is generally believed to be a rarity. Outbreaks of trichinosis are seldom widely publicized. They are seldom even recognized. Trichinosis is the chameleon of diseases. The number and variety of ailments with which it is more or less commonly confused is encyclopedic." [R23B]

Dr. DeSalle reported one case in which a man developed trichinosis after buttering a slice of bread with a knife that had previously been used to slice a trichinae-infected pork sausage. [R23A] A few states have rules preventing feeding raw meat scraps to pig, but enforcement is often lax. ∗ Americans lead the world! Recent autopsies reveal that 1 in 5 Americans have had trichinosis in their lifetime, and it is likely that 1,000,000 Americans are afflicted with trichinosis each year. Ways to kill trichinae include: cooking until pork is bone white (undercooked pork is very risky); refrigeration at 5° C or less for 20^+ days; and scrupulous salting, smoking or pickling pork. [R23C]

(Pig and Trichinae are not drawn to the same scale.)

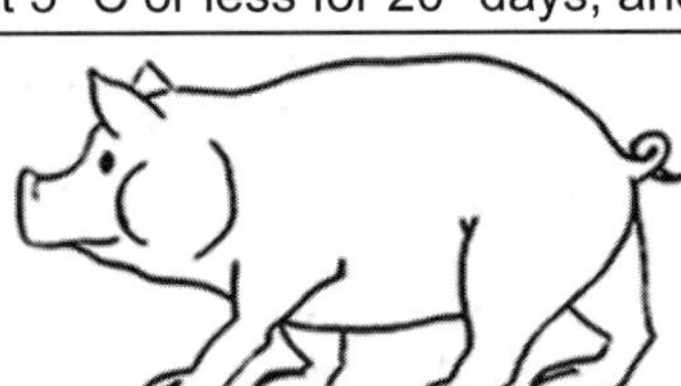

[R23D]

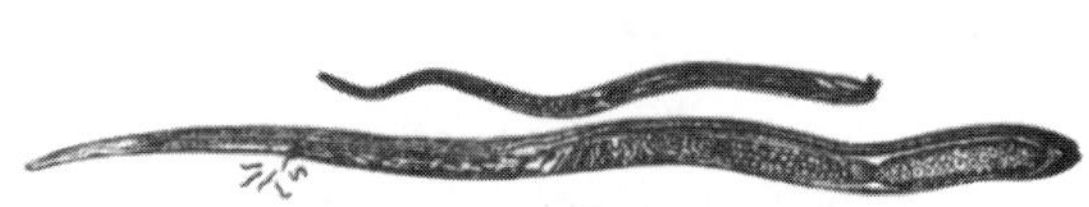

Trichinae – the worms that never die. [R3E]

∗ Pork and trichinosis go hand in hand like rats and plague, or mosquitoes and malaria.

Viruses, Toxins, Trichinosis and Tularemia

Pork contains porcine toxins that cannot be physiologically detoxified through ordinary detoxifying outlets of elimination, such as, urination, fecal secretions, skin secretions or breathing (and coughing up mucus). The only means of detoxifying porcine toxins is through pathological outlets: namely Inflammations. If eaten in small quantities, the porcine homotoxins may be stored until a 'limit is exceeded' and then an inflammatory outlet (illness) becomes necessary. [R2D]

Pig serves the vital function of scavenger and garbage eater. Hog quickly eats organic debris that would become a breeding ground for disease-spreading insects and other microorganisms. Swine maintain an unclean body, helping to keep the world cleaner for clean animals. [R3B]

Dr. Reckeweg stated that just like flu from pork products, certain influenza epidemics can be attributed to eating horse meat, which can also be infected with influenza viruses: [R2B-15]

> "Influenza (flu) is one of the most famous illnesses which pigs share with humans. This illness is harbored in the lungs of pigs and humans in the cooler months. Sausage contains bits of pigs' lungs, so those who eat pork sausage tend to suffer more during epidemics of influenza." [R2B]

The 1918 Flu virus that killed 50$^+$ million people worldwide during WWI epidemic has recently been identified by Jeffrey Taubenberger, MD, PhD of the Armed Forces Institute of Pathology. [R22] Virologists Dr. Robert Webster and Dr. Richard Shortridge theorized that domesticating ducks and pigs together in China allowed a benign duck virus to mutate in pigs and kill men. [R41] Whatever its origins, the terribly lethal 1918 Flu virus closely resembles the 'swine flu' of today. Virologists warn that a similarly lethal virus to the 1918 Flu pandemic could strike again. [R15-22-40]

∗ Viruses responsible for recent flu epidemics may have mutated and multiplied in pig lungs!

∗ People who routinely eat pork products, such as sausage, may be more likely to be infected by flu or succumb to flu (i.e. – The 1918 Flu) than people who do not include pork in their diet. [R2B]

Lions, Tigers and other carnivores have an intestinal tract that is generally short, averaging only three times the length of the body. Carnivores are animals whose primary food is the flesh of other animals, which is full of nutrition, but which can putrefy rapidly. Their food can (must) be digested quickly, and the remains should (must) be eliminated quickly before it rots in the body. Carnivores also have an acidic saliva, an absence of active sweat glands over most of their body surface and specialized sweat glands on the nose and paws. [R7] Pig, like all omnivores, has a digestive tract that is intermediate in length between a ruminant and a carnivore. Trichinosis also affects many other unclean animals besides swine, such as bear, rat, dog, wolf and cougar. [R2E]

Today, public health regulations often require Pig not to be fed raw meet scraps, to attempt to limit trichinosis. But, the regulations are not always followed, and are not entirely effective, because a rat may eat raw meat scraps from a garbage dumpster, and then crawl into a pigsty. If a rat dies, it may quickly become food for a pig. [R14A] Pig is a cannibal as well as a scavenger! A pig infected with trichinosis that dies in a pigpen, may then become meat for an entire herd. [R8]

∗ This scenario makes it virtually impossible to guarantee that a pig herd is free from trichinosis.

Horse is normally a grain eater, rather than a scavenger like pig. Horse however, is capable of carrying trichinae, and transmitting the trichinosis to humans. Horse likely acquires trichinae by eating dead trichinae-infected rodents that find their way into horse feed and then die. [R8A-9] After the recent Mad Cow Disease scare, Europeans are getting trichinosis from eating horse.

> "The disease [trichinosis] is worldwide, and about 15% of the United States population is said to be infected, although the majority of the cases remain asymptotic. The degree of severity of the infection is believed to depend on the number of trichinae contained in the ingested pork ... The majority of symptomatic cases runs from 5 to 40% ...
> Once the trichinae are encysted in the muscle tissue they cannot be dislodged...
> [In severe infections] Death is usually from cardiac or respiratory failure." [R11]

Trichinosis seems to have decreased recently in the US due to a more restrictive diet for pig. However, the proportion of infections from wild game, such as bear, wild boar and walrus has increased. In 1995, an outbreak of trichinosis (10 cases) came from undercooked smoked cougar jerky. [R10]

All meats concentrate nutrients such as proteins and minerals; yet all meats from the unclean animals, fish and fowl also concentrate toxins, and the meat may also harbor pathogenic microbes.

Wild Rabbit, Squirrel, Beaver and other rodents may carry tularemia (rabbit fever). Tularemia is contracted by skinning/dressing infected animals, causing a typhoid-like disease including, fever, diarrhea and pneumonia. Tularemia can be fatal. [R29] Some rodents may also carry trichinae. [R14A]

∗ Toxins abound in unclean meats, whether the meat is contaminated by parasites or not.

Clean 'Ruminant' Animals

Healthy meat is from grazing animals with cloven hooves that also chew the cud (***gerah***).

KJV Deut 14:4 These are the beasts which ye shall eat: the ox, the sheep, and the goat. vs5 The hart, and the roebuck, and the fallow deer, and the wild goat, and the pygarg, and the wild ox, and the chamois.

NIV Deut 14:4 "These are the animals you may eat: the ox, the sheep, the goat, vs5 the deer, the gazelle, the roe deer, the wild goat, the ibex, the antelope, and the mountain sheep."

On the healthy list are clean ruminant plant-eating animals that chew the cud. Ruminants are discussed by Dr. Harold Rosenberg in his book *The Book of Vitamin Therapy*. Their teeth are flat and their jaws move sideways for grinding. Their saliva is alkaline, and they perspire over their entire bodies. Because a ruminant's food requires a lengthy digestion, their intestinal canals average about thirty times the length of their bodies. [R7] Ruminant animals historically put very little fat on their bodies and yield very lean meat. Buffalo eaten by settlers as they crossed the plains was often so lean it could not be fried in a skillet over an open fire without adding fat to prevent the meat from sticking to the pan. [R6] Buffalo, Cow, Deer, Sheep, Goat, Moose, Elk, Ox, Lamb and Antelope are among the ruminant animals that provide clean, healthy nutritious meat. Ruminant grazers have four stomachs, and they are strictly vegetarians. Grasses that grazers eat are low in toxicity and low (25%) in protein. After being regurgitated between four stomachs, requiring many hours of digestion, grasses are digested to become high quality protein muscle. Clean-ruminants require nearly a day for grasses to digested by microbes in their stomachs. [R6]
∗ Ruminants are protein factories, turning low quality plant protein into high quality muscle protein.

> "Where ruminants differ significantly from other mammals is in the microbial pre-digestion of much of their intake in the fore-stomachs, chiefly in the rumen and reticulum. The fore-stomach may be regarded as a fermentation vat in which symbiotic bacteria and protozoa act in a favorable environment to reduce plant products, some of which (cellulose) would otherwise be indigestible, to forms that the ruminant can use. Sugars and starches are fermented rapidly, celluloses less so, the end products being chiefly volatile fatty acids (VFA), CO_2, energy and water.... the ruminant can utilize a larger portion of plant material than can most monogastrics [one stomach – man, pig, bear, horse, lion, etc.] ... as with starches and lipids, conversion of protein by microbes results in nutrients digested by the host animal. Additionally, B vitamins and vitamin K are synthesized by the microbes." [R5]

Protein means that which comes first. [R33] All protein is made from twenty-two amino acids. Eight amino acids (AAs) are called 'essential' because humans must acquire them from food, while the other fourteen amino acids can be manufactured by humans from the essential eight. High quality meat protein contains all eight essential amino acids in ratios that are proper for humans to create and rebuild their own organ, gland and muscle proteins. Sufficient quantity and quality of protein is very important in a healthy diet. All muscles, glands and organs are primarily made of protein. All hormones also have a protein component. It has been said that the human body is as old as its organs and glands. Organs and glands that are protein deficient are not as active, efficient or healthy as younger, protein rich organs and glands. Meat from clean herbivore – ruminant – muscle produces the highest quality protein, which greatly benefits human health. Noah knew the clean/unclean distinction before the Flood, as seven clean and two unclean of each 'kind' came on the Ark. Man and all animals were likely vegetarians before the Flood. [R32] After the Flood, the LORD instructed Noah to include healthy clean protein-rich meat in the diet. Later, instructions for eating meat were formalized by Moses in Leviticus 11 and Deuteronomy 14.

As a result of today's force fed diets for commercially raised animals, the meats too often contain a significant amount of unwanted hormones and antibiotics and fat. So, shop wisely and eat only the highest quality clean meats. If possible, eat meats from animals that are organically raised in open pastures (free-range) and without hormones or antibiotics added to their feed. [R35]

Part of the healthy Hebrew kosher concept of diet includes cooking clean meat, which further eliminates blood from meat and kills any harmful microbes that might occasionally be present. Meat, fish and fowl were always cooked, as the Passover Lamb was roasted over a fire. (Ex 12:9) Mosaic instructions for meat are extraordinarily beneficial for health, especially considering that they were given ≈3500 years ago, when medical and scientific knowledge was nonexistent. [R25] Microwaving meat may increase free-radicals, may not kill parasites and isn't recommended. [R34]

Ovens suitable for cooking meat have been found in most ancient Israeli archeological sites.

∗ Clean animals raised properly produce meat that contains few parasites and few toxins.

Cloven Hooves

Cloven (***shaca***) hooves are found on all clean ruminant animals. Cloven hooves, rather than paws or nails of unclean animals, protect the feet of clean animals. Feet may be paths for many germs or parasites to enter or infest animals from abrasion and injury. [R5] Some parasites, such as hookworm, are able to penetrate the unbroken skin on the feet of a dog, cat or barefoot human. Both 'toes' of clean hooved animals are protected from parasites and microbes by a large keratin sheath that encases the flesh, which is important in a barnyard. Horse and Camel hooves leave the rear exposed and unprotected. Pig hooves are cloven, but pig doesn't chew the cud. Pig has an outlet between the cloven hooves to release a 'vile green ooze' and eliminate some toxins. [3G] Pigs' feet always contains many toxins, but on the butcher's shelf may be considered a delicacy.

PhytoToxicology

David I. Macht, MD, considered the pharmacological action of the 'juices of muscle' on the growth on living plant-physiological test subjects, and conducted these tests using 'juices of muscle' from both clean and unclean animals. This experimentation is capable of detecting toxic constituents and evaluating them according to the level of inhibition of plant growth, which is known as the 'Phytotoxic Index' or 'Index of Growth'. The lower the 'Phytotoxic Index', the greater the inhibition of plant growth, hence the greater the toxicity in the muscle meat. [R1] {see pgs 105 + 111}

CLEAN MEATS	**Index of Growth**	**No. of Experiments**
Ox	91%	20
Calf	82%	20
Sheep	94%	20
Goat	90%	20
Deer (Venison)	90%	20
UNCLEAN MEATS	**Index of Growth**	**No/ of Experiments**
Swine	54%	20
Rabbit	49%	20
Guinea Pig	46%	20
Camel	41%	20
Horse	39%	20
Dog	62%	10
Cat	53%	10
Squirrel	43%	6
Rat (White)	55%	8
Ground Hog	53%	6
Fox (Silver)	50%	6
Opossum	53%	8
Hamster	46%	4
Black Bear	59%	8
Grizzly Bear	55%	8
Rhinoceros	60%	8

{An 'Index of Growth' (PhytoToxic Index) of 100% = Zero reduction of plant growth = No toxicity.}

Once again, the Word of the LORD proves to be a 'rock of refuge' in a 'land of distress'.

The LORD's purpose for the dietary laws is to distinguish between meats (meat, fish or fowl) that are clean, healthy and may be eaten, from the meats that are unclean and unhealthy to eat.

KJV Lev 11:46 This is the law of the beasts, and of the fowl, and every living
creature that moveth in the waters, and of every creature that creepeth upon the earth:
vs47 To make a difference between the clean and the unclean, and between the beast
that may be eaten and the beast that may not be eaten.

Abraham fed the three messengers from the LORD a choice young calf as part of a meal that Sarah prepared. (Gen 18:7) Meats and other foods that the LORD provides are great to nourish the body, and the value of friends for a relaxing atmosphere adds to the value of the meal.

KJV Deut 16:14 Thou shalt rejoice in thy feast.

It is the LORD God that provides the food. When eating in an enjoyable atmosphere, the body is relaxed, digestive enzymes are produced more easily, and the meats are properly digested.

∗ Give reverence and respect to the LORD for His provision during your meals; it's healthy!

----------------------------------- References Ch 11 Meat ----------------------------------

[R1] In the 'Bulletin of the History of Medicine' from Johns Hopkins University (1953)\ by David I. Macht, MD; 'An Experimental Pharmacological Appreciation of Leviticus XI and Deuteronomy XIV';

[R2] The Adverse Influence of Pork Consumption on Health\ by Hans Heinrich-Reckeweg, MD
[R2] pg 1 Lev 11 – Deut 14 – Koran (Sura 16 verse 115) (Biological Therapy; Vol 1, No 2, 1983)
[R2A] pg 2-3 pork – homotoxin (human) poison homotocity – Pig fat is intracellular.
[R2B] pg 4 Pig lungs + Horse meat – influenza virus
[R2C] pg 7 Pig is overall a very sick animal
[R2D] pg 7-8 (cough up mucus, pg 8) Pig (Porcine) toxins require an illnesses for elimination.
[R2E] pg 11 Pig and other scavenger animals harbor trichinosis.

[R3] God's Key to Health and Happiness\ by Elmer Josephson; pg 46-57 Pig eats almost anything
[R3A] pg 58-59 Laird Goldsborough, MD
from Laird Goldsborough, MD; (Readers Digest March 1950); trichinosis quote
[R3B] pg 58-59 Sir James Paget and Thomas Desmond
[R3C] pg 90-91 Jesus talks of spiritual defilement
[R3D] pg 81-86 & 87 Peter's vision & Paul to Timothy
[R3E] pg 60 picture of trichinae
[R3G] pg 50 green ooze from between a pig's hooves

[R4] Did God Change His Mind About Meat?\ by Tim Hegg (w³.torahresource.com) Mark 7 & Peter's vision

[R5] Are the Food Laws Scientific?\ by Harold Hemenway physiology of clean vs unclean animals
from Merck Veterinary Manual (6th Ed 1986); pg 1486 ruminant digestion
Suidae (porcine) family = Boar, Hog, Pig, Razorback, Swine, etc.
Ruminatia (Sub-family) = Buffalo, Cattle, Deer, Elk, Gaot, Lamb, Moose, Sheep, Ox, etc.

[R6] Diet for a Small Planet (1971)\ by Frances Moore Lappe; pg 4-5 Buffalo meat was very lean.
pg 166-169 complete protein and animal protein

[R7] The Book of Vitamin Therapy\ by Dr. Harold Rosenberg with A.N. Felzamen, PhD;
pg 129 compare digestive system of ruminant to carnivore (1974 Berkley Publishing, NY)

[R8] #13 Trichinella and Trichinosis\ ed. by W. C. Campbell; pg 433 rats and trichinosis
[R8A] pg 435-436 Horse meat and trichinosis

[R9] Progress in Clinical Parasitology Vol 4\ by Tsieh Sun, MD; Horse as meat for humans
// pg 117b France // pg 127b Europe

[R10] Outbreak of Trichinosis Associated with Eating Cougar Jerky - Idaho 1995
(Morbidity and Mortality Weekly; March 1996)

[R11] Does the Bible Permit Christians to Eat Unclean Meat in New Testament Times? \ by Steven Collins
[R11A] pg 12 (from Encyclopedia Americana 1988 Ed. Vol22 pg 416) pork consumption and health

[R12] What the Bible Says About Healthy Living\ by Rex Russell, MD
pg 146 Cattle – Ruminant Herbivores (4 pouches to the stomach)
pg 154 digestive system of Pig
pg 155 Pig, pork and viruses
pg 158 Armadillo – eating the meat created an epidemic of Type M Leprosy
pg 159 unclean animals – including birds – can change benign viruses into toxic viruses.
(as was likely evidenced with Pig and the 1918 Flu Epidemic)

[R13] Eat Right for Your Blood Type\ by Peter J. D'Adamo, ND; all blood types should avoid Pig
pg 56 Type O pg 100 Type A pg 149 Type B pg 190 Type AB

[R14] Guess What Came to Dinner\ by Ann Louise Gittleman;
[R14] pg 48-49 quote on trichinosis
[R14A] pg 63-4 Rabbit - small rodents carry trichinae to Pig
[R14B] pg 64-66-67 microwaves do not kill parasites
[R14C] pg 69-77 zooanosis – disease transmitted from animals to humans
[R14D] pg 48-49 trichinae in Walrus

[R15] Man and Microbes \ by Arno Karlen; (1995 Putnam Sons)
[R15] pg 8-38-143-144-145 (swine flu) / (book) – Pale Horse, Pale Rider
[R15A] pg 199; Mad Cow Disease

[R16] What Would Jesus Eat?\ by Don Colbert, MD – pg 49 Pig = glutton // pg 60 ***shehitah***

[R17] Deadly Feasts\ by Richard Rhodes; pg 135 Carleton Gajdusek – Nobel Prize in Medicine 1976
[R17] pg 174-175 quote downer animals
[R17A] pg 228 quote Dr. Richard Marsh - Mad Cow Disease
[R17B] pg 232 quote failing to head the warnings

[R19] Parasites: Who's Eating Who? (audio) (from Enrich International)\ by Brian Carpenter, DVM;

[R20] Parasites: The Enemy Within\ by Hanna Kroeger; minimize the parasite risk

[R21] Atkins Diet\ by Robert C. Atkins, MD emphasizes the importance of proteins for health

[R18] Strong's Concordance\ by James Strong, STD, LLD

pg 228	cud	# 1625	H pg 28	***gerah***	Lev 11:3	
pg 183	cheweth	# 1641	H pg 26	***garar***	Lev 11:7	
pg 183	cheweth	# 5927	H pg 88	***alah***	Lev 11:3	
pg 199	cloven	# 8156	H pg 119	***shaca***	Lev 11:3	
pg 199	cloven-footed	# 8157 (#8156)	H pg 119	***sheca***	Lev 11:3	
pg 490	hoof (cloven-footed)	# 6541	H pg 97	***parcah***	Lev 11:3	
pg 197	clean (pure)	# 2891 # 2889	H pg 45	***taher***	Lev 11:47	
pg 1087	unclean # 2930	# 2931 # 2932	H pg 46	***tame***	Lev 7:21	
pg 175	cattle (collective)	# 929 (clean)	H pg 19	***behemah***	Gen 1:24	(larger)
pg 175	cattle (connotative)	# 6629 (flocks)	H pg 98	***tson***	Gen 30:39	(smaller)
pg 175	cattle (stock)	# 4735	H pg 71	***miqueh***	Gen 13:12 – (Gen 30:29)	
pg 175	cattle (grazer)	# 7716	H pg 113	***seh***	Gen 30:32	
pg 563	kine (*Bovidae*)	# 6510 (Cow)	H pg 96	***parah***	Gen 41:2-4	
pg 477	hefer (female)	# 6510 (#5697)	H pg 96	***parah***	Num 19:2	
pg 154	bullock (male)	# 6499 (#7794) (#1241)	96	***par***	Ex 22:1	
pg 101	beast (wild)	# 2416	H pg 38	***chay***	Gen 1:24	
pg 101	beast (collective)	# 929 (unclean)	H pg 19	***behemah***	Gen 6:7	(either – or)
pg 990	Swine (*Suidae*)	# 2386 (Pig)	H pg 38	***chazyir***	Lev 11:7	
pg 440	Hare (*Leporidae*)	# 768 (Rabbit)	H pg 17	***arnebeth***	Lev 11:6	
pg 167-8	Camel	# 1581	H pg 26	***gamal***	Lev 11:4	
pg 1070	torn (by beasts)	# 2966	H pg 46	***terephah*** (noun)	Lev 22:8	(***treph*** -vb)

Cattle is often used collectively or connotatively to refer to all clean ruminants. (Gen 1:24) {pg 90}
Kine, Bull, Hefer are often used specifically or denotatively to refer to just bovine animals. (Gen 41)

[R22] Virology (Science: vol 275; 21 March 97) \ by Jeffrey Taubenberger, MD, PhD; pg 1739
Genes isolated and sequenced from the deadly 1918 Flu virus 1918 Flu Pandemic

[R23] Epidemic\ edited by Rob DeSalle, PhD; pg 125-131 trichinosis (from – A Pig from Jersey)
[R23] pg 128b pathologist's biopsy of trichinae [R23A] pg 126b-127a Mosaic prohibition of pork
[R23B] pg 127b-128a trichinosis – chameleon of diseases and systems are encyclopedic
[R23C] pg 127a-127b autopsy evidence for incidence of trichinosis and prevention of trichinosis

[R24] Man on Earth\ by John Reader; pg 40-41 pig eats human-like food
from Salmon of Doubt\ by Douglass Adams pig produces more meat for less feed than cow

[R25] Proof Positive\ by Neal Nedley, MD; eat no meat

[R26] Councils on Diet and Food\ by Ellen G. White; eat no meat

[R27] Mad Cow Disease (Dines Newsletter 02-09-2001)\ pg 7-8 & 13-14 Mad Cow Disease = Lethal

[R28] The 28 Day Antioxidant Diet\ by Steve Masley, MD; a vegetarian like Daniel

[R29] Lets Play Doctor\ Joel Wallach, DVM, ND & Ma Lan, MD, MS; pg 162-163 (tularemia-rabies)

[R30] Diet for a New America\ by John Robbins; modern unhealthy animal husbandry - eat no meat

[R31] The Flood (audio cassette)\ by Chuck Missler, PhD; Noah and eating meat after the Flood

[R32] Diseases\ edited by Helen Klusek Hamilton; {from Food Laws [R5]; by Harold Hemenway}

[R33] Webster's Dictionary (1966)/ pg 1170 protein

[R34] HYtBH (Radio Program)\ by Monte Kline, PhD; micro-waved meats ⇒ increased free-radicals

[R35] The Cure for All Cancers\ by Hulda Clark, PhD, ND (1993) Pro Motion Publishers, San Diego, CA

[R36] e-mail (8 March 98)\ from Mark Brigham, PhD rabies carriers - unclean {bats - others}

[R37] Pork The Other White Meat (internet)\ by Alyssa Samadi; pork and viruses

[R38] The Bible Cure\ by Reginald Cherry, MD

[R39] Protein Power\ by Michael R. Eades, MD and Mary Dan Eades, MD

[R40] The Coming Plague\ by Laurie Garrett unclean animals – Rat complicent in Bubonic Plague

[R41] Flu\ by Gina Kolata unclean animals – Pig complicent in Swine Flu

[R42] Hemera Clip Art (CD Rom and Internet)\ photos of Animals – Clean and Unclean {pgs 114-115}

[R43] Outbreak Alert\ by Jason Eberhardt-Phillips, MD; pg 123 German trichinosis outbreak //pg 113 quote
"Innovative, progressive changes introduced by humans can provide advantages to microbes, which, in turn threaten the population. In most cases, advantages are provided unwittingly as a by-product of technology."

[R44] interview with a Pharmacist – Flagel, an anti-parasitic drug to treat trichinosis, was first developed in the 1930-40s. Flagel likely interferes with DNA synthesis, limiting the ability of parasites to reproduce.

[R45] Or Perish in the Attempt (Wilderness Medicine in the Lewis and Clark Expedition)\ by David J. Peck, DO
pg 144-145 trichinosis in wilderness Montana animals: bear, beaver, cougar, coyote, dog, rabbit

---

Genesis 7:2 distinguishes between the clean animals and unclean animals prior to the Flood, while Genesis 9:3 states that 'every moving thing' will be suitable as food for man after the Flood. The author reasons that 'every moving thing' in Mosaic Hebrew implies – only amoung clean animals. Only the clean animals were intended by the LORD to be suitable for sacrifice and as food for man.

Chapter 12 Fish – and other Sea Creatures
Clam, Oyster, Mussel and Scallop

God made the rules for eating seafood easy: all fish (***dagah***) that have fins and scales are clean and healthy; and all sea creatures without fins and scales are forbidden. (Lev 11:9-12 & Deut 14:10)

KJV Lev 11:9 These shall you eat of all that are in the waters: whatsoever hath fins (***cenappiyr***) and scales (***qasqeseth***) in the water, in the seas, and in the rivers, them shall you eat.

JPS Deut 14:10 and whatsoever hath not fins and scales ye may not eat; it is unclean to you.

Shellfish scavenge in water, just as pig, bear and rat scavenges on land. Mollusk shellfish, including bivalves (Clam, Oyster, Mussel and Scallop), barnacle and coral, are all filter feeders. Oysters may filter 1 to 2 gallons of water/hour (≈50 gallons/day) through their digestive organs. [R19] Scallop is a free-swimming, ≈3-inch bivalve that filter-feeds as it propels itself through the water. Marvelous mollusk shellfish filter water, removing harmful microbes, pollutants and filth, and return cleaner water to the sea. What a great service to the sea they perform: clean fish have clean water to swim in because unclean filter feeders take unclean water and make it clean again. I hadn't understood the value of bivalves, until I was sitting on a dock on Hood Canal in Washington State, after I had just gone swimming. Some friends came by and warned me not to eat the mussels (a small clam-like bivalve), attached to the dock. They said the wooden pilings were recently painted with creosote and the mussels tasted like creosote. (Creosote is oil with a pungent odor produced from wood tar or coal tar distillation that is painted on the pilings to protect them from rotting.) [R33] Then, I thanked the LORD for the wisdom of His dietary Law in the ***Torah*** prohibiting shellfish.

For people who want to eat bivalves, shellfish biologist Rita Colwell has some bad news:

"We have very few places left on earth where we can get pathogen-free mollusks." [R50]

Another more frightening problem with eating bivalves (Clam, Oyster, Mussel and Scallop) is the potential that they are contaminated with a poisonous phytoplankton, *Alexandrium catenella* (also called *Gonyaulax tamarensis*), which causes deadly 'paralytic shellfish poisoning' or PSP. PSP is commonly associated with a bloom (large numbers) of phytoplankton that discolor water red, and is also known as 'red tide'. Bivalve shellfish can become highly toxic from PSP with no evidence of red tide water discoloration, and the absence of red tide is no assurance of shellfish that are safe from PSP toxicity. [R2] Red tide is a sign of water pollution, and is an indication of poisonous plankton that rapidly multiply and may release toxins that are stored in bivalves. [R45-46]

PSP toxin may be present at the level up to 80 micrograms/gram, yet bivalve mollusks are still classified as not likely to cause disease, and are acceptable to be harvested according to present U.S. standards. Today, the lowest level of the PSP toxin that can be detected by current assay methods is ≈50 micrograms/gram. Fortunately, most reputable commercial harvesters of clam, oyster and/or mussel will not sell bivalve shellfish with any detectable levels of PSP. [R3-17]

Man's 'R' rule is: harvest bivalves in months containing the letter 'R' when water conditions are <u>hopefully</u> favorable and poisonous plankton aren't in bloom, and avoid harvesting bivalves in the hot summer (May, June, July or August). According to John Wekell, PhD and chemist of the National Marine Fisheries Service: the letter 'R' rule is not very reliable for PSP protection. [R2]

"Detection of the poisons in shellfish can only be done in a laboratory. Reliance on folklore methods like the letter 'R' containing months is extremely dangerous and has no basis in fact."

(Bivalves are often very soft and even less desirable for food during hot summer 'R-less' months.)

The 'R' rule was not protective in September 96, when a potentially lethal plankton bloom exceeding 200 micrograms/gram forced the closure of many beaches in Washington State to harvesting shellfish. [R21] The LORD's rule in the ***Torah*** is perfect, because, determining when water conditions are right for breeding PSP causing phytoplankton is often difficult, if not impossible.

As quoted in *Food and Nutrition* (and the *South African Medical Journal*) N. Sapeika, MD, stated:

"The poison containing plankton (which serves as food for clams, mussels, etc.) may reach shellfish beds in various places and in varying amounts from time to time, sometimes even within a day after such beds have provided non-poisonous specimens." [R14]

"A single specimen [Clam, Oyster or Mussel] may contain a fatal dose. The affected area (of the sea) may remain contaminated for months or weeks. The poison is extremely potent in its central neurotoxic and peripheral neuromuscular action (poisonous to the nervous system) and its depressant action on the circulatory system. There is no specific antidote..." [R14]

∗ Completely avoiding bivalves as food is the only safe answer for avoiding all risk of PSP.

∗ The 'R' rule for harvesting 'safe' bivalve shellfish is not reliable to protect against PSP toxicity.

Bivalve Mollusk Shellfish

In 1793, British Captain George Vancouver was sailing off the British Columbia coast of Canada when several of his men went ashore. The sailors were exploring the shoreline of the clear clean (unpolluted) waters of Mathaison Channel when they came upon a bed of mussels. The temptation of a morning feast on these seafood delicacies was too inviting to pass up.

"... these mussels prove to be of a deleterious quality as all those who had eaten of them in any quantity were, soon after they embarked, seized with sickness, numbness about the mouth, face and arms, which soon spread over the whole body accompanied with giddiness and semi lassitude; ... [crewmember] John Carter became ...very ill ... his pulse becoming weaker and weaker, his mouth and lips appearing black and his face and neck becoming much swelled together with faintness, general numbness and tremor. Under these circumstances he gradually sank without much struggle, and expired ... and this affair happened within five hours from the time of his eating the mussels." [R14] (As recorded by Capt. Vancouver's ship surgeon.)

On 25 Sept 1990, a PSP outbreak was narrowly averted, when a large shipment of oysters contaminated by 300 micrograms/gram was harvested from the waters of Dabob Bay on Hood Canal in Washington State and was sold at the wholesale level. The Oysters were on their way to the retail market before Department of Health officials discovered the level of PSP contamination and the entire shipment of oysters were recalled just prior to reaching the market place. [R17]

"Early symptoms of PSP are tingling of the lips and tongue, which may begin within minutes of eating poisonous shellfish or may take an hour or two to develop. Depending upon the amount of poison, symptoms may progress to tingling of fingers and toes and then loss of control of arms and legs followed by difficulty in breathing. If a person has consumed enough poison, death will result from paralysis of the breathing mechanism in as little as two hours." [R38]

Don Miles of the Kitsap County Health Department in Washington State discussed PSP:

"It's really strange, nobody knows why it [the PSP-causing plankton] does what it does. Sunlight, rain, currents – everything gets in the right proportion, then we get a (plankton) bloom. Toxic shellfish do not look or taste any different, and the toxin is not destroyed by cooking." [R17]

Thus, taste or looks are of no importance in determining whether bivalves contain fatal amounts of PSP, and there is no way of destroying or neutralizing the PSP toxins. In small amounts, PSP causes a tingling or numbness of the lips and tongue and the tips of the fingers, upset stomach, vomiting, weakness or difficulty in breathing; in large amounts, PSP is fatal! The symptoms generally begin within an hour or two of eating contaminated shellfish. PSP is an ongoing problem in Washington State, where large areas of shoreline are annually closed to harvesting of bivalve mollusk shellfish. [R20] PSP can remain at toxic levels for years after a toxic bloom. [R12]

PSP is the best known of a group of shellfish poisons with various neurological effects. [R11A] ASP or amnesuronic shellfish poisoning (domoic acid) may cause permanent (short-term) amnesia; such as – going to a store and forgetting to buy anything and forgetting where the car was parked.

When people eat bivalve shellfish, most of what is consumed are the digestive organs, which filter, absorb and store whatever might be in the water. [R19] No one purposely eats the digestive organs of clean fish, such as cod or salmon, because people intuitively recognize these organs as not being healthy for food. The digestive organs of unclean filter feeders are likely to be even less healthy than the digestive organs of clean fish. Clams are so full of debris that they are often soaked live in clean water in order to 'spit' out stored sand, before they are cooked and eaten.

Dr. Louis Lasagna wrote about these dietary laws of Moses: [R8]

"Many of these make good medical sense.....The prohibition of hare and swine as sources of food certainly must have diminished the incidence of disease, in view of the capacity of these animals to transmit tularemia and trichinosis, respectively. The transmission of gastro-intestinal infections (including typhoid fever) via polluted shellfish or water also testifies to the apparent wisdom of the Hebrews in warning against such seafood and impure water." [R8]

Rex Russell, MD in his book *What the Bible Says About Healthy Living* warns: [R12]

"Viral hepatitis, which leads to cirrhosis, liver failure and liver cancer,
is transmitted through eating shellfish and blood." [R12]

Toxins gathered from filter feeding, apart from PSP, are a part of every bite of bivalves.

"... clams and oysters feed by filtering microorganisms from large quantities of water. Although they [Clam, Oyster, Mussel and Scallop] seek phytoplankton, they also remove bacteria or viruses from the water. Low levels of bacteria in water pollution can be concentrated in shellfish to levels sufficiently harmful to be a health risk in humans." [R17]

The potential for death from PSP requires not ever eating Clam, Oyster, Mussel or Scallop.

Crustaceans

Crustaceans (Crab, Lobster, Shrimp and Prawn) have no fins, no scales, and are scavengers that Moses forbade as food. * Crustacean meat spoils very quickly upon death, due to bacterial decomposition and from proteolytic (digestive) enzyme decomposition of the muscle meat. Crustaceans and all finfish contain similar bacteria and digestive enzymes, however spoilage in finfish is containable, due to a membrane between the muscle meat and the internal organs. [R24]

*** Membranes in finfish prevent digestive enzymes and bacteria from contacting muscle.**

*** Upon death, crustacean muscle spoilage is <u>very</u> fast and pervasive, since the powerful enzymes of the hepatopancreas digestive organ sit directly on the body musculature.**

The hepatopancreas is a yellowish mushy boundless organ that functions like a pancreas and liver in digestion, and is eaten by some people who call it the 'butter' of the crustacean. The lack of a membrane isolating the hepatopancreas is a major cause of crustacean meat spoilage.

Once crustacean muscle spoilage begins, spoilage quickly spreads to the entire musculature. The potential for spoilage <u>requires</u> all crab and lobster to be cooked live or cooked immediately after being cleaned. (Other shellfish such as bivalve mollusks should also be cooked while alive.) Lobster, the 'cockroach of the sea', is especially subject to spoilage. Lobsters swim in a tank of 'fine' restaurants, before being cooked, cleaned and served <u>pronto</u>, to minimize risk of spoilage!

Both shellfish and finfish are subject to the same spoilage, but: [R11]

> "Shellfish normally contains more moisture, greater amounts of free amino acids, and more extractable nitrogenous compounds than finfish. These biochemical characteristics facilitate bacterial growth and deteriorative reactions resulting in rapid spoilage of shellfish." [R11]

Shellfish – Crustaceans and Mollusks – also frequently harbor many pathogenic organisms.

> "Many shellfish grow in estuarine, coastal waters, and aqua-cultural ponds near residential areas and are hence susceptible to contamination by potential pathogenic organisms. Deterioration of shellfish quality results from enzymatic action from both the tissue and the contaminating organisms. Microorganisms that spoil shellfish are similar to those responsible for finfish spoilage. However, such organisms as *Moraxella-Acinetobacter* and *Lactobacillus* are more active in shellfish than in finfish." [R11]

Instructions to shellfish handlers from health agencies are: Crab and Lobster must be cooked live to prevent spoilage, Shrimp can be iced before cooking, but all shellfish are best eaten the day they are cooked. [R24] Today, shellfish harvesters use ice or refrigeration to circumvent God's instructions and minimize health concerns; but avoiding shellfish is better. [R13] If people catch/cook their own, they can be certain shellfish are immediately iced and/or cooked live; but can anyone be certain that all commercial crustaceans (Crab, Lobster or Shrimp) are iced live and/or cooked live?

Crustacean muscle causes some people a serious allergic reaction. Crustacean muscle and enzymes are proteins and antigens that may initiate a life threatening 'anaphylactic' shock. [R24] Crustacean allergies often cause a mild rash, but anaphylactic shock causes bronchial airways to swell, and impairs breathing. People who have experienced this once never go back for seconds. People may not be allergic to one crustacean, but they may develop an allergy to another species. The allergic possibility causes many people to avoid shellfish altogether, which is very wise!

Crustaceans have a layer of potentially infectious bacteria covering their shells, and anyone whose skin is broken by a crustacean's claw or pincher is likely to get a bacterial infection. [R16]

Crab and Lobster scavenge the sea floor. Shrimp scavenge the sea floor or nearer the surface. Eating shellfish that feed on dead, decaying matter; that live on fish feces and urine; and that may ingest spilled petroleum products causes a very high percentage of human cholera. [R12] Cholera bacteria multiply in the colon, causing explosive diarrhea, and rapid dehydration from diarrhea, leading to unconsciousness and even death. [R27] In 1986, a cholera outbreak in Louisiana was attributed to eating meals that included – Shrimp, Pork, Pig blood and salty brine Shrimp. [R12]

Crustaceans accumulate toxins and have poorly developed organs or no organs (no colon) to eliminate toxins. The author theorizes: Crustaceans acquire many toxins that end up in muscle, and toxins give crustacean muscle its characteristic 'delicate', rich flavor. Lobster tail is often considered the 'richest' meat, and is likely where many toxins are absorbed directly from the anus.

Shellfish meat is also high in purines, which may lead to urate crystals in joints causing gout. Urate crystals cause severe irritation of joint tissue. Gout is a very severe arthritis (often involving the big toe) that is usually episodal. Shellfish muscle is a frequent trigger of a gout attack. [R25]

Crustacean meat is always more at risk for spoilage than meat from clean finfish with fins and scales.

Shark

Shark is not a true fish, with cartilage, not bone, as a frame. Shark has fins, but <u>not scales</u>. All clean fish, such as salmon, are 'true fish' that have fins; and scales that <u>overlap</u> one-another. Sharkskin is sandpaper rough and is made of placoids that resemble teeth. Or more correctly: Shark teeth are just a modified form of the skin placoids. Shark gills are open to the sea, which means water passes in or out of the gills to maintain an equal osmotic balance with salt water. Salt water has such a high osmolarity that it would literally draw all the water out of the shark, and the shark would die of dehydration, if it were not for the shark's mechanism of retaining extra electrolytes to balance the osmolarity of the salt water. The electrolytes retained by shark in blood, organs and flesh are: TMAO (trimethylamine oxide) and urea, which regulate/balance an equal osmotic balance with salt water. [R6-9] Urea and TMAO are waste byproducts of nitrogen metabolism, which all clean finfish eliminate through the kidneys as urine. [R6] Urea is formed by combining ammonia (NH_4^-) with CO_2. Sharkskin may also leach some ammonia between the skin placoids. At best, urea in shark is unpleasant to the taste. Without extremely careful handling procedures, urea in shark meat is broken down into ammonia; and TMAO is broken down into TMA (trimethylamine). TMA is reputed to be responsible for the 'stale fish odor' that develops in all spoiling fish. Eating shark meat that contains a large amount of ammonia or TMA can be very unpleasant and very toxic. [R4-9] Ammonia is a neurotoxin that may cause loss of muscle control, paralysis or even death. This huge problem of ammonia development and retention in shark flesh has forced several countries to impose limits on the levels of ammonia that are considered acceptable, before allowing shark meat to be imported. [R9] Researchers are trying to establish procedures to slow the breakdown of urea and TMAO to ammonia and TMA, or purge them from meat, so more shark meat can be sold to the public. Among the common procedures to leach these toxic nitrogenous waste byproducts from shark are: icing shark meat as soon as it dies, washing shark meat several times under running water, salting shark meat by immersing it in brine (a heavy salt solution) and soaking shark flesh in various solutions that have a highly acidic pH, such as lemon juice, tomato juice or vinegar. [R7] Remember that these procedures are just designed to purge obvious toxins from shark flesh, and change fish that the LORD called unclean, to be a little more palatable for people who don't mind too much urine taste in the fish they eat. Or better yet: follow the wisdom of the LORD and Moses, and avoid eating shark meat altogether.

Catfish

Catfish have fins, a thick slimy skin (and rarely poisonous spines), but <u>no true scales</u>. [R10] Catfish may scavenge dead toxin-ridden fish or animal matter from a river or lake-bottom. [R26] Catfish in a fishpond are carnivorous on clean fish, which is a big problem for fish farming. [R30] Catfish may accumulate toxins faster than equal-sized clean fish in the same environment. [R12A] Catfish meat may develop 'off-flavor', causing the meat to not taste good and raisers are urged to wait to harvest until the meat is tastier. The author theorizes: Catfish develop 'off-flavor' when they absorb more toxins than usual, and toxin levels often return to more tolerable levels later. [R31]

Sturgeon

Sturgeon, like Shark and Catfish, has fins, but <u>no true scales</u>. Sturgeon placoids don't overlap; just as shark placoids don't overlap, however, Sturgeon placoids are not teeth-like. Sturgeon is called a 'primitive' fish. Sturgeon feed with an open mouth by sucking in all the filth of a river bottom. Sturgeon has a short straight-tube, relatively simple digestive system that is likely non-selective regarding toxin absorption. Sturgeon eggs, called caviar, are also unclean.

Puffer Fish

Puffer, Porcupine and Globefish have fins but <u>spines rather than scales</u> and contain a deadly neurotoxin – tetrodotoxin. In 1774, Captain Cook nearly died after eating a piece of Puffer fish. [R43] {Today, Puffer fish is sold/served as food in Japan only after poisonous glands are removed by a licensed professional.}

Eel

Eel has fins, a tough leathery skin <u>without scales</u> and may be electric. Eel, just like Sturgeon, has a short, simple, straight digestive system and most likely accumulates many toxins. [R30A-36]

Clean finfish meat is always better suited for human food than meat from unclean sea-creatures. (Although unclean invertebrate sea-creatures are often looked upon as being more primitive than more advanced finfish, there is no evidence of evolutionary change/development from one 'kind' of sea-creature to another 'kind' of sea-creature.)

∗ Some people say: 'Seafood is brain food'; however, Moses urged people to be more selective.

Other Unclean Sea Creatures

---------- **Squid and Octopus** ----------

Squid and Octopus are mollusks without a shell; they feed on other mollusks and crustaceans. Squid and Octopus, just as bivalves, lack a membrane between internal organs and muscle, and the meat has a rubbery-consistency that may be difficult for humans to digest efficiently. [R24]

---------- **Snail** ----------

Snail {Helix (*escargot*) - common garden snail} is considered a true delicacy. But is it really? When eating *escargot*, the internal organs may be eaten along with the muscular foot. Like other shellfish, there is no membrane in the body cavity separating the meat from the internal organs. Snail meat spoilage may be almost as big a problem as it is with crustaceans. Avoid eating Snail!

---------- **Abalone and Limpet and Nautilus** ----------

Abalone, Limpet and Nautilus are one-shell shellfish. Abalone and Limpet attach firmly to a rock by means of a large muscular foot similarly to Snail. Nautilus is free swimming. Abalone, Limpet and Snail are grazers that feed by scraping algae off rock. The same issues of spoilage and accumulating toxins that apply to other shellfish, are also likely important for these shellfish.

---------- **Miscellaneous Marine Invertebrates** ----------

Sea Cucumber, Star Fish, Jelly Fish and Sea Anemone have no backbone and have no shell. Jelly Fish and Sea Anemone have poisonous tentacles for self-defense that no one plans to eat. Sea Cucumber filters mud and/or water for food, in a similar manner to bivalve mollusk shellfish.

---------- **Reptiles** ----------

Reptiles never stop growing through adult life; with one recently found possible exception. Alligator, Crocodile, Dinosaur, Lizard, Snake and Turtle are all reptiles. The author theorizes: Reptiles may accumulate toxins at such a rapid rate and may have such poorly developed organs for elimination that if they ever stop growing, they might be overwhelmed by their own toxins! Reptiles all have a short digestive system for their body size/length. A Turtle's shell is like armor and, like the hide of other reptiles, has no sweat glands. Reptiles may always need more muscle-fat tissues for storing byproducts of their own metabolic waste and the new toxins that they ingest.

---------- **Amphibians** ----------

Frog or Toad may accumulate various toxins in the skin for defense that no one wants to eat. Frog retains, rather than metabolizes, venom/toxins from the insects it fed on most recently. [R41-43A] Frog, like other amphibians, has a relatively short digestive system as compared to its body size.

---------- **Marine Mammals** ----------

Seal, Walrus and Sea Lion are predator/scavengers. Walrus may carry trichinae worms. [R35] These sea creatures are equivalent to pig, bear, rat, cougar, lion, tiger, wolf, etc. on the land. Other than perhaps a water buffalo, there are no true marine ruminants to contrast them to, but many marine mammals have a similar short digestive system to predator/scavengers on land. (It seems likely that Seal and Sea Lion may also carry trichinae, but I have no references for this.)

---------- **Cetaceans** ----------

Cetaceans (Whale, Porpoise and Dolphin) have fins, but no scales. *Orca* is also known as a 'killer whale'. Cetaceans are a 'sentinel' species, since they are atop of a marine food pyramid. Any unhealthy accumulation of toxins low in the food chain will be reflected in poor *Orca* health. If any predator/scavenger atop a food pyramid is in good health, this serves as a good indicator for the health of all lower members of the food pyramid. Petrochemicals, PCBs, insecticides, raw sewage and industrial/agricultural waste have been dumped into Washington's Puget Sound for years without regard to long-term consequences. The real cost of pollution is coming back to haunt *Orca* and other Puget Sound marine residents. *Orca* eats mostly salmon and rarely seal. Salmon/Seal feed on marine life lower on the food pyramid. If toxins are dumped in the salt water, marine algae and other microorganisms will absorb some toxins and pass the toxins on to other creatures that feed on them. ∗ According to the principle of <u>bio-amplification</u>, toxins are usually found in the highest concentrations in the 'sentinel' predator/scavengers atop any food pyramid. *Orca* populations are slowly dwindling in the Puget Sound, and high concentrations of PCBs and other toxins that are found in the tissues of dead *Orca* are being blamed for their demise. [R40] People that eat any unclean sentinel animal atop any food chain, such as *Orca*, become the new top predator for that food pyramid and incur the risk of absorbing the highest toxin concentrations. The same toxins that are accumulating in and killing *Orca* will surely also cause human illness. The LORD called all sentinel predator/scavengers unclean; and Moses wrote not to eat them. [R39]

∗ More scientific research may yield more reasons to avoid eating unclean sea creatures.

Clean Fish

Clean fish have both fins and scales. Fins (***cenappiyr***) are common to all clean fish and many unclean fish. Fins allow mobility away from polluted waters. True scales (***qasqeseth***) overlap one another and act as tough plating that is protective against abrasion, predators and parasites. Protection from trauma and damage prevents wounds that predispose fish to microbial infection. Salmon, Cod, Tuna, Perch, Halibut, Pike, Bass, Smelt, Trout and many sport fish are grouped as clean finfish. Clean fish contain healthy oils, including cod liver oil, that are rich in essential linolenic – omega 3 fatty acid. Clean fish are also rich in essential protein, minerals and vitamins.

----------- **Discussion distinguishing the Clean Fish from the Unclean** ----------

Clam, Mussel, Oyster and Scallop are filter feeders. Crustacean, Shark, Catfish and Eel are predator/scavengers. These unclean sea-creatures all have a relatively short, straight digestive system for their body size. The relatively short, straight, digestive system compared to body size for unclean sea-creatures is similar to the relatively short, straight digestive system compared to body size for predator/scavenger land animals, as discussed in *The Book of Vitamin Therapy*.

∗ The only physical characteristic that appears to be consistent among all clean creatures (animal, fish, or fowl) is a long coiled digestive system as compared body size; while all unclean creatures seem to have a short straight digestive system compared to body size!

Clean ruminant land animals have a very long, twisted digestive system for their body size, in a similar manner to the relatively long, twisted digestive system of all clean finfish. This long 'sophisticated' digestive system is what makes a ruminant land animal a living protein factory that is able to convert low-protein grasses into protein-rich muscle mass of the highest quality for food.

<u>The author's theory</u> is: the relatively short straight digestive system of unclean filter feeders and predator/scavengers causes them to digest, absorb and assimilate their food very quickly. There is little time or space for a long digestion. Predator/scavengers often eat a few big meals in haste while on the go. Sharks need to eat quickly now and set off searching for their next large meal. The digestive system of all unclean sea creatures is relatively short, straight and unsophisticated; digestion is accomplished almost exclusively by acids and enzymes produced by the sea creature. Food ingested by unclean predators, scavengers and filter feeders is likely absorbed in a relatively non-selective manner. Toxins that may ingested by unclean sea creatures as part of food are likely absorbed and stored 'as is', with little time to be neutralized or brokendown; and harmful byproducts of quick digestion are likely absorbed easily, stored in tissues, and not very efficiently eliminated.

The long(er) digestive system of clean finfish and all clean creatures may allow friendly symbiotic bacteria to substantially participate in the digestion! While unclean creatures rely almost exclusively on their own production of acids and enzymes, clean creatures rely on their own acids and enzymes, <u>plus</u> enzymes from numerous symbiotic bacteria. A longer more coiled digestive system may also be more specialized. A healthy human digestive system must maintain at least seven distinct pH levels for efficient digestion. Food often requires a very narrow pH range for proper digestion, and nutrients frequently have a very narrow pH range for ideal absorption. Keeping multiple digestive pH levels by clean finfish may allow for greater efficiency of digestion, greater activity by symbiotic bacteria, greater selectivity of absorption; and requires more time. ∗∗∗ A clean animal's digestive system may allow more nutrients and fewer toxins to be absorbed.

∗ Another physical characteristic that appears to be consistent among all clean creatures (animal, fish, or fowl) is better developed and/or more efficient glands of elimination, while all unclean creatures seem to have poorly developed and/or absent glands of elimination.

Shellfish and all marine invertebrates lack a true colon. The author theorizes: that the colon and sweat glands of clean ruminant land animals, such as cattle, are more efficient in removing toxins than the colon and absence of sweat glands of predator/scavengers, such as lion. The colon of clean finfish, such as salmon, is likely more efficient in eliminating toxins that the absent colon of a crustacean and bivalve, or the poorly developed colon of a shark, catfish and sturgeon. ∗ Less sophisticated glands of elimination in unclean creatures, may result in more retention of toxins.

∗ More time and a more specialized digestive system to absorb only what is wanted from food and to either neutralize or eliminate unwanted toxins: this is likely the essence of why all clean creatures are freer from toxins, and healthier as food than all unclean creatures.

More research and more data from anatomy and physiology will be needed to confirm or disprove the authors' theories concerning the differences between clean and unclean animals, fish and fowl.

PhytoToxicology

Dr. David I. Macht prepared a 'juice extract' of the muscles of various clean and unclean fish and then introduced the 'juice extract' to a growth medium of seedlings of *Lupinus albus*, in order to determine whether there is any effect on plant growth. Any inhibitory effect on plant growth compared to a control is considered to be caused by some inherent toxic element within the meat and was called the 'Phytotoxic Index of Growth'. The higher the 'Phytotoxic Index', the lower the inhibitory effect on plant growth. All clean fish had a statistically significant higher 'Phytotoxic Index' than unclean fish, indicating less inhibition of plant growth and less retention of toxins. [R1]

CLEAN FISH	**Index of Growth**	**No. of Experiments not given**
Black Bass	80	—
Butterfish	81	—
Carp	90	—
Cod	90	—
Flounder	83	—
Halibut	82	—
Herring	100	—
Pike	98	—
Rainbow Trout	81	—
Smelt	90	—
Sea Bass	103	—
Tuna	88	—

UNCLEAN FISH	**Index of Growth**	
Catfish	48	—
Eel	40	—
Sand Skate	59	—
Shark	62	—
Toad Fish	49	—

{An 'Index of Growth' (PhytoToxic Index) of 100% = Zero reduction of plant growth = No toxicity.}

Salmon, Trout, Cod, Bass, Perch, Halibut, Sole, Pike, Flounder, Smelt or Tuna are clean finfish that provide excellent, nourishing muscle tissue for food. Clean fish are healthy for any diet. Shark, Catfish and Sturgeon do not have true scales and they are classified as unclean to eat.

Again God's commandments prove to be an 'island of safety' in a 'sea of trouble'.

--- **end of text Ch 12 Fish** ---

{Surimi (imitation Crab) = Pollock or Haddock (clean fish) + white table sugar} – and is not recommended.

----------- Theory and Speculation concerning unclean fish, shellfish and invertebrates ----------

The author theorizes: much of what makes unclean meat (land, sea, or air) so 'flavorful' are the toxins they contain. The taste of toxins in all unclean meats seems to be almost addictive. There is definitely some food value to unclean meat, but the food value is always compromised by increased toxicity compared to clean meat. The primary food value from any meat is protein and the mineral content of meat is also very important. The author also theorizes: protein from unclean meat may not be as easy for humans to digest as compared to protein from clean meat; and minerals from unclean meat may also be bound in such a manner as to make the minerals more difficult to absorb. Digestion functions because of enzymes. The author also theorizes: enzymes needed for efficient digestion of protein from unclean meat may be difficult to produce by humans. Poor digestion of unclean meat may lead to a heavy sluggish feeling after eating a big meal, and may often lead to residues of unclean meat becoming impacted in the colon. The author theorizes: Any meat, clean or unclean, cooked or warmed in a microwave may also make digestion difficult.

The author believes more evidence for the physiological uncleanness of all unclean animals will only be found on the biomolecular level. The author welcomes dialogue with Veterinarians, Physicians, Pathologists, Biochemists, Biologists and other scientists who study health or tissue toxicity, to better understand the uncleanness of animals such as Pig, Horse, Bear and Rabbit; unclean sea creatures including Shellfish, Shark, Catfish, Sturgeon, Eel, Reptiles, Amphibians, Marine Invertebrates and Marine Mammals; and all unclean birds including Raptors, and Bats.

Please send information or discussion via e-mail to: Moses5in1Torah@msn.com .

---------------------------------- References Ch 12 Fish ----------------------------------

[R1] 'An Experimental Pharmacological Appreciation of Leviticus XI and Deuteronomy XIV' \by David I. Macht, MD
[R2] Personal Correspondence (18 June 91) \ with John C. Wekell, PhD; Chemistry – NW Fisheries Center
[R2A] Personal Interview (May and Nov 91) \ with John Wekell, PhD; PSP toxin in Clam, Oyster & Mussel
[R3] God's Key to Health and Happiness\ by Elmer Josephson unclean fish = unhealthy to eat
[R4] Personal Correspondence and Interview (17 May 91) \ with Richard W. Nelson, PhD; Shark & urea
Northwest Fisheries Center / 2725 Montlake Boulevard East / Seattle, Wash
[R5] Are the Food Laws Scientific?\ by Harold Hemenway scales overlap + protect
[R6] Commercial Fisheries TL-16 (pamphlet); pg 1-2 Urea and TMAO in Shark
US Dept of Interior /Fish and Wildlife Service /Washington 25, D. C. Feb 1961
[R7] Sharks and Their Utilization (Marine Fisheries Review; Vol 40, No 2; Feb 1978)\ pg 7; purge urea from Shark
[R8] The Doctor's Dilemma\ by Louis Lasagna; pg 85 quoted from Principles of Healthy Living;- WorldWide Church of God
[R9] Laboratory Reference Document # 83-15 \ from National Marine Fisheries Service; pg 3-5 Shark
[R9] pg 3-4-5 ammonia and TMAO in Shark meat
[R10] Conversations (from 1990 through 2002)\ with Don Seavy, PhD (Marine Biology); unclean shellfish
[R11] Encyclopedia of Food Science and Technology - Vol 3 (1-P)\ \edited by Y. H. Hin; pg 870 – Domoic Acid
(Domoic Acid and PSP closes Shellfish in Wash. – 09-19-03 – PI {B1-2}) – $75 million/year Wash. Shellfish harvest
[R12] What the Bible Says About Healthy Living\ by Rex Russell, MD; pg 157 cholera from shellfish
[R12A] pg 160 catfish – accumulate toxins
[R13] Edible Incredible\ by Marjorie Furlong and Virginia Pill marine invertebrates as food
[R14] Food and Nutrition\ ed. by Rodale Press; pg 257-258 Dr. Sapeika – Bivalves and PSP
[R15] Man and Microbes\ by Arno Karlen; pg 54 shellfish likely to transmit hepatitis to man
[R16] Conversation (27 Dec 96) \ with Kevin Bright , (Fisheries Biologist) – bacteria on shells of all Shellfish
[R17] Horse Waste Land Management \ pg 4; bivalve mollusks [Clam, Oyster, Mussel] concentrate bacteria–virus
[R18] Strong's Concordance\ by James Strong, STD, LLD

pg 354	fish	# 1710	H pg 29	***dagah***	Num 11:5
pg 350	fins	# 5579	H pg 83	***cenappiyr***	Lev 11 & Deut 14
pg 890	scales	# 7193	H pg 105	***qasqeseth***	Lev 11 & Deut 14

[R19] Growing an Oyster Garden\ (The Sun – Kitsap County newspaper – Saturday 12 August 2000); pg B1
Oysters can filter up to 50 gallons of water per day. (≈1 to 2$^+$ gallons of water per hour)
[R20] Shellfish are Safe Again (Central Kitsap Reporter – Saturday 13 Dec 1997)\ pg A10; – no 'detectable' PSP
[R21] Beaches Closed\ (The Sun – Sept 96) some Kitsap beaches closed to shellfish harvesting; while nearby beaches remain open
[R22] Oysters and Paralytic Shellfish Poisoning {The Sun (newspaper) 25 Sept 90 & 10 Oct 90} \ PSP in Oysters
[R23] Reptile and Amphibian Parasites\ by Eric Rundquist; many internal & external parasites transmissible to man
[R24] Conversations (04-02 -97)(02-08-2001)\ with Harold Barnett, (NWMFC Fisheries Chemist) Shellfish spoilage
[R25] Gout and Shellfish (various Internet articles) \ shellfish often trigger episodes of gout
[R26] Frame by Frame (movie)\ (½ way through the movie); Catfish scavenge a dead body in a river
[R27] Mapping Epidemics\ by Brent Hoff and Carter Smith III; pg 16-21 Cholera // pg 21 shellfish (Crab)
[R28] Molecular Identification of the Lobster Muscle Protein Tropomysin as a seafood allergen\ by Leung, Chen
Mykles, Chow, Li, and Chu; in Molecular Marine Biology Biotechnol (Mar 1998); 7(1):12-20 Lobster protein allergy
[R30] Freshwater Fish Pond Culture and Management (Peace Corps)\ pg 171 Catfish /[R30A] pg 140 Eels
[R30B] pg 101 food for freshwater fish in a pond [R30B] pg 94-99 compost and different manure's
[R31] Catfish Farming Handbook\ pg 140 insects won't harm Catfish //- pg 141 'off-flavor' of Catfish meat
[R33] Webster's New College Dictionary\ pg 347 creosote
[R34] Marine Invertebrates\ by Martyn Hawood and Sue Wells; pg 28 color picture of Crustacean anatomy
[R35] Dangerous Marine Animals\ by Bruce Halstead, MD various marine toxins
[R36] Outbreak of Trichinosis Associated with Eating Cougar Jerky \ in (Morbidity and Mortality Weekly; March 1996)
In 1995, in Idaho a trichinosis outbreak from undercooked smoked cougar jerky. Trichinae also in Walrus.
[R37] What Would Jesus Eat?\ by Don Colbert, MD; pg 37-46 clean and unclean fish
[R38] Gunkholing in the San Juans\ by Joanne Bailey and Carl Nyberg; pg 293 shellfish - PSP quote
[R39] Cry of the Orca (Nov 2000)\ on King 5 TV; Orca and Eagle are sentinel species // PCBs – polychlorinatedbiphenols
[R40] Spirit of the Sound (video)\ Orca and pollution in the Puget Sound // PCBs – used in electrical transformers
[R41] The Eleventh Plague (audio) \ by John Marr, MD & John Baldwin (side2) Frog retains insect venom.
[R42] Hemera Clip Art (CD) and Microsoft Clip Art (Internet) \ – Clean & Unclean Sea Creatures {pgs 116-117}
[R43] Murder, Magic and Medicine\ by John Mann; pg 36-37; Puffer, Porcupine, Globe fish – tetrodotoxin
[R43A] pg 39-40 Reptile & Amphibian poisons //pg 121 – Aspirin – 1st isolated 1897 – 1st synthesized – 1899
[R44] The Serpent and the Rainbow (DVD-movie #11 & #20)\ by Wes Craven – Tetrodotxin is used in vodoo.
[R45] Flu\ by Gina Kolata; pg 201 'Red Tide' is a sign of pollution and a big risk for PSP
[R46] Reptiles and Amphibians\ by William Lamar; pg 182 & 202 Amphibian toxins
[R47] Poisonous Marine Animals\ by Findlay E. Russell pg 12-23 PSP – paralytic shellfish poisoning
[R48] Toxic Fish and Mollusks (Air Force Manual)\ by Edith Keane, Sharee Pepper & Diane Aline
[R49] Shellfish and Seaweed Harvests of Puget Sound\ by Daniel P. Cheney and Thomas F. Mumford, Jr.
[R50] The Coming Plague\ by Laurie Garrett; pg 562 few pathogen-free mollusks to be found
[R51] Passage to Juneau (audio)\ by Jonathan Raban; (sd 2B) In 1792, HMS Discovery's sailor, Carter, died from PSP.

(A healthy alternative to clam chowder, which I used to eat often, is corn chowder.)

Chapter 13 Fowl
Unclean Bird Lists

Moses divided the healthy clean birds for food, from the unclean birds that aren't fit for food. The ***Torah*** lists predator/scavenger fowl as unclean; and all fowl that are not so-listed are clean. Clean birds include all gallinaceous 'game' birds: Pigeon; Quail; Pheasant; Grouse; poultry (Duck, Goose, Swan, Chicken and Turkey); as well as all 'songbirds' (Robin, Sparrow, Swallow, etc.).

Unlike the land animals that must chew the cud and part the hoof to be classified as clean or sea creatures that must have both fins and scales to be classified as clean, there are no easy to distinguish characteristics to separate clean from unclean flying creatures. There just two lists of the unclean flying creatures, any bird not on the unclean list is automatically classified as clean.

Lev 11:13-19 **Unclean Birds** (Lev 11:46 – ***owph*** – flying or winged creature ^#)

	NIV	KJV	JPS (1917)	NJPS	NASB	1901 SE	RSV	Jay Nelson			
13)	eagle	eagle	great vulture	eagle	eagle	eagle	eagle	Eagle	*****	#01	(13
	vulture	ossifrage	bearded vulture	vulture	vulture	gier-eagle	vulture	Vulture	** **	#02	
	black vulture	osprey	osprey	black vulture	buzzard	osprey	osprey	Buzzard	*	#03	
14)	red kite	vulture	kite	kite	kite	kite	kite	Kite	** **	#06	(14
	black kite	kite	falcon	falcon	falcon	falcon	falcon	Falcon	** **	#05	
15)	raven	raven	raven	raven	raven	raven	raven	Raven	*****	#07	(15
16)	horned owl	owl	ostrich	ostrich	ostrich	ostrich	ostrich	Owl	* * *	#08	(16
	screech owl	night hawk	nighthawk	nighthawk	owl	nighthawk	nighthawk	Nighthawk	*****	#09	
	gull	cuckow	sea-mew	sea gull	seagull	sea-mew	sea gull	Seagull	*****	#10	
	hawk	hawk	hawk	hawk	hawk	hawk	hawk	Hawk	*****	#11	
17)	little owl	little owl	little owl	little owl	little owl	little owl	owl	Little Owl	*****	#12	(17
	cormorant	cormorant	cormorant	cormorant	cormorant	cormorant	cormorant	Cormorant	*****	#17	
	great owl	great owl	great owl	great owl	great owl	great owl	ibis	Great Owl	*****	#13	
18)	white owl	swan	horned owl	white owl	white owl	horned owl	water hen	White Owl	** **	#14	(18
	desert owl	pelican	pelican	pelican	pelican	pelican	pelican	Pelican	*****	#15	
	osprey	gier eagle	carrion vulture	bustard	carrion vulture	vulture	carrion vulture	Osprey	**	#16	
19)	stork	stork	stork	stork	stork	stork	stork	Stork	*****	#18	(19
	heron	heron	heron	heron	heron	heron	heron	Heron	*****	#19	
	hoopoe	lapwing	hoopoe	hoopoe	hoopoe	hoopoe	hoopoe	Hoopoe	*****	#20	
	bat	bat	bat	bat	bat	bat	bat	Bat	*****	#21	
	NIV	KJV	JPS	NJPS	NASB	1901 SE	RSV	Jay Nelson			

Deut 14:12-18 **Unclean Birds** (Lev 11:46 – ***owph*** – flying or winged creature ^#)

	NIV	KJV	JPS (1917)	NJPS	NASB	1901 SE	Hebrew	Jay Nelson			
12)	eagle	eagle	great vulture	eagle	eagle	eagle	***nesher***	Eagle	*****	#01	(12
	vulture	ossifrage	bearded vulture	vulture	vulture	gier-eagle	***peres***	Vulture	** **	#02	
	black vulture	osprey	osprey	black vulture	buzzard	osprey	***ozniyah***	Buzzard	*	#03	
13)	red kite	glede	glede	kite	red kite	glede	***ra'ah***	Glede	* * *	#04	(13
	black kite	kite	falcon	falcon	falcon	falcon	***ayah***	Falcon	** **	#05	
	falcon	vulture	kite	buzzard	kite	kite	***dayah***	Kite	** **	#06	
14)	raven	raven	raven	raven	raven	raven	***oreb***	Raven	*****	#07	(14
15)	horned owl	owl	ostrich	ostrich	ostrich	ostrich	***ya'anah***	Owl	* * *	#08	(15
	screech owl	night hawk	night-hawk	nighthawk	owl	night-hawk	***tachmas***	Nighthawk	*****	#09	
	gull	cuckow	seamew	sea gull	seagull	sea-mew	***shachpah***	Seagull	*****	#10	
	hawk	hawk	hawk	hawk	hawk	hawk	***nets***	Hawk	*****	#11	
16)	little owl	little owl	little owl	little owl	little owl	little owl	***kowc***	Little Owl	*****	#12	(16
	great owl	great owl	great owl	great owl	great owl	great owl	***yanshuph***	Great Owl	*****	#13	
	white owl	swan	horned owl	white owl	white owl	horned owl	***tinsemet***	White Owl	** **	#14	
17)	desert owl	pelican	pelican	pelican	pelican	pelican	***qa'ath***	Pelican	*****	#15	(17
	osprey	gier eagle	carrion-vulture	bustard	carrion vulture	vulture	***racham***	Osprey	**	#16	
	cormorant	cormorant	cormorant	cormorant	cormorant	cormorant	***shalak***	Cormorant	*****	#17	
18)	stork	stork	stork	stork	stork	stork	***chaciydah***	Stork	*****	#18	(18
	heron	heron	heron	heron	heron	heron	***anaphah***	Heron	*****	#19	
	hoopoe	lapwing	hoopoe	hoopoe	hoopoe	hoopoe	***dukipat***	Hoopoe	*****	#20	
	bat	bat	bat	bat	bat	bat	***atalleph***	Bat	*****	#21	
	NIV	KJV	JPS	NJPS	NASB	1901 RE	Hebrew	Jay Nelson			

^# For simplicity, Bat may be referenced as a 'bird', although Bat is a mammal. ***Owph*** is best translated: flying or winged creatures, which groups Bat and birds together. ***Tsippor*** is also translated little bird or fowl.

The symbol * indicates (1-5) how certain Jay Nelson is that the bird names on his list are correctly identified.

Word Study on Clean and Unclean Birds

The first problem is, since no two translations have the same list: Which list is correct? All translators had some difficulty in equating modern bird names to bird names used by Moses. First: realize all predator/scavenger birds, such as: Eagle, Vulture, Buzzard, Falcon, Kite, Raven, Owl, Seagull, Hawk, Pelican, Osprey, Cormorant, Stork, Heron, Hoopoe; and all Bats are unclean. The only two instances in which there is a question about which family of birds are unclean are: ***tinsemet*** (***tanshemeth***), which the KJV translates Swan, and other versions translate White Owl, Water Hen or Horned Owl; and (***bat***) ***ya'anah***, which the KJV translates Owl, the NIV translates Horned Owl, and all other versions translates Ostrich. Second: Does Swan or Ostrich belong on the unclean bird list? A word study of Hebrew bird names is required to help resolve this controversy. To help decide whether Swan or Ostrich belongs on the list of unclean birds, the next issue is: What, if any, are the common characteristics of birds on the unclean list? And a similar issue is: What, if any, are the common characteristics of birds that are clean? Scatology is the study of the dung, feces or scat of an organism. Since the scat of an animal, fish or fowl is contingent upon: 1) what the animal eats, and 2) how efficiently the food is digested. A future study of the scat of Swan and Ostrich will help group these Hebrew bird names as being either clean or unclean fowl. Dr. David Macht used the phytotoxic index to group Swan with several other birds that are clean. Swan, Goose and Duck are members of the same bird family. Since Goose and Duck are known to be clean, my bias before starting any study was that: Swan did not belong on the unclean list. The KJV translates ***tanshemeth*** as Swan, and Strong says Water Hen is an alternate translation. Stone's ***CHumash*** commentary on the ***Torah*** discusses the unclean bird list in Leviticus 11.

"Leviticus 11:13-19 The Torah names the twenty non-kosher species of birds, but as a result of various exiles and dispersions, the language of the Torah fell into relative disuse, and exact identities of the non-kosher birds became doubtful. Therefore, the *Shulchan Aruch* (*Yoreh Deah 82:2*) rules that it is forbidden to eat any species of bird unless there is a well-established tradition that it is kosher. We follow the lead of R' Hirsch in transliterating the names, but the commentary offers possible translations." [R23]

The *Anchor Bible Commentary* on Leviticus by Rabbi Jacob Milgrom discusses ***tinsemet*** as being the White Owl, Barn Owl, Little Owl or Screech Owl, but certainly not the Swan. The author is confident that some variety of Owl is the proper translation of ***tinsemet***. (Lev 11:16 – Deut 14:15) The author follows the NIV and translates ***tinsemet*** as White Owl, although other Owl types are also possible. One possible explaination for the KJV error in translation of ***tinsemet*** as Swan may be related to the common white color of Swan being confused with the white color of White Owl.

The difficulty in the proper translation of (***bat***) ***ya'anah*** is much more complex and intriguing. ***Ya'an*** is a Hebrew root that means 'to pay attention'. ***Ya'an*** has a feminine form ***ya'anah*** that is found on the unclean lists. (Lev 11:16a and Deut 14:15a) ***Ya'an*** also has a masculine form ***ya'en*** that isn't found on the unclean lists, but the plural of ***ya'en*** is always translated Ostriches. (Lam 4:3) Another Hebrew word ***notsah*** is translated Ostrich by all versions. (Job 39:13) ***Notsah*** comes from the root ***nuwc,*** which means to 'vanish' or 'flee'. The notion of 'to flee' from which ***notsah*** is derived seems to fit Ostrich well, as ostrich can run 40^{+} mph. [R22] The notion 'to pay attention' also seems to fit Owl well, as an Owl often sits quietly in a perch (tree) for hours observing everything. Ostrich also has great vision, which may cause confusion over the proper translation of ***ya'anah***. Ostrich, Emu, Rhea and Kiwi are members of the ratite bird family and are considered together.

Rabbi Jacob Milgrom wrote in the *Anchor Bible Commentary* about identifying unclean birds.

"The identifications [of the unclean birds] are, in many cases, educated guesses, as the many alternative suggestions readily indicate." [R8]

Rabbi Milgrom also discusses the sense of ***ya'anah*** as used by Isaiah, Jeremiah and Micah is that of 'daughter of the desert', as in desolate places after judgment, which fits Owl perfectly. [R8-39]

"The usual rendering [of (***bat***) ***ya'anah*** as], 'ostrich' must be abandoned because ostriches do not haunt ruins, as do owls." [R8]

KJV Is 34:13 And thorns shall come up in her palaces, nettles and brambles in her fortresses thereof: and it shall be a habitation of dragons, and a court for owls (***ya'anah***).

∗ The Hebrew language seems to indicate that ***tinsemet*** should be translated (White) Owl; ***ya'anah*** should be translated Owl; and ***notsah*** should be translated Ostrich. The LORD may have anticipated the difficulty in properly translating ***ya'anah*** from the unclean bird lists, by using ***ya'anah*** four other times in the ***Tanakh*** in a sense that's designed to clarify its translation as Owl.

∗ Scatology, biochemistry and phytotoxicity should confirm that Swan and Ostrich are clean birds.

Unclean Birds

Eagle, Vulture, Buzzard, Falcon, Kite, Raven, Crow, Seagull, Hawk, Owl, Pelican, Osprey, Stork, Cormorant, Heron and Hoopoe are unclean predator/scavenger birds. Many unclean birds may feed on dead, decaying, diseased, rotting flesh and survive, primarily, by having a highly acidic stomach.

John Hendrickson in his book *Raptors* discusses carrion, microbes and a highly acid stomach:

> "The food preferences and digestive system of vultures are truly amazing. How anything can live on a diet of rotting and often-diseased carrion (dead decaying flesh) is a wonder, and a service to all. Vultures lack the sharp talons of other raptors, and so, rather than killing their own prey, they live entirely on carrion. By quickly disposing of infected carcasses, vultures help to reduce the spread of diseases. A [Raptor's] highly acid digestive system kills many viruses and some of the most virulent strains of bacteria." [R7]

Like predator/scavenger land animals, all unclean birds have a very short digestive system, as compared with their body size, and they must process spoiled meat (carrion) very quickly. Predator/scavenger can't always count on regular meals, so they are prepared to eat large meals on the fly. Raptors have a highly acid stomach and a rapid secretion of digestive enzymes can make a quick job of digestion. Scavenging fowl often can't take the time for a long, slow digestion. High stomach acidity kills most microbes that birds of prey eat, but may not degrade/destroy toxins.

∗ Raptors, and all other carnivores, are the top 'sentinel' predator of a biological ecosystem.

The biological principle of bio-amplification or bio-multiplication discusses that toxins from the environment are absorbed by life near the bottom of a food chain and increase in concentration as the toxins move higher up the food pyramid. Rachel Carson in her book *Silent Spring* discussed that bio-accumulation of DDT often destroyed eagle eggs. Pesticides, such as DDT, were absorbed by plants in small concentrations, were absorbed by small plant eaters and by fish from water runoff in yet higher concentrations, and were often found in the highest concentration in eagle eggs. [R6-27]

Small 'clean' songbirds have a much higher metabolic rate than larger 'unclean' raptors. [R27-28] Dennis Paulson, PhD and Sharon Walters discussed that songbirds and predator/scavengers are often susceptible to the same infections. Yet the small 'clean' birds have a much higher metabolic rate, often causing them a rapid demise; where the much larger birds of prey have a much slower metabolism, which may prolong their time before death. [R9-27] When challenged with an infectious microbe, smaller songbirds tend to die very quickly (often within hours) from infections, while larger birds of prey can often survive and fly for many weeks. As the author understands the facts: Eventually, larger birds of prey will likely also succumb to the infection, but during the time between initial exposure until death, a raptor may fly quite normally for weeks without appearing diseased. Birds of prey, if challenged with an infection, appear to be flying incubation chambers for microbes, and, presumably, would be very likely to spread disease or disease toxins to people eating them. One author also theorized: That some birds of prey, if afflicted by an infectious microbe, respond with a supraproportional increase of red blood cells (RBCs) that allows them to appear healthy on the outside and keep flying until death, while the microbe is multiplying out-of-control internally. [R31]

∗ Raptors often accumulate toxins and may incubate microbes, while small clean birds are likely dead from an infection or toxic accumulation before they could be eaten.

The effect of environmental poisons on raptors, as opposed to small songbirds, is similar, in that the high metabolic rate of clean songbirds causes them to succumb quickly to toxins, while for larger birds of prey with a much slower metabolism, the same poisons are much slower acting. Birds of prey may accumulate toxins internally, while they soar and appear healthy on the outside. Most discussion about birds of prey accumulating toxins, deals with health detriments to the birds. If people ate raptors, more discussion would likely focus on health problems for people who eat them.

Bat

Bat has a short digestive system for its body size. Fruit Bat lives exclusively on the ripest fruit. Fruit Bat eliminates undigested seeds from ripe fruit in ≈20 minutes, which is ideal for seed dispersal. Bat produced enzymes, plus enzymes and yeast in the ripe fruit likely perform most of the digestion. All mammals of the land, sea or air have bacteria that participate, to some extent, in digestion. [R15] Bat rapidly digests food, which may not allow symbiotic bacteria to work as efficiently as in clean birds. Bat guano (feces) contains nitrogen waste – saltpeter, resulting from incomplete protein digestion. Vampire Bat drinks blood, which presents risk for contracting or carrying disease, such as rabies. Bat often eats exclusively insects, the same insects as many small clean birds, such as swallow. The author theorizes: Bat will absorb more toxins from food than a similarly sized 'clean' songbird.

∗ Little data exists about health risks from eating unclean birds, since few people eat unclean birds.

Clean Birds

Clean birds include poultry (Chicken or Turkey), Duck, Goose; all gallinaceous 'game' birds (Pigeon, Quail, Pheasant, Grouse) as well as all 'songbirds' (Robin, Sparrow, Swallow, etc.) ...

Pheasant, Grouse and Quail are gallinaceous birds that primarily eat grain, have a relatively long digestive system, spend much time on the ground, and likely retain few toxins in muscles. Most clean birds spend a good deal of time on the ground or on water looking for food and eating, which means clean birds can devote much time and energy for a long slow efficient digestion. Clean game birds often migrate long distances, but they don't spend flying time looking for food. Clean swallow-like birds feed on insects in the air. Many clean birds include grains in their diets. Duck and Goose are both called a clean bird by everyone, and swan is of the same bird family. Duck, Goose and Swan eat a primarily a vegetable diet and all have long coiled digestive system. Along with gallinaceous birds and poultry, these clean birds are frequently hunted for human food.

∗ **Many clean animals, fish and fowl are primary targets for predation, as well as food for humans.**

One question that often is asked is: Why is chicken clean? Chicken eats almost anything. Chicken is not found on anyone's unclean list. Chicken often eats some poor quality food, as do scavengers, but they also have a longer more coiled digestive system than predator/scavengers. The author theorizes: A longer more coiled digestive system for poultry allows greater activity by healthy symbiotic bacteria, which likely means that more food-borne toxins can be neutralized. Poultry digestion is also likely more discriminating in terms of the absorption of food-borne toxins.

Ratites poised big questions. 1st Are Ratites clean or unclean? 2nd If Ratites are clean: Why? Ratite anatomy/physiology and physical habits/characteristics seemed, after a brief study, to more nearly resemble poultry than predator/scavengers. Before the author closely studied the ***Tanakh***, my inclination was: Ratites appear to be clean, but nearly all modern scholars call them unclean. After reading Rabbi Milgrom's commentary on Leviticus 11 concerning ***ya'anah*** in a theological library, and then reading the related Scriptures in the ***Tanakh***, a verdict of clean was rendered. (Shouting 'Yes!' in a theological library was somewhat inappropriate, but the library was emptied for vacation.)

∗ **Ratites have a long, coiled digestive system compared to their body size, as do poultry.**

Ratites, especially ostrich, are able to digest plant cellulose similarly to ruminant land animals. Ratites are virtual eating machines for their first 6 months, as they do little else than eat or sleep. Ostrich often weighs 2 or 3 pounds at birth, and may weigh 200 or 300 pounds in 6^{+} months. Ratite meat is red, virtually indistinguishable from beef in taste and very low in fat/cholesterol. Grains and grasses are the majority of the ratite diet, although ratites rarely eat small animals. Plant cellulose is a very complex food that requires a long slow digestion facilitated by microbes. Ratites, especially ostrich, digest cellulose in the colon, rather than in the stomachs of ruminants.

∗ **The author believes: Ratites are the bird equivalent of land animal ruminants, and are clean!**

The author frequently pondered clean and unclean birds, by watching pigeons and seagulls. Pigeon is clean and seagull is unclean, yet they are of a similar size, and they often eat a similar diet from people who feed them in a park. When paddling my kayak around the Puget Sound, the author has occasionally seen a seagull scavenging a dead salmon carcass or the carcass of a dead seal, which puts seagull more at risk of obtaining toxins and parasites than pigeon. Questions often arise from people who are skeptical about the importance of the clean/unclean distinction, such as: What if a seagull was kept in cages, fed a vegetarian diet and ate no meat? The author theorizes: like pig on land, and shellfish in water, an unclean seagull processes food and absorbs toxins in a less selective, less sophisticated, less specialized manner than a clean pigeon.

∗ **Even if Pigeon and Seagull were fed an identical diet, Pigeon would necessarily absorb fewer toxins**.

A woman who visited South America and ate pig that was exclusively fed a diet of bananas, said, the pork tasted delicious, and the taste was different then grain-fed pork that she was used to. People who hunt bear tell say, the time of year that they kill the bear affects the meat's flavor. The taste of any clean/unclean creature's meat may be affected by food that was recently eaten.

∗ **Most unclean creatures eat a significantly more toxin laden diet than the diet of most clean creatures.**

∗ **The author theorizes: meat from clean animal, fish or fowl, always absorbs, stores and contains fewer toxins than meat from unclean animals, fish and fowl.**

The Flood drastically altered Earth's climate and placed new demands on human health that did not exist before the Flood. Protein means: that which comes first. Meat from clean animals, fish and fowl is a nutritious and highly concentrated source of protein, minerals and other nutrients. A variety of clean meat, fish and fowl are often a valuable and important part of a healthy diet.

{Anyone may send data or insights concerning clean/unclean meats to: Moses5in1Torah@msn.com .}

PhytoToxicology

According to Dr. David I. Macht's phytopharmacology study, clean birds consistently scored significantly higher on the 'Index of Growth' scale, indicating less toxicity, than unclean birds. [R1]

---------- Phytotoxic Indices of 2% Solutions of Fresh Muscle Juices -------------

CLEAN BIRDS	**Index of Growth**	**No. of Experiments**
Chicken	83%	20
Duck (*Mallard*)	90%	10
Goose (*Anser albifrons*)	85%	6
Turkey	85%	10
Pigeon	93%	10
Quail (*Coturnix communis*)	89%	20
Canada Goose (*Branta canadensis*)	85%	7
Coot	88%	8
Wild Duck (*Aytha americana*)	85%	8
Swan	87%	6
UNCLEAN BIRDS	**Index of Growth**	**No. of Experiments**
Sparrow Hawk (*Falco parverius*)	63%	6
Red Tail Hawk (*Bulco brcalis*)	36%	8
Owl	62%	8
Crow	46%	10

Insects

KJV Lev 11:20 All fowls (***owph***) that creep, going upon all four, shall be an abomination unto you. vs21 Yet these may yet eat of every flying creeping thing that goeth upon all four, which have legs above their feet, to leap withal upon the earth; vs22 Even these of them may ye eat; the locust (***arbeh***) after its kind, and the bald locust (***colam***) after its kind, and the beetle [cricket] (***chargol***) after its kind, and the grasshopper (***chagab***) after its kind.

Spiders, Bees, Wasps, Flies, Cockroaches and Mosquitoes are included as unclean insects that are unacceptable as food, and they all inflict venomous wounds or carry human disease. [R4] Feeding on feces puts unclean insects at risk for carrying infectious diseases to mankind. [R2-8] Mosquitoes carry *Malaria plasmodium* that cause human malaria, or microbes causing yellow fever. Cockroaches and Flies carry *Entamoeba histolytica* that may cause human amoebic dysentery. [R2] Wasps, Spiders and Bees all produce venom that is harmful to humans. There is great wisdom from Moses in not eating unclean insects, and in avoiding contact with these insects altogether.

Grasshoppers or Locusts were common food in ancient times in Canaan, Asia and Africa. [R39] When conditions are proper, 'gregarious grasshoppers' congregate to become a locust swarm. [R41] Locusts are strict vegetarians, as opposed to unclean insects, which are often scavengers. [R4-39] Locusts are often roasted on a plate over hot coals – head, wings and legs aren't usually eaten. [R37] Locusts are boiled and mixed with other food, roasted with flour or honey, strung on a chord and preserved for later eating by drying [R36] or ground into powder and made into cakes for roasting. Locusts are digestible and low in toxicity, and contain 62% protein, 17% fat and many minerals. [R33] Locusts enable the poor to inexpensively get enough quality protein to stay healthy and allowed Hebrews to get a healthy protein meal, if they ran out of other provisions while traveling. [R38-39] Grasshoppers as food might reduce the incidence of locust swarms that periodically eat valuable grain crops and/or green plants. Locusts are still common as food today in the Middle East. [R39] Cricket is in the same family (*Orthoptera*) as locust/grasshopper, and is similarly nutritious. [R39]

Once again, God's commandments are a 'nest of shelter' amidst an 'air of uncertainty'.

∗ No statements, events or visions in the history of the world have changed animals that the LORD called unclean, to make them clean. In fact, just the opposite may be true. As human history has progressed there are now more toxins in the Earth's environment than at any time in the past. Since the unclean animals, fish and fowl are for the most part predator/scavenger type animals, these creatures may be collecting toxins within their flesh at a much more substantial rate today than they did in the days of Noah or even in the days of Moses. (Gen 7:2 – Lev 11 and Deut 14)

∗ Today, the difference between the clean and the unclean has been blurred to the point of becoming nearly unrecognizable, until only shades of gray remain, instead of maintaining the clear crisp clean healthy distinction that the LORD God intended.

---------------------------------- References Ch 13 Fowl ----------------------------------

[R1] An Experimental Pharmacological Appreciation of Leviticus XI and Deuteronomy XIV \by David I. Mach, MD; in 'Bulletin of the History of Medicine'; from Johns Hopkins University (1953)
[R2] Guess What Came to Dinner\ by Ann Louise Gittleman; pg 38 Cockroach may carry disease.
[R3] Gods Key to Health and Happiness\ by Elmer Josephson; pg 45-47 Does gizzard kept Poultry clean?
[R3C] pg 91-96 Levitical Dietary Law concerning meat, fish and Fowl
[R4] Destructive and Useful Insects\ by Metcalf, Flint & Metcalf; pg 906 vegetarian Grasshopper – Locust
[R5] Are the Food Laws Scientific?\ by Harold Hemenway predator/scavenger birds = unclean
[R6] Silent Spring\ by Rachel Carson; pg 108 Eagle often accumulates DDT to death.
[R7] Raptors (Birds of Prey)\ by John Hendrickson; pg 7 definitions // pg 28 highly acidic stomach of Raptors
[R8] The Anchor Bible Commentary on Leviticus\ by Rabbi Jacob Milgrom; pg 662-664 ***ya'anah*** as Owl
[R9] conversations (1995 SARDUS Wildlife Center)\ with Sharon Walters; Raptors vs Songbirds die quickly
[R10] conversations (Sept-Oct 2000)\ with Singh Dhillion, DVM, PhD; Ratites, Poultry and Raptors
Sept-Oct 2000 Avian Health Laboratory; WSU Co-Operative Extension (all bird gizzards nearly same).
[R11] Environmental Science\ by G. Tyler Miller Jr.; pg A26, 398-399 bio-amplification as a principle
[R12] What the Bible Says About Healthy Living\ by Rex Russell, MD; pg 148-149 clean birds // pg 151&153 unclean birds
[R13] Protein Power\ by Michael R. Eades, MD and Mary Dan Eades, MD
[R14] Stone Edition of the Tanakh\ pg 268 commentary and quote on Lev 11:13-19
[R15] Those Amazing Bats\ by Cheryl Mays Halton; pg 4-5 bacteria in digestion / saltpeter in guano
[R16] Husbandry and Medical Management of Ostriches, Emus and Rheas\ by Jensen & Johnson
[R17] The Ratite Encyclopedia\ pg 43-48 digestion of cellulose in the colon
[R18] Strong's Concordance\ see next page of References
[R19] Ratite Management, Medicine and Surgery\ pg 4-6 cellulose digestion by Ostrich
[R20] The Plague Killers\ by Greer Williams; pg 101 *plasmodium* protozoan of *Anopheles* mosquito – causes malaria
[R21] Davis Dictionary of the Bible\ pg 584 Davis considers both Ostrich and Owl to be unclean.
pg 791 Swan - ***tinshemeth*** - RV calls it a Horned Owl – same name as an unclean Lizard
[R22] Mutual of Omaha's Wild Kingdom (Ostrich)\ with Marlin Perkins; Ostrich is voracious eater – runs 40$^+$mph
[R23] Stone Edition of Chumash; (Torah plus half-Torah)\ pg 600 - (Lev 11:16) - bird names forgotten
(pg 1013 - Deut 14) - identification of bird names on the unclean lists is often uncertain
[R24] The Genesis Diet\ by Gordon Tessler, PhD; pg 58 Raptors as unclean birds
[R25] Expositors Bible Commentary\ by Frank Gaebelein; pg 569-572 Clean and Unclean birds
[R26] The Pentateuch (vol 1&2) \ by Keil and Delitzch; pg 362 ***ya'anah*** // pg 366-367 Locust as food
[R27] e-mail Dennis Paulson (Slater Museum Natural History) (Feb 2001)\ Eagles – toxins – metabolic rates
[R28] Veterinary Aspects of Captive Birds of Prey\ by John Eric Cooper; pg 136-137 metabolic rates
[R29] Lets Play Doctor\ by Joel Wallach, DVM, ND and Ma Lan, MD, MS; pg 163 Vampire Bat & rabies
[R30] Compton's Pictured Encyclopedia (vol 3 -1963 Ed)\ pg 423 Cockroach NaFl as insecticide
[R31] Internet Article \- I didn't print this and when I went back to find it, it wasn't there. -\
(I haven't found any corroborating evidence to support this. – This concept is currently unsubstantiated.)
[R32] Encyclopedia Americana 2000: (Islam)\ pg 495
Koran was finished between 644 and 656 AD by the 3rd successor Caliph to Mohammed.
[R33] The Koran\ by Mohammed // (translated by William Watt); pg 45 The Cow – Surah III – #173 &
pg 280 The Bee – Surah XVI – #115 Koran prohibits Islamics from eating carrion, blood and Swine-flesh.
[R34] The IVP Bible Background Commentary: Old Testament\ by Walton, Matthews & Chavolas; pg 128
[R35] BUGINFO + Insects as Food for Humans (both Internet)\ Locusts often boiled before being cleaned.
Desert Locust Information Service of FAO: Locust FAQs – dried weight: 62% protein, 17% fat + minerals
[R36] Encyclopedia of the Bible (vol 1)\ ed by Walter A. Elwell; pg 804 Locusts fried in flour/honey – dried.
[R37] Grzimek's Animal Encyclopedia Vol 2: Insects\ pg 112 Locusts (w/o head, wings) as human food
[R38] Eerdman's Handbook of the Bible\ pg 176 Locusts as common ancient food – and on a desert trip.
[R39] Leviticus An Introduction and Commentary\ by R. K. Harrison, PhD, DD; pg 128 ***ya'anah*** as Owl
pg 129 Locusts – Middle East food for centuries – high in protein, fat and minerals – *Orthoptera* family
pg 129 Unclean insects feed on filth, rubbish or carrion – and may carry or transmit disease to people
[R40] All the Birds of the Bible\ by A. Parmalee (from [R39])
[R41] Locusts, Teeth of the Wind (National Geographic 136 Aug 1969)\ Locust swarm eats anything green
pg 202-226 solitary Grasshoppers become gregarious – as a Locust swarm in Canaan, Asia and Africa
[R42] Hemera Clip Art (CD Rom and Internet)\ photos of Birds & Insects – Clean & Unclean {pgs 118-119 & 120}
[R43] Jerusalem's Locust Plague (National Geographic Dec 1915)\; pg 547 Locust (w/o legs) roasted, dried, stored
[R44] What Would Jesus Eat?\ by Don Colbert, MD; pg 66-67 poultry are clean
[R45] A Time of Angels\ by Karen Hesse ***treph*** from – animal 'torn' = non-kosher food
[R46] 'Mystery' Marine Toxin Found – (09-19-03 – *Seattle PI* – B1-pg 2) Alfred Hitchcock's (1963 movie) — The Birds was based on shorebirds that were likely poisoned by 'domoic acid' and that subsequently attacked townspeople of Capitola, Calif.
[R47] ***Mishnah*** \ by Jacob Neusner (translation into English) ***Talmud*** = ***Mishnah*** + ***Gemarah*** {pg 90 & 98}
Talmud means 'study' / ***Mishnah*** means 'retelling' {Oral Law or Oral ***Torah***} / ***Gemara(h)*** means 'conclusion'

The Babylonian ***Talmud*** of ≈550 AD with it's completed ***Gemarah*** is more widely referenced than the Palestinian ***Talmud*** of ≈400 AD, while both the Palestinian ***Talmud*** and Babylonian ***Talmud*** contain the identical ***Mishnah***. The ***Mishnah*** was written in unique, ***Mishnaic*** Hebrew, while both ***Gemarah's*** were primarily written in Aramaic.

---------------------------- References continued Ch 13 Fowl ----------------------------

[R18] Strong's Concordance\ by James Strong, STD, LLD

				unclean bird (fowl) lists		transliterations	L 11:13-19	D14:11-18
pg 371	fowl	cover with wings		# 5775	H pg 86	***owph – oph***	L11: 13&20&46	---------
pg 128	birds	little hopping (bird)		# 6833	H pg 100	***tsippor – tsippowr***	---------	D14:11
	KJV	Jay Nelson				plus alternatives		
pg 288	Eagle	Eagle	#01	# 5404	H pg 81	***nesher – neser***	L11:13	D14:12
pg 760	Ossifrage	Vulture	#02	# 6538	H pg 96	***peres – perec***	L11:13	D14:12
pg 760	Osprey	Buzzard	#03	# 5822	H pg 87	***ozniyah – ozniyya***	L11:13	D14:12
pg 391	Glede	Glede	#04	# 7201	H pg 106	***ra'ah***	---------	D14:13
pg 573	Kite	Falcon	#05	# 0344	H pg 11	***ayah – ha'ayya***	L11:14	D14:13
pg 1102	Vulture	Kite	#06	# 1772	H pg 30	***dayah – daa***	L11:14	D14:13
pg 827	Raven	Raven	#07	# 6158	H pg 91	***oreb – kol-owreb***	L11:15	D14:14
pg -----	daughter of			# 1323	H pg 24	***bath – bat***	L11:16	D14:15
pg 766	Owl	Owl	#08	# 3284	H pg 50	***ya'anah – hayya'ana***	L11:16	D14:15
pg 717	Night Hawk	Nighthawk	#09	# 8464	H pg 123	***tachmas – tahmac***	L11:16	D14:15
pg 228	Cuckow	Seagull	#10	# 7828	H pg 114	***shachpah – sahap***	L11:16	D14:15
pg 464	Hawk	Hawk	#11	# 5322	H pg 80	***nets – netz***	L11:16	D14:15
608-766	Little Owl	Little Owl	#12	# 3563	H pg 54	***kowc – kos***	L11:17	D14:16
419-766	Great Owl	Great Owl	#13	# 3244	H pg 50	***yanshuph – yanshowph***	L11:17	D14:16
pg 989	Swan	White Owl	#14	# 8580	H pg 125	***tinsemet – tanshemeth***	L11:18	D14:16
pg 777	Pelican	Pelican	#15	# 6893	H pg 100	***qa'ath – qa'at***	L11:18	D14:17
385-288	Gier Eagle	Osprey	#16	# 7360	H pg 108	***racham***	L11:18	D14:17
pg 219	Cormorant	Cormorant	#17	# 7994	H pg 117	***shalak – salak***	L11:17	D14:17
pg 978	Stork	Stork	#18	# 2624	H pg 41	***chaciydah – hasida***	L11:19	D14:18
pg 480	Heron	Heron	#19	# 0601	H pg 15	***anaphah – ha'anapa***	L11:19	D14:18
pg 586	Lapwing	Hoopoe	#20	# 1744	H pg 30	***dukipat – dukiyphath***	L11:19	D14:18
pg 099	Bat	Bat	#21	# 5847	H pg 87	***atalleph – atalep***	L11:19	D14:18
pg -----	to pay attention			# 3282	H pg 50	***ya'an***	---------	---------
pg 760	Ostriches	all translations	(mas)	# 3283	H pg 50	***ya'en***	Lam 4:3	
pg 766	Owl	Owl	(fem)	# 3284	H pg 50	(***bat***) ***ya'anah***	L11:16	D14:15
pg 766	Owl	Owl		# 3284	H pg 50	(***bat***) ***ya'anah***	Isaiah 13:21 & 34:13	
pg 766	Owl	Owl		# 3284	H pg 50	(***bat***) ***ya'anah***	Jer 50:39	Micah 1:8
pg 760	Ostrich	all translations		# 5133	H pg 77	***notsah – nowtsah***	Job 39:13	
--------	to flee			# 5127	H pg 77	***nuwc***	---------	---------
pg 225	creeping	swarming flying		# 8318	H pg 121	***sherets***	Deut 14:19	
pg 371	fowls (KJV)	flying insect (NKJV)		# 5775	H pg 86	***owph***	L11:20	D14:--
pg 611	locust – (all translations)			# 697	H pg 16	***arbeh***	L11:22	D14:--
pg 611	bald locust (KJV)	katydid (NIV)		# 5556	H pg 83	***colam***	L11:22	D14:--
pg 108	beetle (KJV)	cricket (all other)		# 2728	H pg 43	***chargol***	L11:22	D14:--
pg 418	grasshopper – (all)			# 2284	H pg 37	***chagab***	L11:22	D14:--
pg 1070	torn (by animals)			# 2966	H pg 46	(noun – ***terephah***) (***treph*** – to tear – verb)	Lv 22:8	
pg 668	meats			# 1033	G pg 18	*broma*	I Tim 4:3	

Numerals (#01-#21) used to identify unclean birds are based on the list in Deuteronomy. The unclean bird ***ra'ah*** (#04) is only found on the Deuteronomy list. All unclean birds are not in same order on both lists.

KJV Lev 11:20 All fowls (***owph***) that creep (***sherets***), going upon all four, shall be an abomination unto you.

NKJV Lev 11:20 'All flying insects [fowls] (***owph***) that creep (***sherets***) on all fours shall be an abomination to you. vs21 Yet these you may eat of every flying insect (***owph***) that creeps on all fours which have jointed legs above their feet with which to keep on the earth. vs22 'These you shall eat: the locust (***arbeh***) after its kind, the destroying locust (***colam***) after its kind, the cricket (***chargol***) after its kind, and the grasshopper (***chagab***) after its kind.

NIV Lev 11:20 All flying insects (***owph***) that walk (***sherets***) on all fours are to be detestable to you. vs21 There are, however, some winged creatures (***owph***) that walk on all fours that you may eat: those that have jointed legs for hopping on the ground. vs22 Of these you may eat any kind of locust (***arbeh***), katydid (***colam***), cricket (***chargol***) or grasshopper (***chagab***).

JPS Lev 22:8 That which dieth of itself, or is torn (***terephah***) of beasts, he shall not eat ...

KJV Deut 14:19 And every creeping thing that flieth (***owph***) is unclean to you: they shall not be eaten.

JPS Deut 14:19 All winged (***sherets***) swarming things (***owph***) are unclean to you; they shall not be eaten.

NIV Deut 14:19 All flying (***sherets***) insects (***owph***) that swarm are unclean to you; do not eat them.

(Compared to documentation in other chapters, some arguments in Chapter 13 are unsubstantiated and speculative.)

Animal, Fish, Bird or Insect pictures that may be used by the author can e-mailed to: Moses5in1Torah@msm.com .

Clean Animals

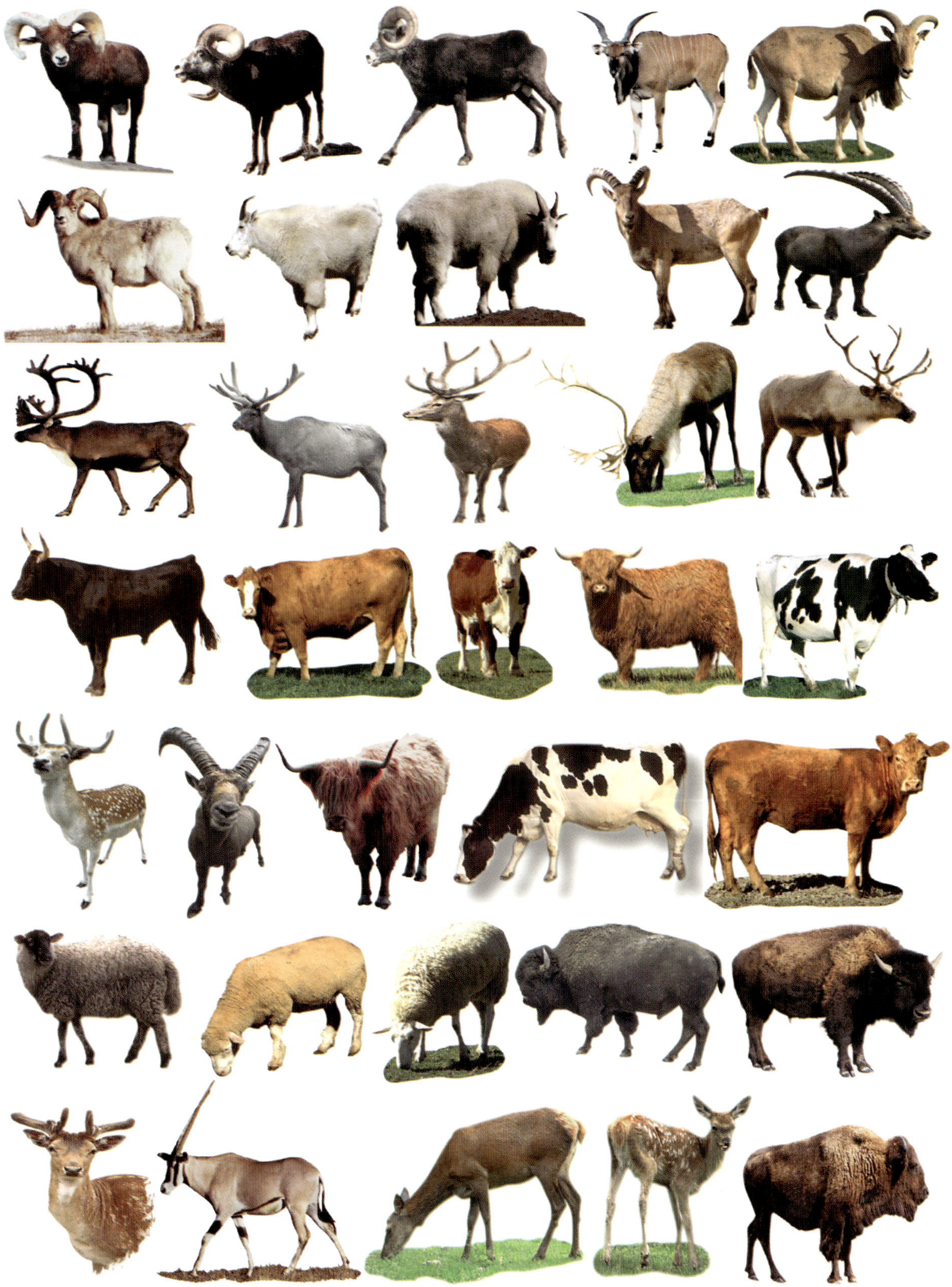

[R42]

Unclean Animals

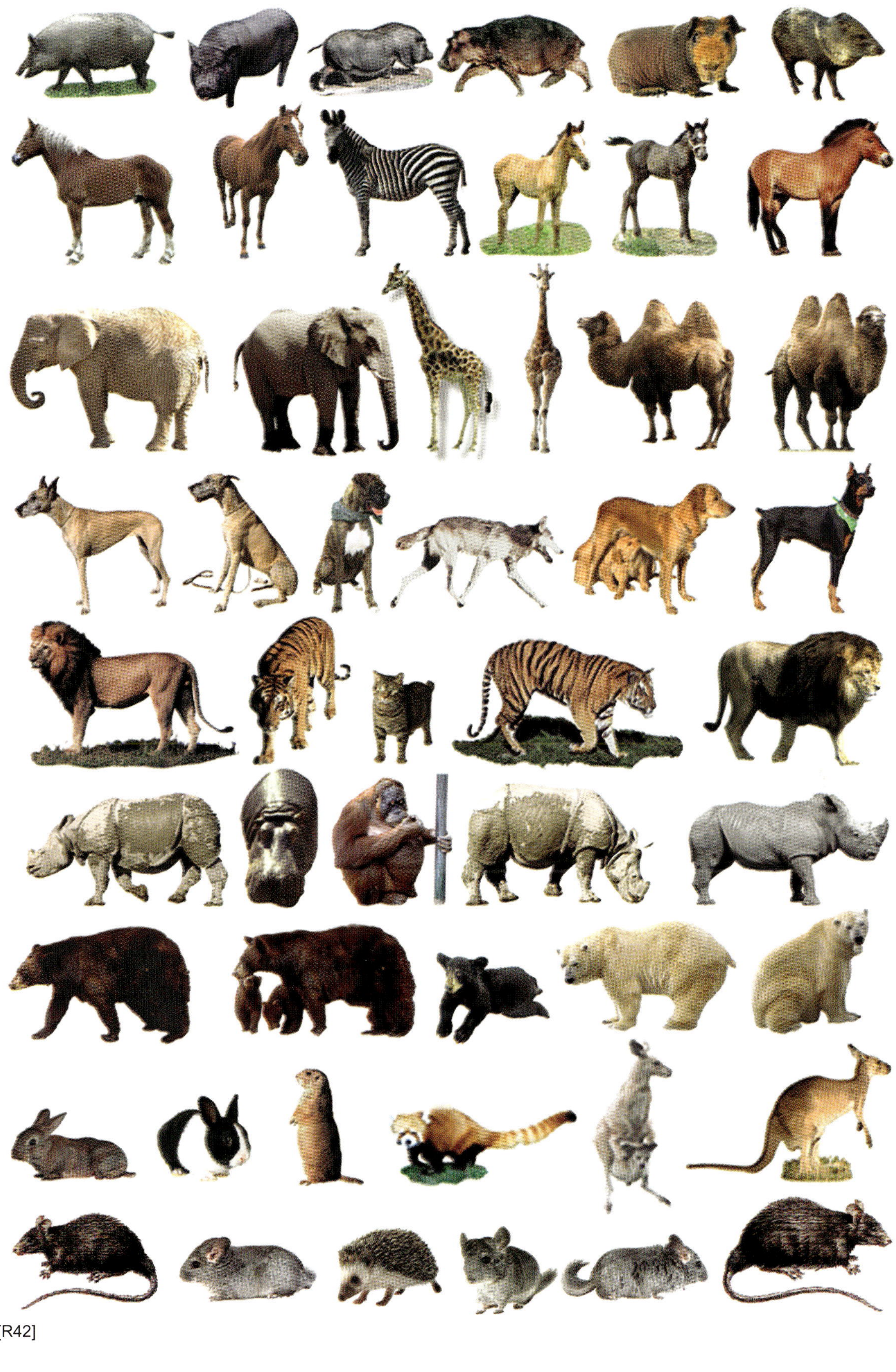

[R42]

Clean Fish

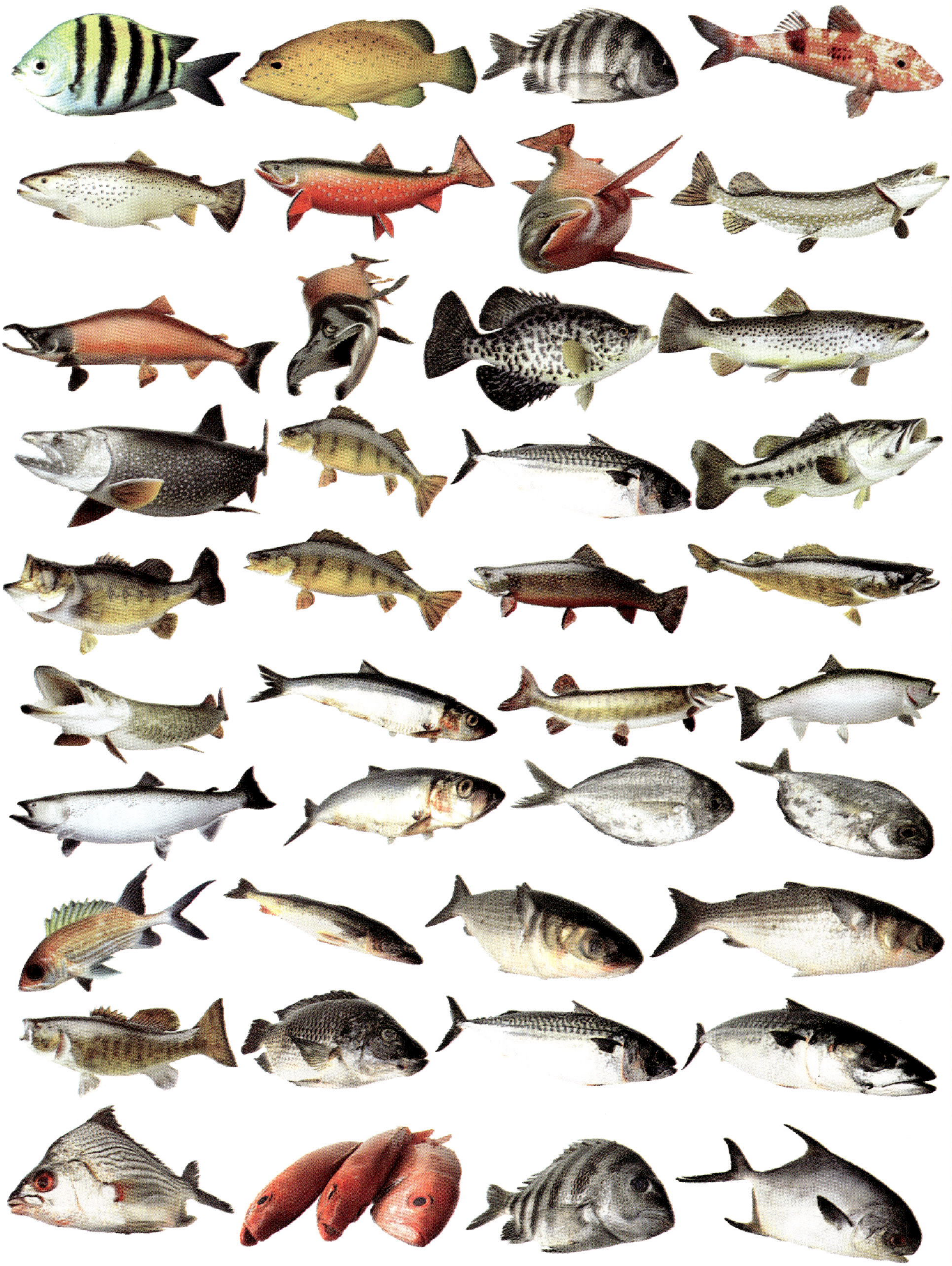

[R42]

Unclean Fish and other Unclean Sea Creatures

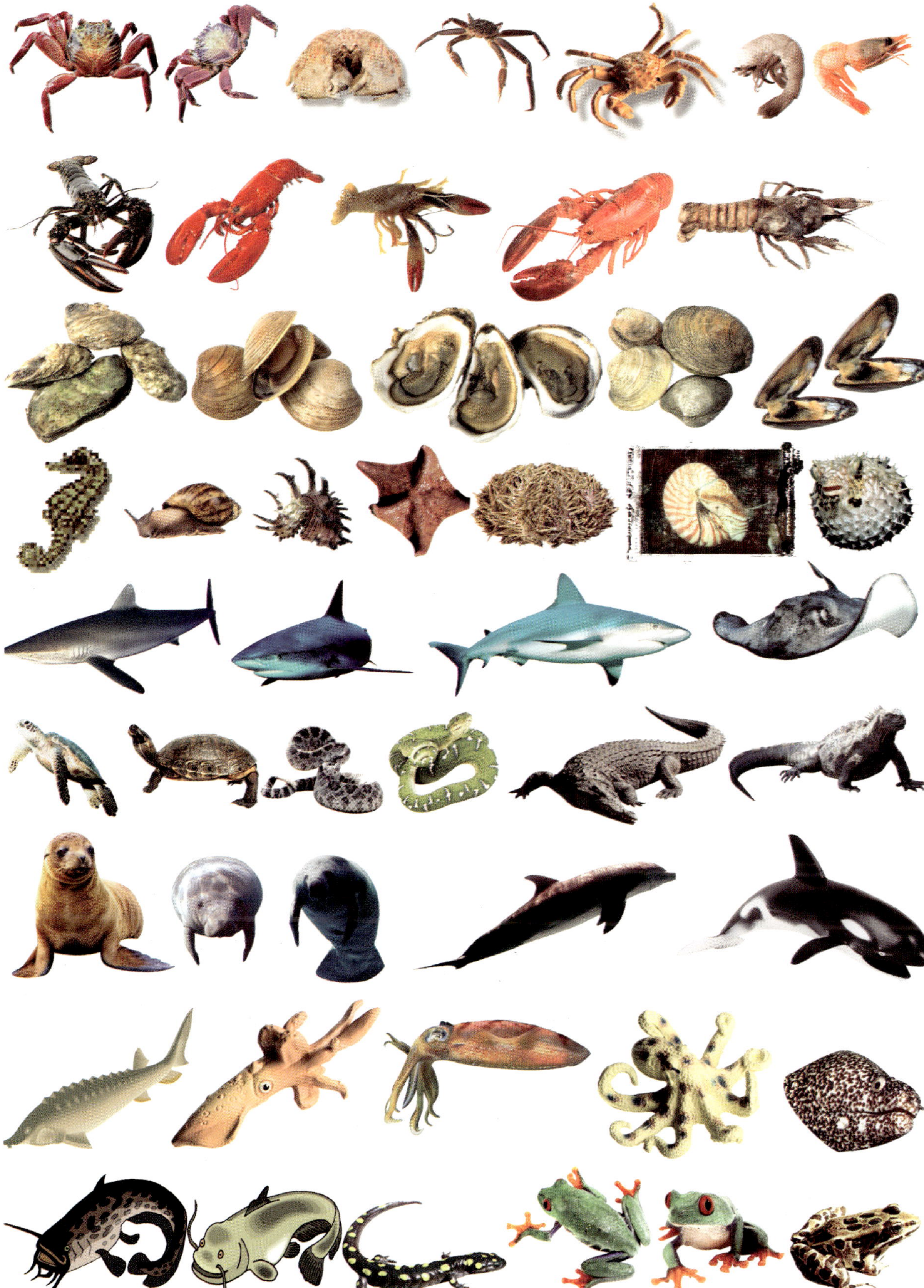

[R42]

Clean Birds

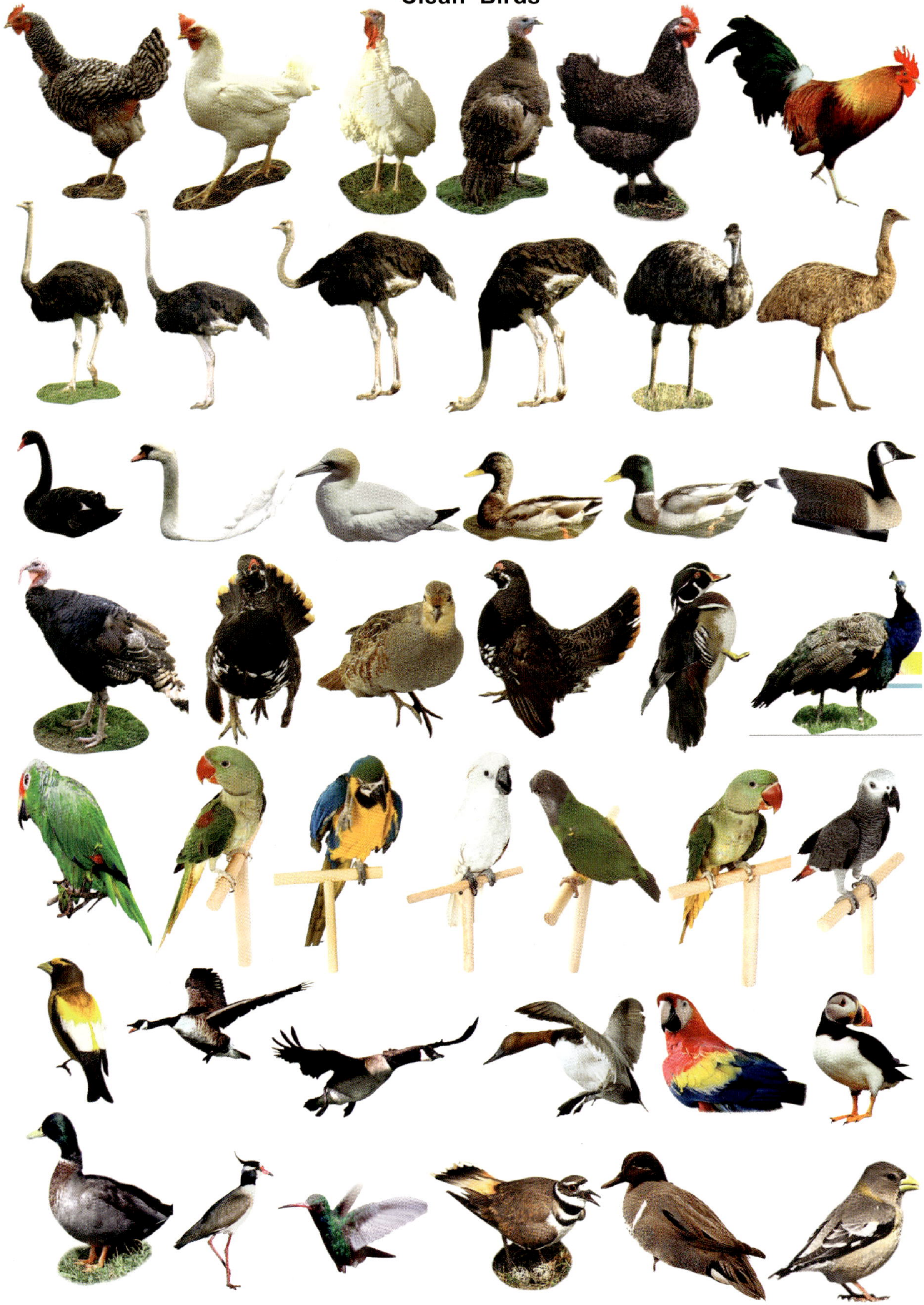

[R42]

Unclean Birds

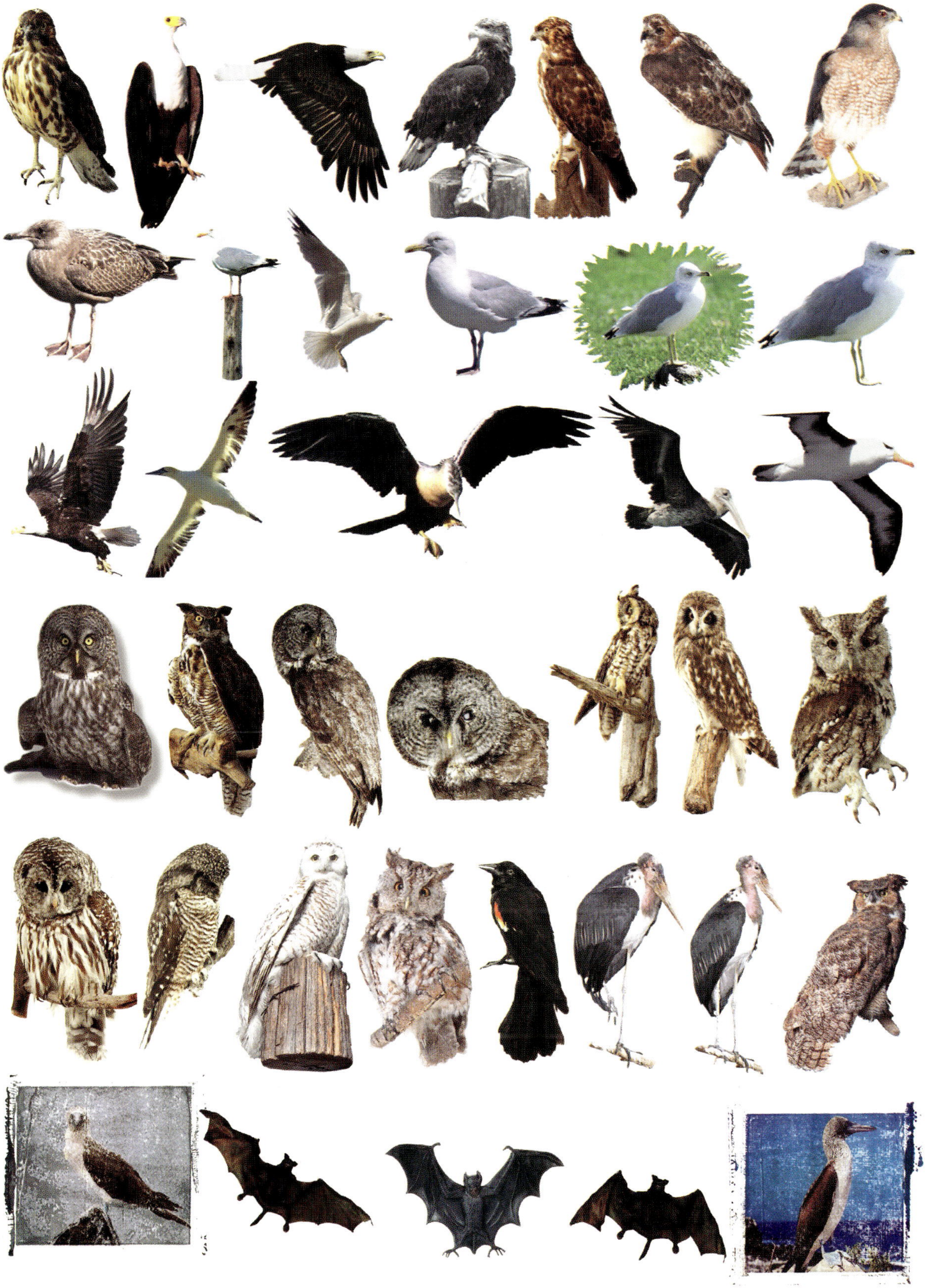

[R42]

Clean Insects

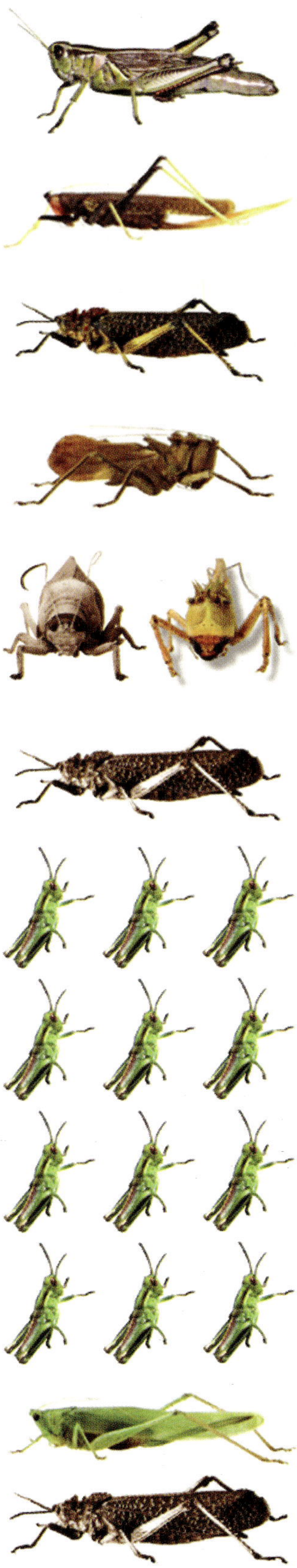

Unclean Insects

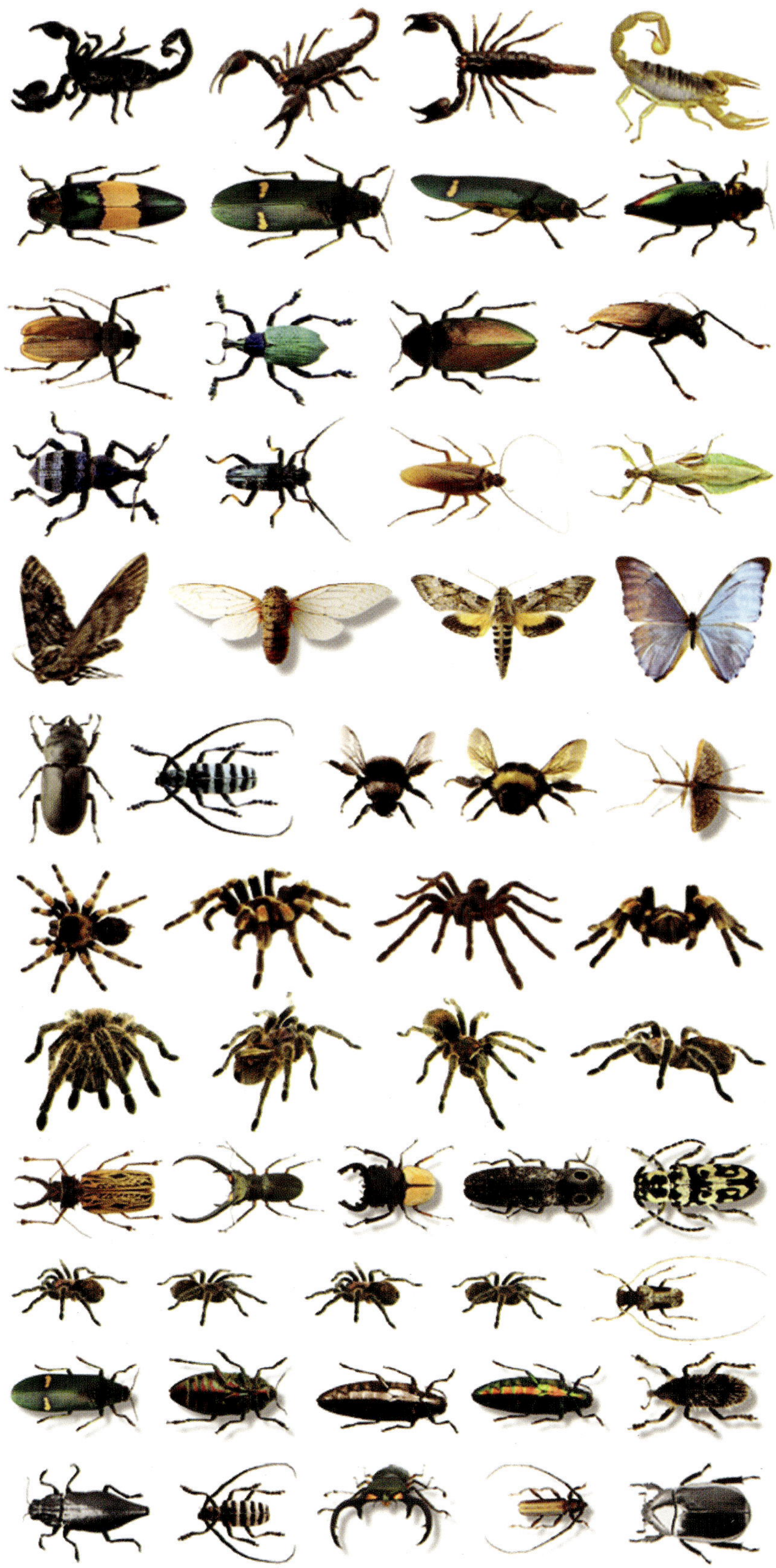

[R42]

Should People Follow the Dietary Laws Today?

Jews follow the ***Torah*** and ***Tanakh***, and their health has been consistently good as a result. Christians follow the ***Torah***, the ***Tanakh*** plus the teachings of Jesus, Paul and the New Testament. In 325 AD, the Nicean Council canonized the New Testament (***B'rit CHadashah***). In ≈96 AD, John, the last living Apostle, died. Muslims follow the teaching of Mohammed in the Koran, which was finished, in ≈650 AD, by Mohammed's third successor Caliph. Mohammed wisely included some teachings of Moses from the ***Torah*** in the Koran, such as the prohibition against eating pork. [R33]

---

1) The parenthetical statement that declares all foods clean is translated in the NIV to give the impression that Jesus encouraged abandoning the Mosaic dietary law; which is very misleading.

KJV Mark 7:18 And he [Jesus] saith unto them, Are ye so without understanding also?
Do ye not perceive, that whatsoever thing [food: such as meat] from without entereth
into the man, it cannot defile him; vs19 Because it entereth not into his heart,
but into the belly, and goeth out into the draught, purging all meats?

NIV Mark 7:18 "Are you so dull?" he [Jesus] asked. "Don't you see that nothing [food: i.e. - meat]
that enters a man from the outside can make him 'unclean'? vs19 For it doesn't go into his heart
but into his stomach, and then out of his body." (In saying this, Jesus declared all foods "clean.")

"... as Jesus relates that food (the literal translation of the word 'meats' in verse 19, is 'food' - he is not speaking of flesh) cannot defile the man "Because it entereth not into his heart." ... Would Jesus break any part of the law or suggest such to us? It is true that breaking the dietary law does not defile the spiritual heart but it certainly can defile the human flesh." [R3C]

Jesus said that eating any food (including meats) will not cause people spiritual defilement; but spiritual defilement comes from evil thoughts of a sinful man's heart, of which all are guilty. [R3C]

2) Peter's vision is often regarded as justification to dismiss the importance of the dietary laws.

NKJV Acts 10:10 ... he [Peter] fell into a trance vs11 and saw heaven opened and an object
like a great sheet bound at the four corners, descending to him and let down to the earth. vs12 In
it were all kinds of four-footed animals of the earth, wild beasts, creeping things, and birds of the
air. vs13 And a voice came to him, "Rise, Peter, kill and eat." vs14 But Peter said, "Not so, LORD!
For I have never eaten anything common or unclean." vs15 And a voice spoke to him again the
second time, "What God has cleansed you must not call common." vs16 This was done three
times. And the object was taken up into heaven again. vs17 Now while Peter wondered within
himself what this vision which he had seen meant, behold, the men who had been sent from
Cornelius had made inquiry for Simon's house, and stood before the gate. ... vs28 Then he said
to them, "You know how unlawful it is for a Jewish man to keep company with or go to one of
another nation. But God has shown me that I should not call any man common or unclean."

Peter was initially perplexed as to the meaning of the vision. Peter didn't immediately rise and eat pork, instead he visited Cornelius and fellowshipped with gentiles. [R3D] Then, Peter reasoned correctly that the vision was to show him that he, a Jew, should no longer call gentiles unclean.

3) Daniel and his three friends, while living in Persia, were encouraged to eat clean meat along with unclean meat. They chose to eat no meat at all, rather than to eat clean and unclean meat. After 10 days on a vegetarian diet, the health of Daniel and his friends was judged to be superior to others who ate both clean and unclean meat. (Dan 1:8-16) Seventh Day Adventists have often followed a similar vegetarian dietary program for the last 100^{+} years, with similarly good results.

4) The Apostle Paul, in his 1st letter to Timothy, stated that meat *[broma*] which was created for food was appropriate to eat; but not all meat (i.e.-unclean) was created to be received as food. (1 Tim 4:1-5)

Food for thought: Do the dietary laws in Leviticus 11 and Deuteronomy 14 pertain to health?
If there was a hygienic aspect to the dietary laws in the day of Moses, has this changed today?
Was a hygienic aspect of the Mosaic dietary laws part of the ***havdala*** separation that the LORD intended between Hebrews in the Promised Land, and heathens in the surrounding nations?
If the kosher dietary laws were originally intended in part for health, and this book documents a health benefit to following them: What, if any, are the reasons not to follow the dietary laws?

*** To follow, or not to follow Mosaic Law for clean/unclean meat, that is the health question.**

Standard American Diet

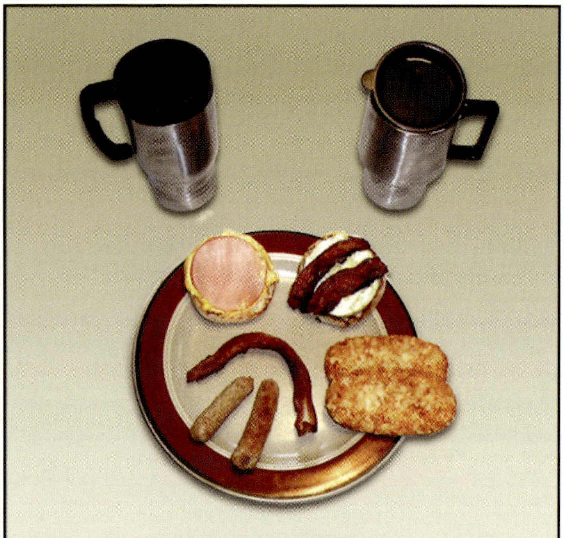

Egg-Pork Muffin – Fried Hash Brown
Coffee

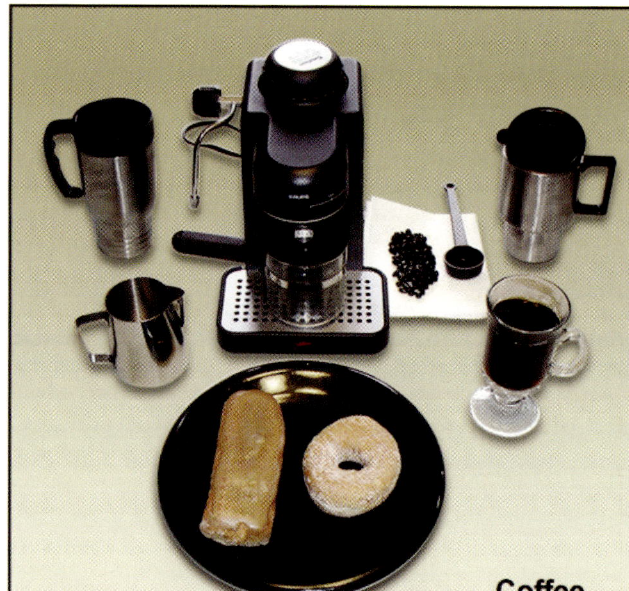

Coffee
Donuts

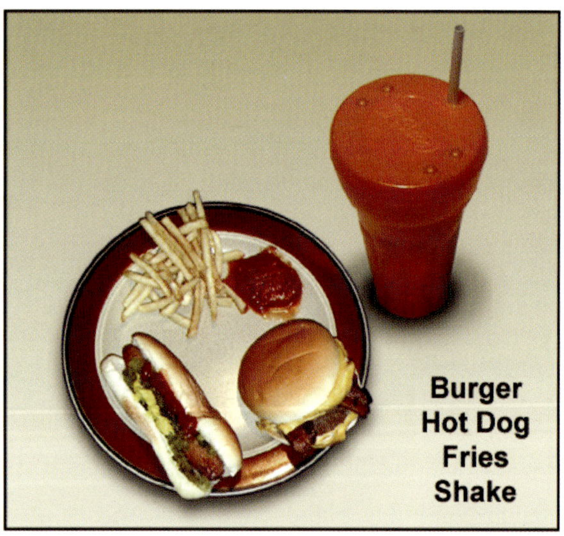

Burger
Hot Dog
Fries
Shake

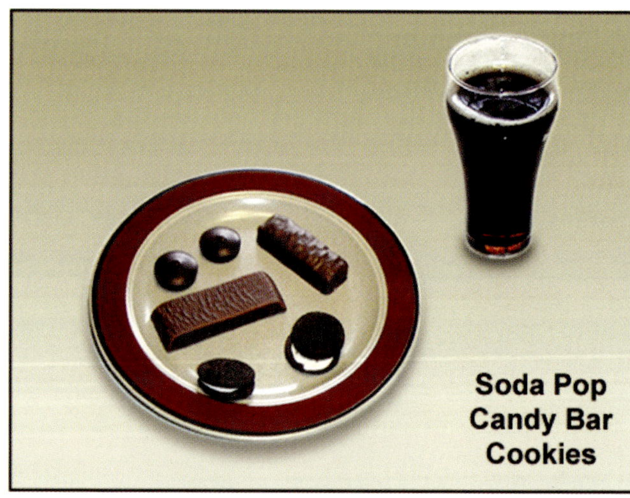

Soda Pop
Candy Bar
Cookies

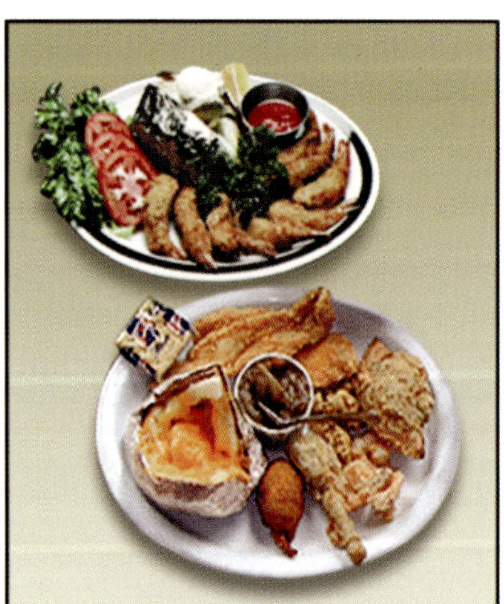

Shellfish Combo

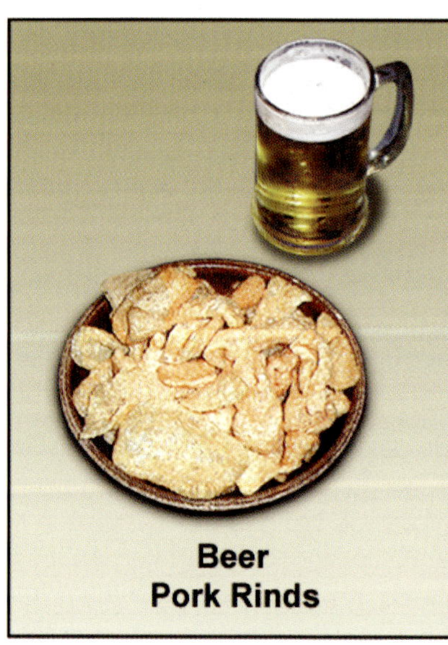

Beer
Pork Rinds

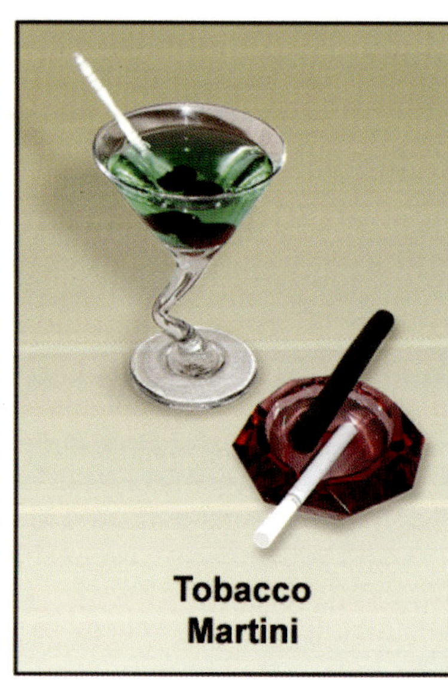

Tobacco
Martini

Jay's – Favorite Fast Fitness Foods

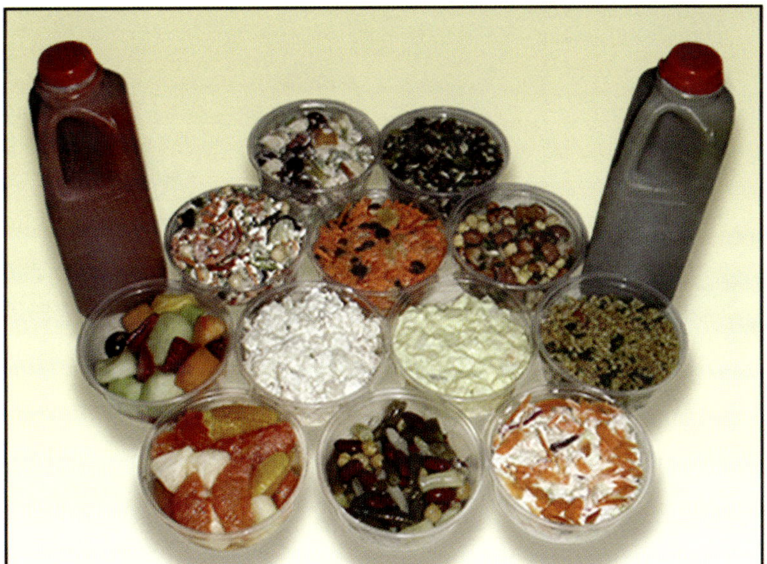

Tomato/Vegetable Juice Blend & Deli Salads & Green Juice Blend

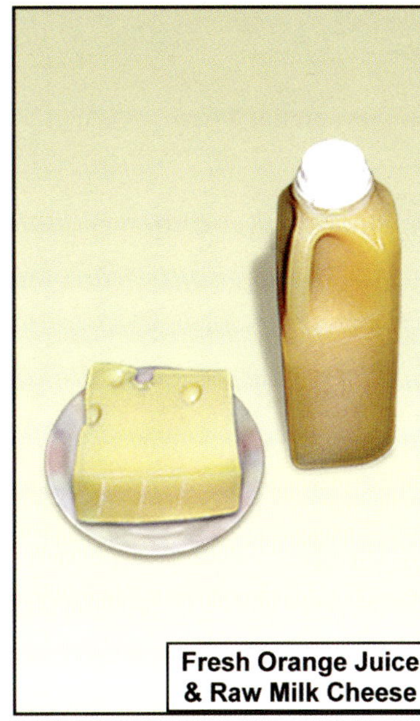

Fresh Orange Juice & Raw Milk Cheese

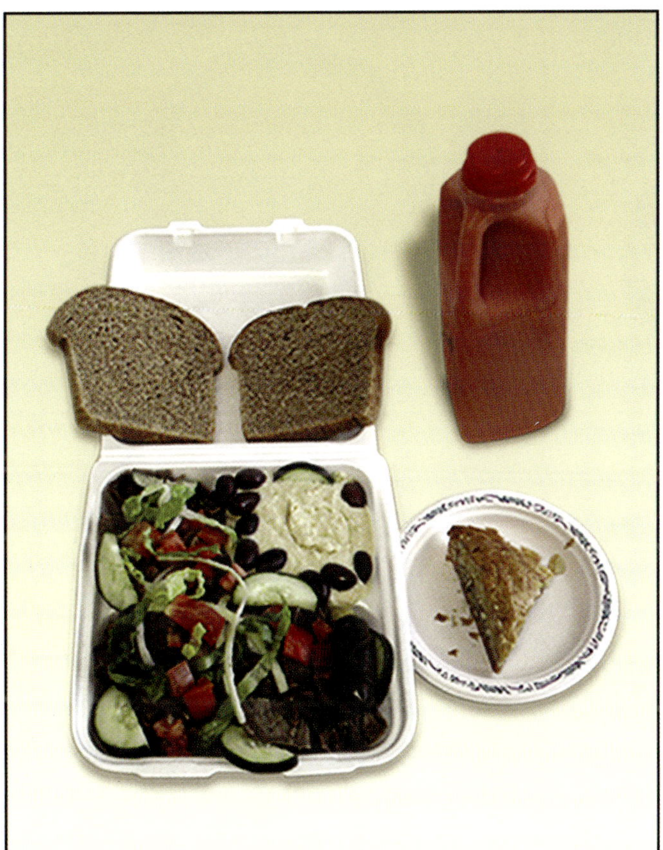

Beef & Lamb with Vegetables – Whole Whole Wheat Bread
Hummus – made of Chickpeas, Tahini, Olive oil and Garlic.
Carrot juice — Baklava made of Honey, Wheat flour & Nuts

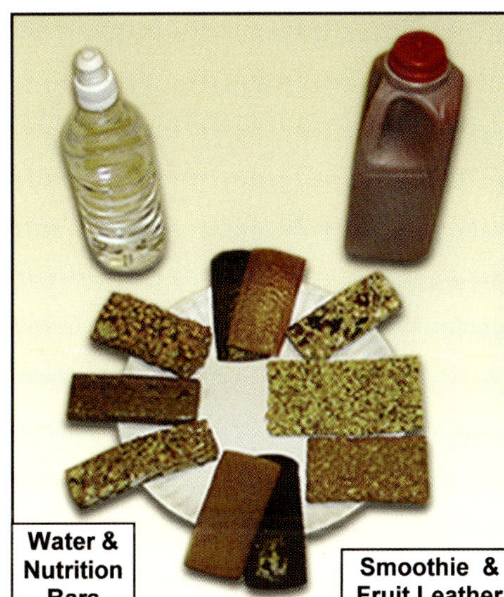

Water & Nutrition Bars

Smoothie & Fruit Leather

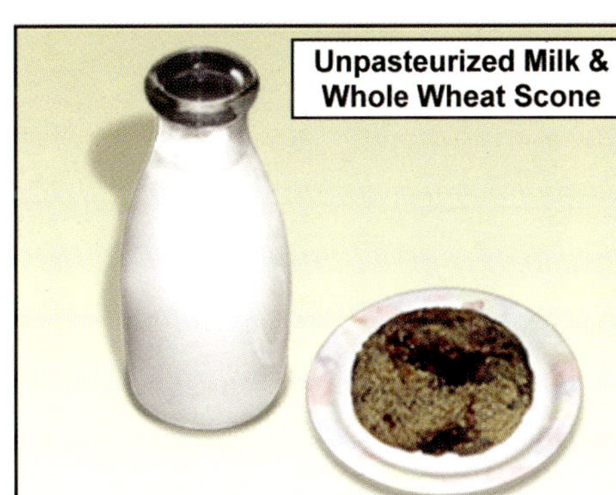

Unpasteurized Milk & Whole Wheat Scone

Quick meals and snacks for active people can be healthy and scrumptious, if people make wise choices. Great snacks that aren't pictured include: raw nuts, raw seeds, ripe fruit, dried fruit and fresh vegetables.

Kosher Food photos – pg 1

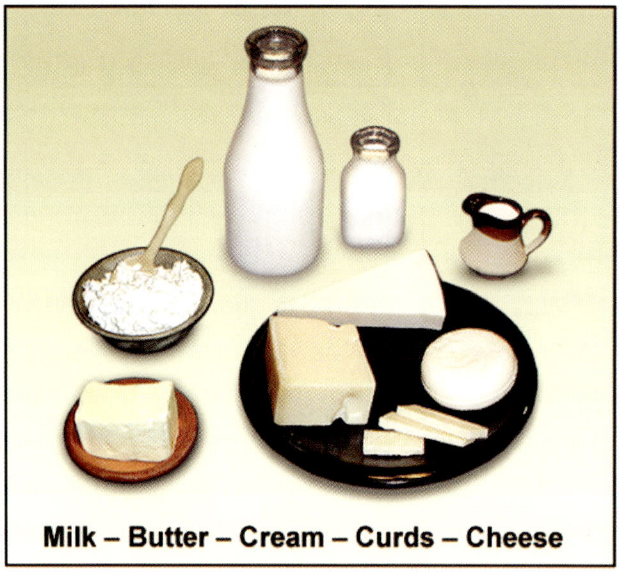

Milk – Butter – Cream – Curds – Cheese

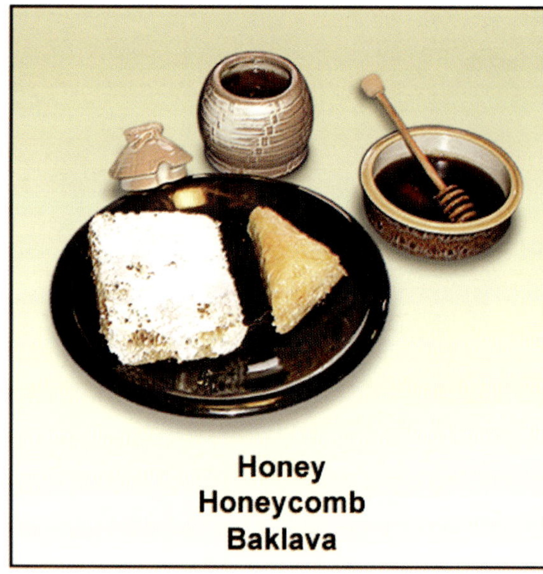

Honey
Honeycomb
Baklava

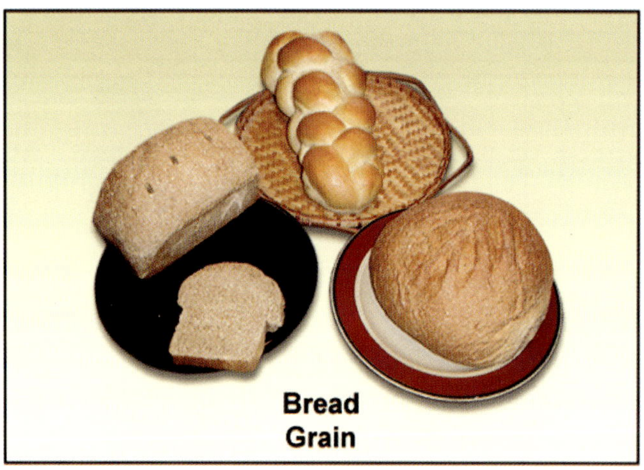

Bread
Grain

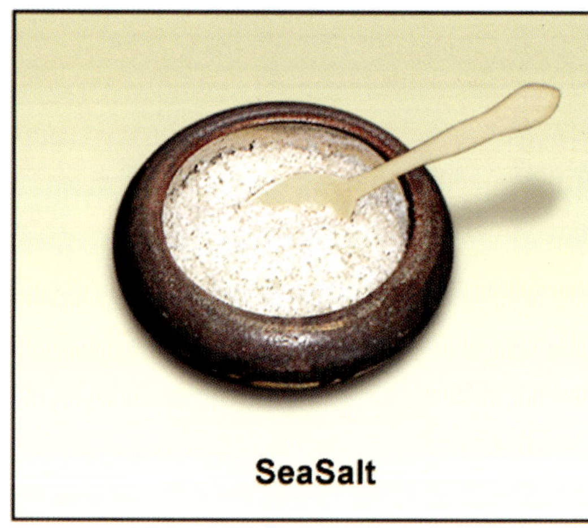

SeaSalt

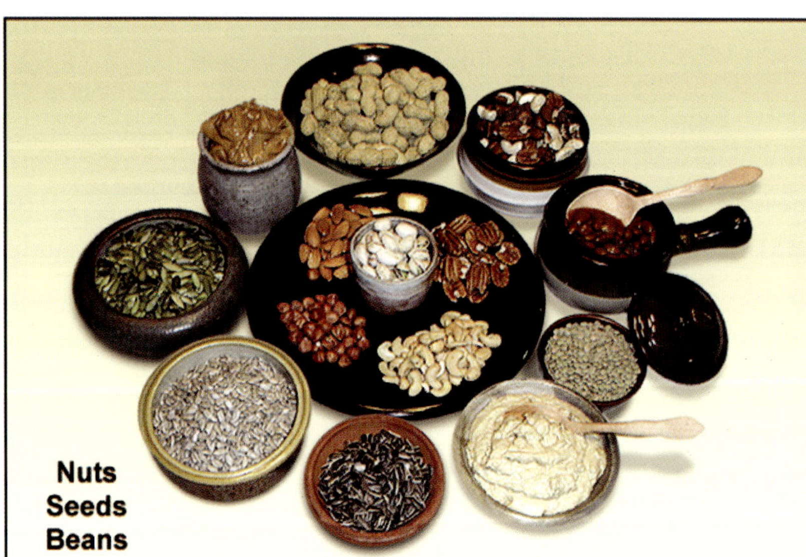

Nuts
Seeds
Beans

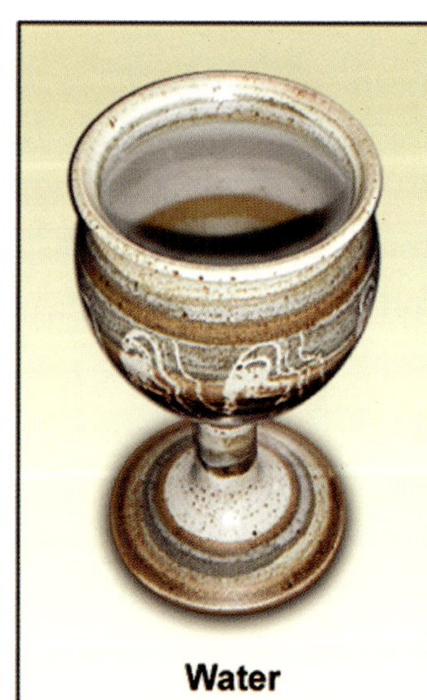

Water

Seven Days without *Kosher* food makes one weak.

Kosher Food photos – pg 2

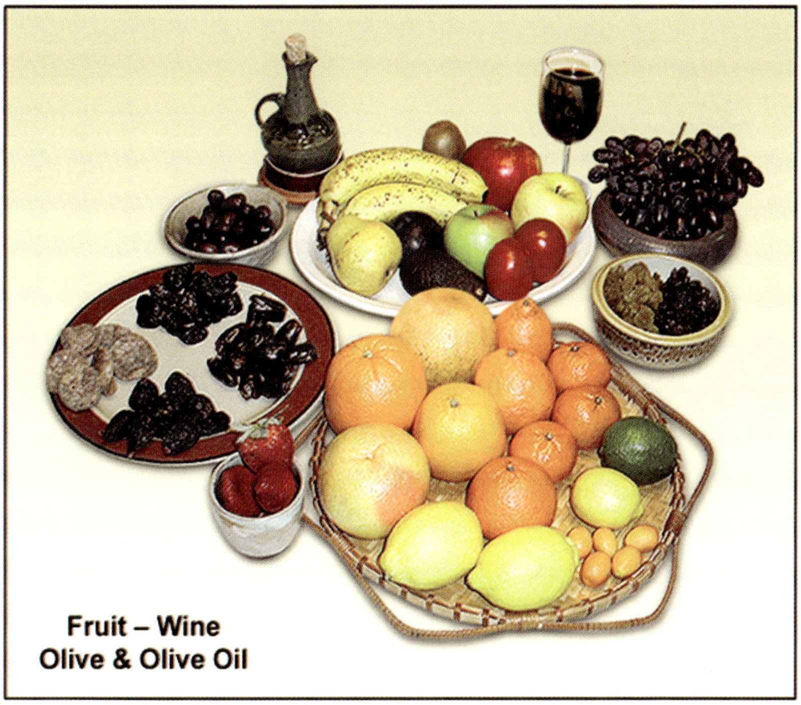

Fruit – Wine
Olive & Olive Oil

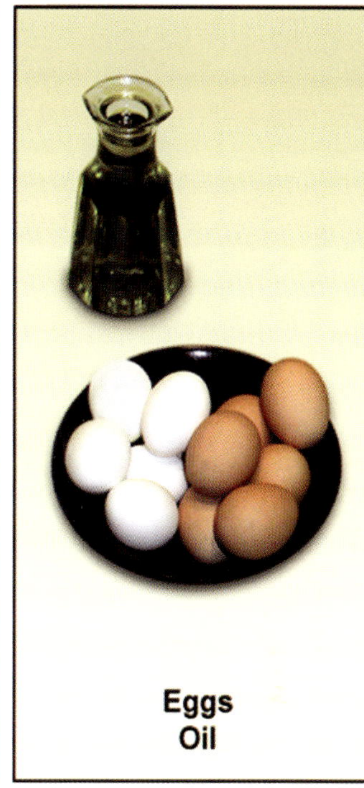

Eggs
Oil

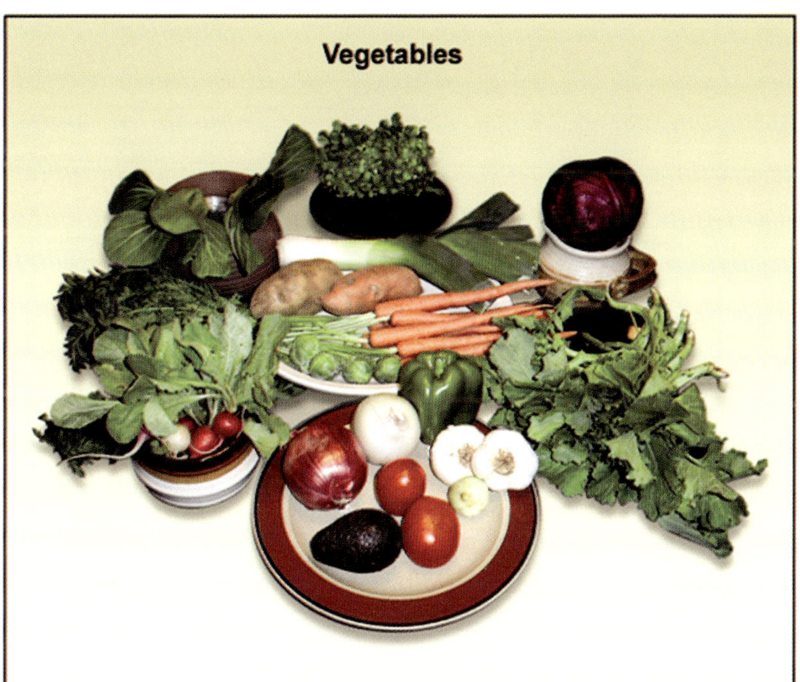

Vegetables

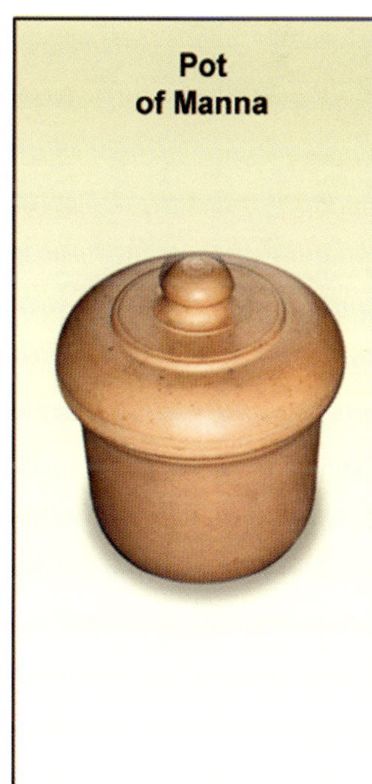

Pot
of Manna

Seven Days without *Kosher* food makes one weak.

Section V: KOSHER (Fit and Proper) FOOD
Chapter 14 Milk and Dairy Products
Raw Milk

The 'Rest of the Story' continues by examining foods in the Hebrew diet. Milk has been a staple of man's diet since Abel was a keeper of the flocks. (Gen 4:2) Milk (***chalav***) is first directly mentioned as food in Genesis 18, when Abraham served it to God's three messengers.

KJV Gen 18:8 And he [Abraham] took butter (***chemah***), and milk (***chalav***), and the calf which he had dressed, [prepared] and set it before them [the three messengers of God] ...

Moses was a keeper of flocks, as were all the Patriarchs and many other Hebrews. (Ex 3:1) (Gen 46:32-34) Milk from their herds was undoubtedly a normal part of the healthy Hebrew diet, and gave the Hebrews in Goshen a huge health edge over the Egyptians, who often preferred beer.

KJV Gen 46:32 And the men are shepherds, ... vs34 ... Thy servants' trade hath been about cattle from even until now, both we and also our fathers

KJV Ex 3:1 Now Moses kept the flock of Jethro his father in law, the priest of Midian: ....

Calcium is needed by the body in abundance and dairy products are the only foods that can meet this need. [R12] Carl Pfeiffer, PhD, MD in his book *Mental and Elemental Nutrients* states that in addition to calcium, milk contains phosphorous and magnesium in a balanced ratio for the needs of the body, and everyone should drink at least one glass per day. [R11] Today, in most 'civilized' countries, the majority of milk is pasteurized, and cows' milk is also often homogenized. Milk that is <u>not pasteurized</u> is labeled: 'Raw Milk', and it is often banned by law from public sale. (Understanding animal husbandry and dairy hygiene is needed to comprehend the health issues of milk processing.)

As nutritionally perfect as milk is, the production of clean healthy pathogen-free milk is still dependent upon dairies following proper biblical standards of hygiene for their animals. In recent times, including today, cleanliness of dairy cows has often been neglected or has been largely ignored states William Campbell Douglass, MD in his book *The Milk Book*. Up to the late-1800s, Dr. Herman E. Hillaboe, the commissioner of the New York State Health Department reported that cows were milked in a mixture of 'manure, mud, dust, dirt and filth' and disease–causing germs were as much the total product that people drank as was the milk itself. On farms, pails that were used to carry slop to pigs were also used without first being cleaned to convey milk to human consumers. [R2] Dr. Douglass also said that cows produce two things in great abundance: one is milk; the other is manure. A cow's legs and udders are frequently caked with mud and manure. Unfortunately, many people drank an unhealthy mixed product of milk, mud and manure. [R2A]

Dr. Park of the New York City Health Department reported: [R2B]

"Cholera infantum was a dreaded disease of children in the early 20th century.
Five thousand babies died annually from this summer diarrhea. The cause was found to be milk contaminated by an excessive number of 'ordinary dirt bacteria'. <u>Just plain dirty milk!</u>" [R2B]

In 1984, the author observed a lack of proper dairy hygiene, while visiting Cali, Colombia in South America as part of a VOSH (Volunteer Optometric Service to Humanity) trip to distribute used eyeglasses to needy people. One morning, I noticed a dairyman walking his cow in a field. **∗ The cow had every manner of mud, manure, dirt and filth caked on its udders and teats.** My hosts got their morning milk from this farmer, and the milk was put in a pot on the stove and brought to a boil 3 times, to kill the 'bad amoebae'. The microbes and milk were now both dead!

The association between drinking raw milk and human disease is not properly linked to any imperfection or uncleanness in raw milk itself. Health problems from drinking raw milk are always related to poor animal husbandry and/or contamination of milk after the milk leaves the cow, often by not keeping the legs, udders and teats of the cow clean. [R2] The milker may also become the agent by which mud or manure from the cow's legs and udders or just plain dirt and filth may contaminate healthy milk. The milker may also carry his own disease–causing germs to the milk, as was occasionally the case with tuberculosis (TB). Milkers with contagious diseases might not be quarantined until after they become observably ill. When infectious workers are allowed to milk cows, they can transfer disease to consumers who drink milk. Other ways to contaminate healthy milk frequently came from distributing milk in unsanitary containers. [R2T] Paramount health problems from drinking milk developed in the 1800s, when many people moved away from rural farms, to live in crowded cities with poor standards for dairy husbandry, sanitation and hygiene.

∗ The health value of fresh 'raw' dairy products in the Hebrew diet cannot be over emphasized.
∗ Dirty, unhygienic handling of otherwise healthy raw milk can produce deadly human disease.

Louis Pasteur Never Pasteurized Milk

In 1864, Louis Pasteur heated beer and wine (≈145°F for ≈30 minutes) to arrest fermentation. Wine and Beer could now be bottled and kept without spoiling. In the mid-1800s, bacteria were discovered everywhere, including in food. Bacteria are central to the 'germ theory' of disease. [R2F] Diseases such as leprosy, malaria, tuberculosis and cholera were found to be 'caused' by germs. Since infants were getting ill from drinking milk, bacteria were sought as the cause of this disease. Pasteurization of milk solved the cholera infantum disease and other diseases of dirty milk by killing all bacteria in milk. [R2-2G] Pasteurization allowed dirty milk to be consumed without the consumer immediately becoming sick, but pasteurization did nothing to make dirty milk clean.

Louis Pasteur never pasteurized milk! In 1891, milk was first 'flash pasteurized' in Germany. The 30 minutes at 145°F that Pasteur used to pasteurize wine and beer didn't work for milk; as the low heat and long time resulted in milk that was unpalatable and not all bacteria were killed. [R7F] 'Flash pasteurization' of milk for 30 seconds at 184°F resulted in milk that people would drink. [R7F-30]

In the early 1900s, pasteurization of milk could have a temporary expedient, to allow the dairy industry time to eliminate 'swill milk' and institute strict dairy hygiene standards for delivering fresh wholesome milk from the farm to the city. [R2D] However, the effort required for safe collection and transport of raw milk soon showed many profit-minded dairyman that lax standards of dairy hygiene followed by flash pasteurization was by far easier, less expensive and more convenient. Flash pasteurized milk can remain at the market for a much longer time without apparent spoilage. Pasteurization of milk reduces the amount of milk that spoils and is thrown out, which maximizes a dairyman's profit. ∗ One-week-old raw milk sours, while, two-week-old pasteurized milk rots. [R2D]

In 1891, after Dr. Henry Coit's 2-year-old son died from contaminated milk, Dr. Coit set out to ensure high standards of dairy husbandry and hygiene, so people could drink the best quality milk.

> "Dr. Henry Coit, the father of certified milk, recognized clearly that top quality milk depended upon getting the milk fresh from the cow and not heating it as is done in the pasteurization process. He recognized that the best way to present the best and most nutritious product to the public was to deliver it as made by nature from a completely clean environment." [R2A]

'Raw Certified' dairies such as Mathis in Georgia and Steuve in California conduct inspections of cows by physicians, and they produce milk certified to meet rigid standards of cleanliness. [R2A]

Professor Fosgate, of the Dairy Science Department of the University of Georgia, discussed the notion that pasteurization has been preached as a 100% safeguard for milk. [R2G]

> "If milk gets contaminated today, the chances are it will be after pasteurization. Pasteurized milk and raw milk are equally susceptible to contamination by pathogenic bacteria ..." [R2G]

Dr. Douglass says because raw milk contains enzymes and antibodies that are destroyed by pasteurization, raw milk is less susceptible to bacterial contamination than pasteurized milk. [R2Q] While *salmonella* contamination of raw milk has never been a problem for raw certified dairies, *salmonella* contamination has occasionally been a health problem for pasteurized dairy products. Once healthy bacteria normally present in milk are destroyed by flash pasteurization, as is always the case, milk is much more vulnerable to *salmonella* contamination than when it was 'raw'. [R2P]

> "It [salmonella] is ubiquitous. Salmonella is in your nose; it is in your living room rug. There is salmonella in your gut and plenty in your hair. It is also in your food — all your food that hasn't been sterilized and sealed in a container. The CDC reported an outbreak [1979] of salmonella food poisoning in Arizona. Twenty-three people sick – from pasteurized milk." [R2S]

A 1985 episode of milk contamination by *salmonella* in the Midwest United States led to 7,000 reported cases of illness and 70,000 suspected cases of gastrointestinal disease. [R29] The culprit was milk contaminated by improper dairy hygiene after pasteurization, not one case from raw milk.

Many people have allergies to pasteurized milk, due to milk proteins altered by heat. [R2F] Raw milk in the USA contains as much vitamin C as the entire citrus crop, but most vitamin C in milk is destroyed during pasteurization. [R2Q] The enzyme phosphatase is also destroyed in pasteurization. Phosphatase is necessary for milk calcium absorption, which may explain why osteoporosis is such problem in elderly women. Osteoporosis, a loss of calcium, causes bones to lose size and strength. Similar problems exist with the loss of other milk enzymes after pasteurization: no galactase for milk sugar digestion, no lipase for fat digestion, and no diatase, peroxidase or catalase either. [R2Q]

Pasteurization has had a huge impact on milk consumption by extending the 'shelf life of milk', which transformed the dairy industry from relative obscurity to a food industry giant in about a century.

In *The Milk Book* summary, Dr. Douglass says pasteurized, homogenized milk is biochemically, enzymatically and nutritionally as close to raw milk, as non-dairy creamer is to raw cream. [R2G]

∗ No wonder Dr. Douglass in 'The Milk Book' describes pasteurization of milk as 'udder destruction'.

Swill Milk

In the 1830s, the problem of unclean milk causing salmonella or cholera infantum went way beyond the contamination of milk by an unwashed milker or the collection of milk in an unsanitary container or the transport of unhygienically kept milk from the farm to the city on a hot summer day.
∗ In the 1830s, the biggest culprit in milk-borne disease was unscrupulous dairy husbandry. ∗
In the 1830s, distillers were in the cities, where they made whiskey from rye and corn. ∗ 'Swill' is the watery remains of rye or corn after whiskey-making that became cheap feed for dairy cows. By the 1880s, most dairy cows moved out of the cities to rural farms, and milk was delivered by wagon to cities in large metal cans. Milk was often distributed to consumers by a milk wagon, or by a milkmaid, who carried two large buckets of milk suspended from a yolk over their shoulders. [R2-7]

"The cattle stood in rows of seven to ten across the building. Most of the stalls were no more than three feet wide by eleven feet long. But most of the cows in the swill-milk dairies never left their stalls from the time they entered them. An average cow in one of these dairies consumed about thirty-two gallons of swill a day. The animals drank no fresh water, since the distillers figured they were getting enough water from the swill. Nor were most of them given any hay or other solid fodder to eat. As a result their teeth began to go bad because they had nothing to chew on. Although the animals were weak, unfit specimens, they were milked daily, ... These cows produced more than five million gallons of swill milk each year. [Robert] Hartley described the milk as being 'very thin and of a pale bluish color'. To make it [swill milk] look richer and whiter, he [Hartley] claimed that the distillery dairymen frequently added starch, flour, plaster of Paris and chalk. In some of the dairies the mixing was done in unclean cans, and the milkmen who handled the job were dirty too. Because of this, Hartley suggested, there might well be a connection between swill milk and the startling rise in infant deaths." ∗ [7B]

In 1848, the New York Academy of Medicine found that most swill milk they sampled had far less nutritional value than pure milk from upstate New York, and the swill milk was positively ... [R7A]
"... detrimental, especially to young children, and is a probable cause of many fatal diseases."

Swill milk was much cheaper than farm milk, and was often all that poor people could afford. Swill fed cows were often too weak to stand and were supported by a rope harness so they could be milked. Children who drank swill milk often suffered from terrible diarrhea and were often fatal victums of ordinary childhood diseases such as chicken pox or measles. Long low-ceilinged wooden swill dairy stables often housed hundreds of cows, summer temperatures often reached 110° F, and manure piled up until it had to be moved. Swill fed cows seldom lived more than 6 months. [R7C] Swill milk was nutritionally bankrupt and likely deficient in friendly bacteria. Unhealthy bacteria likely grew at will in swill milk, without competition from friendly bacteria. In 1910, 'swill milk' led Nathan Straus on his campaign to <u>pasteurize all milk</u> – his moto was: 'to save the babies is my religion'. [R7E]

In 1853, Gail Borden first produced canned 'Condensed Milk' and Civil War soldiers drank it. [R7G] Borden produced disease-free milk, but for canned milk to preserve nutritional value is impossible. Borden must have heated the milk, similarly to pasteurization, to preserve the milk as canned.

Milk and Meat

Moses wrote no instruction that required heating or processing milk in any manner. Cooking a calf in its mother's milk was part of heathen idolatrous worship of their false gods. [R3-13] Moses commanded three times that this was not to be done, as the LORD required the Hebrews to set themselves apart spiritually and physically (– ***havdala*** –) from their wicked, ungodly neighbors.

JPS Ex 23:19 Thou shalt not seethe a kid in its mother's milk.
NKJV Ex 34:25 or Deut 14:21 "You shall not boil a young goat in its mother's milk."

Based on these three verses, Orthodox Judaism requires that all meat and all dairy products be eaten at separate meals and many Jews have separate dishes/utensils for meat and dairy products. Today, 'Kosher' approved food requires inspection by a Rabbi to give assurance that meat and milk are not found in the same product, nor were any meat and dairy products cooked in the same oven.

There is no nutritional reason that dairy products and meat cannot be eaten together.

Abraham served the three messengers meat, milk and a cultured dairy product at the same meal.

NIV Gen 18:8 He [Abraham] then brought some curds and milk and the calf that had been prepared, and set these before them [the messengers of God].

Abraham knew the three messengers were from the LORD, and he served them the best food.

∗ How 3 key *Torah* verses are interpreted has a huge impact on 'Kosher' food/meal preparation.

Cultured Dairy Products

The Hebrews consumed cultured, churned milk products (***chemah***) in their diet. (Gen 18:8) The Hebrew word ***chemah*** could be properly translated as either curds or butter.

NIVDeut 32:13 He nourished him [Jacob]... vs14 with curds (***chemah***) and milk from the flock, ...

KJV Deut 32:14 Butter (***chemah***) of kine, and milk of sheep, ...

Churned dairy products are produced by agitating milk at a constant warm temperature for several hours, which allows bacteria within milk to 'culture' or multiply. Churning or agitating milk ensures that growing bacteria will culture all milk within the animal skin. As bacteria multiply they digest or partially breakdown the complex of carbohydrates, proteins and fats in the milk to more simple molecules, which results in a cultured or 'predigested' dairy product. [R2D] Since the bacteria in milk are also the same bacteria that normally populate the healthy human intestines, cultured dairy products are rich in 'friendly' bacteria. Curds are the solid portion of cultured dairy products, and are called cottage cheese; and whey is the liquid portion of cultured dairy products. Today, there is very little demand for fresh liquid whey, so whey is often powdered and added to other food products. Whey is great for maintaining intestinal flora and as a protein supplement.

Laben was cultured dairy product. Laben may have been used similarly to yogurt today. [R30] Laben as a drink was made by keeping milk and yeast warm in a covered dish for one day. [R10] Laben as cultured milk may have been similar to buttermilk. Laben may have been preserved like cheese. Laben may have been added to raw milk and churned to culture milk into buttermilk. [R26] Laben means the color 'white', as in milk. Laban was also the name of Jacob's father-in-law. [R18]

Butter is a solidified cultured dairy product made by churning cream. Cream is pure milk fat.

Today, most milk is pasteurized, which destroys both healthy and unhealthy bacteria. Yogurt is one of many dairy products that are cultured with friendly bacteria not normally present in milk. Yogurt may be very valuable in helping to maintain a healthy balance of bacteria in the intestines. (For live friendly healthy yogurt bacteria be certain the yogurt is not pasteurized after the milk is cultured.) People who cannot easily digest pasteurized milk can often digest cultured dairy products such as: cottage cheese, cheese, yogurt, kefir, whey, butter or buttermilk, etc. Milk from an unclean animal, such as camel, is considered unclean, and is difficult, if not impossible, to culture. (Gen 32:15 {16})

Mother's milk is always the perfect food for every newborn. Most babies do well when nursed for several months up to a couple of years. After or during the weaning time from mother's breast, fresh 'raw' goat, sheep or cow's milk should become part of the diet. Raw fresh milk is healthy from the cradle to the grave. Unfortunately, feeding newborns a commercial formula rather than mother's milk, may overly tax the developing pancreas, and put the infant at a higher risk for developing type-2 diabetes in later years, than for an infant nursed on healthy breast milk. [R20]

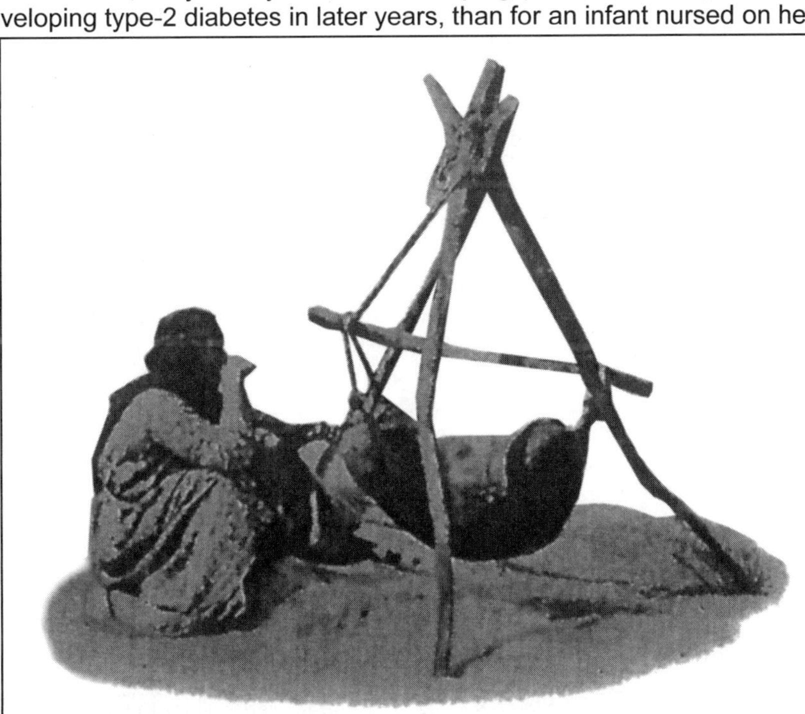

∗ Cultured raw milk dairy products such as cottage cheese, cheese, buttermilk, butter and kefir, as well as yogurt are often beneficial for good digestion.

Churning milk produces 'curds'. Churinng cream produces 'butter'.

Picture of a person churning milk in an animal skin or in an animal stomach on a stick supported by a tripod to make butter or curds. [R3A] DLiBT

Homogenization

Fat-soluble elements in whole milk, also called cream, include: lecithin; vitamin A; and EFAs. Water-soluble elements that make up the largest volume of whole milk include: proteins; sugars, such as galactase; vitamins such as B complex and C complex; and minerals, such as calcium. [R19] Milk fat (cream) is lighter than the water elements, causing much of the cream to rise to the top of and float on the water-soluble portion of the milk. Milk cream gives whole milk its rich, wholesome taste and is where the saying: 'the cream rises to the top' originates. The cream atop milk can be skimmed off the water portion of the milk, then, the cream can be churned and solidified as 'butter'.

The uniform mixing of water and fat-soluble portions of milk is called 'homogenization'. Goat's milk has smaller fat molecules that are more easily mixed within the water-soluble part of milk. Because goats' milk is naturally homogenized, the cream is largely intermixed within the water portion of the milk, and only a small amount of the cream will rise to the top of goats' milk. [R2H] Cow's milk contains mostly larger fats that are not easily intermixed within the water-soluble portion. Homogenization of cows' milk is produced when the long chain fat molecules are broken down into miniscule fat molecules of less than one millionth of a meter (or yard) in size by forcing the milk through very fine pores. [R2F] These extremely small, extremely artificial fat molecules in milk are now artificially homogenized or mixed within the water-soluble elements of cows' milk. The only reason to homogenize cows' milk is so the consumer can drink a uniform mixture of water-soluble elements and fat-soluble cream without needing to shake (i.e.– mix) milk each time before drinking.

∗ **Homogenization of cows' milk promises that cream will no longer rise to the top of milk.**

The normal pattern of digestion, assimilation and utilization of milk fat by the human body is disrupted for the miniscule homogenized milk fats. Dr. Kurt A. Oster has advanced a theory that homogenization of milk is closely related to atherosclerosis (plaque build-up on artery walls), which is very common for citizens in the developed countries of the world, where large quantities of pasteurized homogenized milk products are consumed. The reduction in size of the fat molecules caused by homogenization permits them to be assimilated directly through the stomach lining into the bloodstream in a manner that is not intended by nature. These miniscule homogenized fats along with xanthine oxidase are now unnaturally absorbed into the bloodstream directly from the gut (stomach) instead of first being metabolized by the digestive system and absorbed through the intestines. Xanthine oxidase is normally found within all milk, but is not absorbed under normal conditions (before the pasteurization and the homogenization of milk). Xanthine oxidase may disrupt the normal biochemistry in arteries, causing breaks or scarring of the artery walls. [R8] Injured artery walls may allow cholesterol plaques to form and may encourage vascular disease.

Jacob (Israel) likened the whiteness of teeth to (drinking white) milk. This was wise, as only milk and dairy products can provide the quantity and quality of calcium that is ideal for teeth.

KJV Gen 49:12 .. and his teeth white (***laben***) with milk.

Today, legislation often tries to ban the sale of fresh raw milk, while some physicians, such as, Dr. Douglass, Dr. Oster, Dr. Bieler and Dr. Jensen recognize the value of raw milk for good health and they recommend most people drink raw milk as part of a nutritional program. [2H-16A]

Statistics today suggest that in our old age (50s? 60s? 70s? 80s?), clogging of the arteries is inevitable and/or expected. Autopsies on American soldiers killed in the Korean War showed that 12% had a 50% blockage of some arteries of the heart and 5% had a blockage of 90%. [R2H] Is this the fate that God intended for mankind, when we consider that Abraham lived to be 175 years and Noah lived to be 950 years? Dr. Douglas suggests that pasteurized, homogenized milk may contribute to chronic degenerative disease, which are new modern-civilization diseases that are not prominent in the medical literature until the middle 19th or/and the 20th century. [R2E] Certainly, life spans after the Flood were considerably shorter than Methuselah's 969 years, but Moses was in perfect health when he was 120 years old. Could a change in dietary habits from Moses' time to today be partially responsible for today's declining health and shorter life span?

Which do you choose? Milk the way God designed it and the way Noah, Abraham, Isaac, Jacob and Moses consumed it, and the way milk was consumed for thousands of years since the time of Abel without any health problems; or the currently popular pasteurized homogenized fortified milk of the last 110 years, which seems to be at least partly responsible for many of the chronic degenerative health problems that plague our society in epidemic proportions today?

Mother's breast milk is the formula for health for all infants; while cow, goat or sheep furnish milk for longevity.

References Ch 14 Milk

[R1] Nutrition and Your Body\ by Benjamin Colimore, MA & Sarah Stewart Colimore, LPT;
pg 17-19 raw milk compared to pasteurized, homogenized milk

[R2] The Milk Book\ by William Campbell Douglass, MD; pg 4 germs in milk (swill) – Nathan Straus

[R2A] pg 5&64 need for cleanliness = Raw Certified Milk for today – Dr. Henry Coit

[R2B] pg 9 udders coated with mud, manure – 5,000 deaths from cholera infantum – Dr. Park

[R2C] pg 66-75 Chart comparing Raw Milk to Pasteurized Milk

[R2D] pg 10-11 Dairy Industry transformed – Pasteur + (pg 9&25) Pasteurization – a temporary expedient.

[R2E] pg 9&105 pasteurized/homogenized milk linked to modern chronic degenerative disease (CVD)

[R2F] pg 9-25 poor dairy hygiene – Pasteurized milk rots – Raw milk sours – (22) allergies

[R2G] pg 27&31 Professor Fosgate quote – Douglass quote: non-dairy creamer vs cream

[R2H] pg 103-110 homogenization of cow's milk

[R2P] pg 19&53 healthy bacteria lost from pasteurization of milk

[R2Q] pg 12-19&34 osteoporosis – loss of enzymes – loss of vitamin C

[R2S] pg 52-53 to 61 salmonella is ubiquitous in food, including pasteurized milk – but never in raw milk

[R2T] pg 58 infected workers brought TB to milk – modern hoses eliminate this risk

{old title} The Milk of Human Kindness is Not Pasteurized; by William Campbell Douglass, MD; // 1-800-728-2288

[R3] Daily Life in Bible Times\ by Albert Edward Bailey; pg 36 food & pg 44 herds of cattle, sheep

[R3A] pg 45 picture curds churning on tripod

[R4] Eat, Drink and Be Ready\ by Monte L. Kline, PhD and W.P. Strube Jr.; pg 203-206

[R5] Which Do You Choose?\ by Alta Dena (now Steuve) Dairy Raw and Pasteurized Milk Chart

[R6] Don't Drink Your Milk\ update by Dr. Monte Kline – allergy common to pasteurized milk {1-800-255-4246}

[R7] Milk The Fight for Purity\ by James Cross Giblin; pg 10 milkmaid picture – pg 13 milk wagon

[R7A] pg 19 NY Academy in 1948

[R7B] pg 16-19 – swill milk – quote concerning distillery

[R7C] pg 27 cows lived 6 months in swill dairy

[R7D] pg 29 children + swill milk = disease – pg 28 cow on hoist – pg 29 swill milk

[R7E] pg 56 In 1910, Nathan Straus led the campaign for pasteurization of all milk.

[R7F] pg 40-43 Pasteur heated beer & wine to 145° F-30 min // milk is 'flash pasteurized' to 184° F-30 sec

[R8] The X O Factor\ by Kurt Oster, MD; harmful to health xanthine oxidase – homogenization

[R9] Article in the A.J.C.R., vol II, No 1, April 1971\ by Kurt Oster, MD homogenization

[R10] Manners and Customs of Bible Lands\ by Fred H. Wight; pg 49-51 milk and dairy

[R11] Mental and Elemental Nutrients\ by Carl Pfeiffer, MD, PhD; pg 274-5 milk and calcium

[R12] What the Bible Says About Healthy Living\ by Rex Russell, MD; pg 213-221 milk – dairy

[R13] Don't Drink Your Milk\ by Frank Osky, MD what's wrong with milk today

[R14] Food is Your Best Medicine\ by Henry Bieler, MD; pg 208-213 raw milk as a healthy food

[R14A] pg 210-211 raw milk as a nutritional therapy

[R15] What Would Jesus Eat?\ by Don Colbert, MD; pg 71-77 milk – pasteurization reduces nutrition

[R16] LaLeche League – discusses the health value of breast milk for infants

[R17] Making the Best of Basics\ by James Talmage Smith; Ch 12 pg 135-136 powdered milk

[R18] Strong's Concordance\ by James Strong, STD, LLD (***cheleb*** – as 'meat fat' – pg 82)

pg 681	milk	# 2461	H pg 39	***chalav***	Gen 18:8
pg 158	butter	# 2529	H pg 40	***chemah***	Deut 32:13-14
pg 158	curds - cottage cheese	# 2529	H pg 40	***chemah***	Deut 32:13-14
pg 578	Laban - Rachel's dad	# 3837	H pg 58	**Laban**	Gen 29:10
pg 1148	white	# 3835	H pg 58	***laben***	Gen 49:12
--------	cultured milk drink	# 3836	H pg 58	***laben***	-------------------
pg 229	curdled (cheese)	# 7087	H pg 104	***qapha***	Job 10:10
pg 846	right	# 3787	H pg 58	***kasher – kawsher***	Esther 8:5

{***Kasher*** is often transliterated as *kashrut* or kosher. ***Kasher*** can also mean: clean, fit or proper.}

[R19] Nutrition Almanac (1979 Ed) \ pg 204-207 nutritional value of milk

[R20] 700 Club - Health Facts Video\ - formula feed babies are more likely to become diabetics

[R21] Pasteurization\ Encyclopedia Americanica 2000; Vol 21, pg 518; - 1864 Wine & Beer

[R22] Pasteurization\ Britanica Encyclopedia 1997; Vol 9; pg 190 - 1860s Wine & Beer – 145° F for 30 min

[R23] Help Yourself to Better Health\ by Monte Kline, PhD; (10-07-2000) 'Don't Drink Your Milk'

[R24] Pottenger's Cats\ by Francis M. Pottenger Jr., MD; cats feed raw milk verses heated milk

[R25] Proof Positive\ by Neil Nedley, MD; Ch 11 pg 237-255 milk

[R26] Encyclopedia of Bible Life\ (see nutrition); pg 313 laben drink

[R27] Food and Nutrition\ by Rodale Press; ch 34 milk and dairy

[R28] The 28 Day Antioxidant Program\ by Steven Masley, MD

[R29] Newspaper articles from 1985 mid-west outbreak of *salmonella* from pasteurized milk

[R30] Microbiology\ by Alice Lorraine Smith (7th Ed); pg 587 – 'flash pasteurization' of milk – 184° F for 30 sec

[R31] Milk the Deadly Poison\ by Robert Cohen // [R32] The Yogurt Cookbook; by Kay Shaw Nelson

[R33] Milk, Butter, and Cheese\ by Carolyn Meyer; pg 22 pasteurization

[R34] Judaism 101: Kashrut: Jewish Dietary Laws http://www.jewfaq.org/kashrut.htm

Milk Chart – Raw Certified Milk compared to Pasteurized Milk

CATEGORY	RAW CERTIFIED MILK	PASTEURIZED MILK
1. Enzymes:	**1.** All available.	**1.** Less than 10% remaining.
2. Protein: (All natural protein -bearing foods contain fats.)	**2.** 100% available, all 22 amino acids, including 8 that are essential.	**2.** Proteins - lysine and tyrosine are altered by heat with serious loss of metabolic availability. This results in making the whole protein complex less available for tissue repair and rebuilding.
3. Fats:	**3.** All 18 fatty acids 'metabolically available', both saturated and unsaturated fats.	**3.** Altered by heat, especially the 10 essential unsaturated fats.
∗ Research indicates:	∗ Fats are necessary to digest milk proteins and milk calcium.	∗ Fats are necessary to metabolize both protein and calcium from milk.
4. Vitamins:	**4.** All 100% available.	**4.** Among the fat-soluble vitamins, some are classed as unstable and therefore a loss is caused by heating above blood temperature. This loss can run as high as 66%. Vitamin C loss usually exceeds 50%. Losses on water-soluble vitamins are affected by heat and can run from 38% to 80%.
5. Carbohydrates:	**5.** Easily utilized in metabolism. Still associated naturally with elements.	**5.** Tests indicate that heat has made some changes, making elements less available metabolically.
6. Minerals:	**6.** All 100% metabolically available. Major mineral components are Calcium, Chlorine, Magnesium, Phosphorous, Potassium, Sodium and Sulfur. Vital trace minerals, all 24 or more, 100% available.	**6.** Calcium is altered by heat, and loss in metabolism may run 50% or more, depending on pasteurization temperature. Losses in other essential minerals, because one mineral usually acts as a synergistic for another element. There is a loss of enzymes that serve as leaders in assimilation of minerals.
7. Cleanliness:	**7.** Milk tested daily at an independent laboratory for the Certified Milk Commission in all states.	**7.** Never tested over twice per month by the Department of Health.
8. Bacteria count for standard plate count: Milk and cream	**8.** MILK : 10,000/millimeter maximum at all certified dairies. CREAM: 10,000/millimeter maximum in all states.	**8.** MILK: In Georgia, 100,000/ml before pasteurization and 30,000 after. In New York, 100,000 before and 30,000 after pasteurization. In California, 75,000/ml maximum before pasteurization and 15,000 after. CREAM: 25,000/ml maximum.
22. Milk Quality	**22.** Bacteria-Maximum allowable bacteria per millimeter of milk --- 10,000. Maximum allowable coliform bacteria per milliliter --- 10. Milk is considered excellent quality when the concentration of leukocytes does not exceed 500,000 per milliliter.	**22.** Generally tested 4 times each 6 months by the health department. Bacteria - Maximum count 100,000 per milliliter before pasteurization. 20,000 per milliliter maximum after. Not exceeding 300,000 per milliliter as commingled milk prior to pasteurization. Coliform bacteria count not checked on raw, but cannot exceed 10 per milliliter after pasteurization. Leukocyte count may not exceed 1,500,000 per milliliter.

Milk Chart from The Milk Book by William Campbell Douglass, MD – [R2C] pages 66 - 75

William Campbell Douglass, MD // Second Opinion Newsletter // PO Box 467939 // Atlanta, Georgia 31146 // 1-800-728-2288

Which Do You Choose?

D. NUTRITIONAL VALUES	RAW CERTIFIED MILK	PASTEURIZED MILK
** Wulzen and Bahrs reported that guinea pigs fed raw whole milk grew excellently and at autopsy showed no abnormality of any kind. Guinea pigs fed pasteurized milk rations did not grow as well and developed a definite syndrome, the first sign of which was wrist stiffness.	**1.** Enzymes, catalase, peroxidase and phosphatase are present. a) Phosphatase is needed to split and assimilate the mineral salts in foods that are in the form of phytates. b) Wulzen Factor (anti-stiffness) available. ** c) X Factor in tissue repair available.	**1.** Pasteurization destroys the enzyme phosphatase. a) Absence of phosphatase indicates that milk has been pasteurized. b) Wulzen Factor destroyed (anti-stiffness nutrition factor lost).** c) No evidence of alteration by pasteurization.
	2. Protein—100% metabolically available: all 22 amino acids, including the 8 that are essential, for the complete metabolism and function of protein.	**2.** Protein— Digestibility reduced by 4%, biological value reduced by 17%. From the digestibility and metabolic data it is concluded that the heat damage to lysine and possibly to histidine and perhaps other amino acids destroys the identity of these amino acids and partly decreases the absorbability of their Nitrogen.
	3. Vitamins —all 100% available **a)** Vitamin A —fat soluble **b)** Vitamin D —fat soluble **c)** Vitamin E —fat soluble **d)** Vitamin K —fat soluble **e)** Vitamin B —complex Vitamin Bw —Biotin Vitamin B —Choline Vitamin Bc —Folic Acid Vitamin B1 —Thiamine Vitamin B2 —Inositol Vitamin B2 —Nicotinic Acid Vitamin B2 —Riboflavin Vitamin B2 —Pantothenic Acid Vitamin B3 —Niacin Vitamin B6 —Pyridoxine Vitamin B12 —Cyanocobalamin **f)** Vitamin C g) Antineuritic vitamin	**3.** Vitamins **a)** Vitamin A —destroyed **b)** Not altered **c)** Not altered **d)** Not altered **e)** Vitamin B–complex — Pasteurization of milk destroys about 38% of the vitamin B complex. **f)** Vitamin C is weakened or destroyed by pasteurization. Infants fed pasteurized milk exclusively will develop scurvy. **g)** Testing of pasteurized milk indicates destruction of this vitamin.
	4. Minerals —all 100% available metabolically **a)** Major mineral components: Calcium, Chlorine, Magnesium, Phosphorous, Potassium, Sodium and Sulfur. **b)** Vital trace minerals, all 24 or more, 100% available.	**4.** Minerals —After pasteurization the total of soluble Calcium is very much diminished. The loss of soluble Calcium in regards to infants and growing children must be a very important factor in growth and development, not only in the formation of bone and teeth, but also in the Calcium content.
	5. Carbohydrates—easily utilized in metabolism. Still associated naturally with elements (instable).	**5.** Health inspector visits dairy monthly.
Which Do You Chose Chart from Steuve's Dairy	**6.** Fats-all 18 fatty acids metabolically available, saturated and unsaturated.	**6.** Fats— Pasteurization harms the fat content of milk.

Research indicates that fats are necessary to assimilate protein and calcium from milk.

Over-eating proteins, especially meats, may lead to acidosis – blood pH below the normal 7.34 pH. Calcium is useful as a 'buffer' for blood acidosis and to re-establish the required 7.34 pH for the blood. Overly acid blood may obtain extra Calcium to buffer acidosis from its Calcium bank – bones and teeth. Calcium from raw milk products and vegetables (especially greens) helps protect blood against acidosis.

Chapter 15 Honey
Nutritional Value of Honey

Honey (***devash***) was a special food gift that Jacob gave the Prime Minister of Egypt (Joseph).
KJV Gen 43:11 … take the best of the fruits in the land in your vessels, and carry the man [Joseph] a present, a little balm, and a little honey (***devash***), spices, and myrrh, nuts and almonds.

To make honey honeybees gather nectar from the flowers and process it in their digestive system. One pound of honey requires about 37,000 round trips of honeybees from the hive to the flowers and back. [R11] After breaking down complex carbohydrates in the nectar into the simple, 'predigested' sugars levulose and dextrose, honeybees deposit honey in the comb of their hive. [R1A-4-5] Honey is a valuable source of water-soluble vitamins B and C and a few minerals. [R3-4] The B vitamins found in the highest quantities in honey are - thiamine, riboflavin, pyridoxine, pantothenoic acid, biotin, and niacin. [R11A-5A] Although the total mineral content of honey is not high as compared to meat or milk, the minerals can be important when honey is used daily as a sweetener. [R1-2A-4A-5A] Minerals often found in honey include - aluminum, calcium, chlorine, copper, iron, magnesium, manganese, phosphorus, potassium, silicon (silica), sodium and zinc. Bodog Beck, MD in his book *Honey and Health* discusses the nutritional value of honey. [R2B-3-5]

Content of Honey	Percentage
Levulose (fructose)	40.50%
Dextrose (glucose)	34.02%
Water	17.70%
Sucrose	1.90%
Dextrins* and gums	1.51%
Ash-Minerals (Silicon, Iron, Copper, Manganese, Chlorine, Calcium, Potassium, Sodium, Sulfur, Phosphorus, Aluminum, Magnesium)	0.18%
Indeterminate Elements	4.19%
[R1-2-R4]	100.00%

The honey chart is an 'average' composition of American honey by percentage. [R1-2C-4]

Honey and Spice and all that's nice.

The indeterminate elements in honey include minute quantities of pigments, flavorings, sugar alcohols and inhibine – which is a substance that kills bacteria (bactericidal). [R5C]

(*Dextrin is a gum that is important in making honey easily digestible.) [R1B]

The sugars in honey are called 'invert' because the honeybee has taken the more complex carbohydrates in nectar and has broken them down into the simple monosaacharides: levulose (also called fructose) and dextrose (also called glucose). This pre-digestion of the nectar by the honeybee means the human digestive system does not have to do this work, and the sugars of honey are absorbable directly by the gastrointestinal tract. [R4] **Honey is predigested food!**

Pollen is found in honey. Honeybees gather pollen from plants at the same time as nectar. Pollen is rich in protein, is unprocessed by honeybees and is suspended within honey. [R2-5A]

"The pollen of many flowers has a higher vitamin C content than almost any fruit or vegetable. Honey with the largest amount of pollen will have more vitamin C than other honeys." [R4]

Honeybee larvae developing inside the hive live entirely on honey and pollen. Honey/pollen must be complete food for honeybees. [R1C] Pollen in honey is also important for human health. Processing drastically reduces the nutritional value of honey. Filtering, done under high-pressure, removes pollen and ash (i.e. – minerals – colloidal elements suspended within honey). [R2A-2C-3A] Commercial honey may often be allowed to absorb water, which increases profits for the vender. Honey that is watered down may lose its bactericidal property and is not better for human health. All unfiltered, unheated honey will eventually granulate or 'sugar' as the dextrose crystallizes. Granulation of honey is normal and does not change its nutritional value. Heating honey, which eliminates crystals, can prevent granulation of honey. If honey is heated above 150°F the nutritional value is considerably reduced and it will never granulate. Heating honey to prevent granulation has become common, since people often consider granulation a sign of spoilage. [2B] Warming granulated honey at low heat will return raw honey to its normal semisolid consistency.

∗ Heated, filtered, commercial honey is golden clear, easy flowing and looks appealing on a shelf, but contains extra water and lacks protein, enzymes, vitamins B & C and minerals; while pollen and ash makes raw unfiltered unheated honey unequaled as a sweetener. [R2B]

∗ Honey (and honeycomb), especially unfiltered and unheated honey, is the premier sweetener.

White Table Sugar

Although honey is one of the most perfect foods known to man, it has been largely replaced in modern society by white, processed sugar as a sweetener. White table sugar is technically a food, because it provides calories that the body can use for energy; however, the effect of sugar on the body, and the digestive system in particular, is more like a drug than a food! [R2F]

A publication from the sugar industry *Sugar As A Food* justifies their refining of sugar: [R6A]

"Refined, granulated sugar contains almost no vitamins or minerals. Assays, however, show that neither the sugar cane or sugar beet is sufficiently rich as a natural source of vitamins and minerals to justify the effort to retain them in the finished product. Besides, the small quantities that are lost are ordinarily amply supplied by many other foods with which sugar is used in the diet." [R6A]

However, the enlightened scientific community has recognized the danger of consuming these processed sugars for a long time. In 1929, Dr. F. G. Banting, the discoverer of insulin, delivered a forthright warning on the subject of artificial sugar (white table sugar):

"In the United States the incidence of diabetes has increased proportionately with the per capita consumption of cane sugar. In the heating and recrystalization of natural sugar cane, something is altered which leaves the refined product a dangerous foodstuff." [R2F]

Dr. Harvey Wiley, chief chemist of the US Dept. of Agriculture and director of the Bureau of Food, stated that daily use of refined sugar was hazardous to health. [R2F-3] Dr. Wiley also wrote about processing food, using dangerous chemicals to preserve canned food, putrefied meat in sausages and potted meats, and other ways that food manufacturers damaged human health. Unfortunately, Dr. Wiley's voice against processed foods and sugar was largely ignored. [R2-3-6-7]

Dr. Beck discussed ill health from eating white, table sugar as does Monte Kline, PhD: [R2-6]

"Refined sugar has a calorie content that will provide heat and energy; but it does not provide nourishment. All of the artificial sugars and syrups, whether cane, corn, beet or maple, are manufactured by a process in which all of their nutritive properties are destroyed. In the manufacture of cane sugar, for instance, the cane is heated with fumes of burning sulfur, or else heated with bisulfide of lime – a process in which all of the fats, proteins, minerals, vitamins and enzymes of the natural cane juice are extracted. The sugar crystals that form are sterile. Because sugar is a devitalized product, it will keep almost indefinitely. These sugars in their final highly concentrated form become powerful stimulants. These processed sugars oxidize violently in the human stomach upon the slightest contact with oxygen which obliges the vital organs suddenly to work harder and faster." [R2F]

William Dufty in his book *Sugar Blues* wrote that sugar cane is native to India, was isolated to crystals that didn't ferment by Persians in ≈600 AD, and was carried to the world by Islam. [R3] About 1500 AD, sugar cane plantations began in the Canary Islands off the NW coast of Africa. Sugar plantations began Black African slavery, genocide of native peoples, and organized crime. Rum is made from fermented sugar. In the 1600s, fortunes were made selling sugar and rum. [R3]

Pulitzer prize winner William Longgood in his book *The Poisons in Your Food* wrote about how food, such as sugar, is treated by <u>wizards who can beguile, deceive and defraud</u> consumers:

"... with chemicals including; dyes, bleaches, emulsifiers, antioxidants, preservatives, flavors, buffers, noxious sprays, acidifiers, alkalizers, deodorants, moisturizers, drying agents, gases, extenders, thickeners, disinfectants, defoliants, fungacides, neutralizers, sweeteners, anticaking agents, antifoaming agents, conditioners, curers, hydrolizers, hydrogenators, maturers, fortifiers, and many others. These are the tools of the food technician, a wizard who can beguile, deceive and defraud the housewife by making her think she is getting something she isn't. His alchemy can make stale products appear fresh, permit unsanitary practices, mask inferior quality, substitute nutritionally inferior or worthless chemicals for more costly natural ingredients. The chemicals, almost without exception, perform their mission at the cost of destroying valuable vitamins, minerals, and enzymes, stripping food products of their natural life giving qualities." [R7]

In his book *Sweet and Dangerous* John Yadkin, MD states that sugar consumption accounts for about one-fifth of the caloric intake of wealthy countries and may promote type-2 diabetes. [R8] Dr. Yadkin also writes that consuming large amounts of 'empty calorie' foods, including sugar, may contribute to cardiovascular disease (CVD). [R8A] Physicians at the Wiemar Institute discuss methods for diabetics to control blood sugar without medication, and to regain good health. [R26]

∗ Sugar isn't as sweet as honey, is void of nutrients and may contribute to chronic health problems.

Aspartame

Aspartame is a man-made, non-food sweetener that doesn't exist in nature. Aspartame is produced by a chemist in a laboratory and is often marketed as NutraSweet, Equal or Spoonful. Although expensive to make, manufacturers claim that aspartame does not promote tooth decay, provides the same sweetness as sugar at a fraction of the calories and doesn't have the bitter aftertaste associated with other synthetic sweeteners. A prominent food wizard and manufacturer that often includes aspartame in their products said, 'consumers have fallen in love with the stuff'.

However, a 10-year study of the sweetener may soon turn aspartame's initial promise's sour. The chemical structure of the sweetener is two amino acids (Aspartic Acid and Phenylalanine) linked together by a molecule of methanol (methyl alcohol). [R10] A group of scientists insist that large amounts of aspartame may cause everything from depression and aggressiveness to epileptic seizures or even brain lesions in humans. Once ingested, the deadly poison 'methanol' is metabolized into formic acid (ant sting poison) or formaldehyde, which may cause blindness. Formaldehyde is a neurotoxin, embalming fluid and a 'class A Carcinogen'. Aspartame may cause neurological symptoms, including: headache, dizziness, seizure, depression, etc. [R14], and may exacerbate neurological diseases such as: lupus, multiple sclerosis, Parkinson's disease, Alzheimer's, fibromyalgia and diabetes. **Aspartame can change the brain's biochemistry.** [R37] Phenylalanine and aspartic acid are found in food, but in excess their effect on the body can be like a drug: lowering the seizure threshold in the brain and blocking seratonin production. [R14] Aspartame may encourage carbohydrate bingeing, which may negate weight-loss benefits. [R46] (People with a rare metabolic disorder, PKU, can't metabolize phenylalanine and <u>must</u> avoid aspartame.) [R45]

> "There has been substantial proof that ingesting large amounts of aspartame changes the levels of neurotransmitters in the brain thereby affecting behavior." [R10A] "In pregnancy the effects of aspartame can be passed directly on to the fetus, even in small doses." [R33]

Several prominent researchers have spoken out against consuming aspartame, including: Washington University chemist Dr. James Olney, who conducted many animal tests; attorney James Turner author of *The Chemical Feast*; and the co-authors Dennis Remington, MD and Barbara W. Higa, RD in their book *The Bitter Truth About Artificial Sweeteners*. [R8-9-10-37]

> "The ingredients [of aspartame] stimulate the neurons of the brain to death, causing brain damage of varying degrees." [R37]

A recent article described methanol toxicity from aspartame as: a slow poison that destroys the brain a little bit at a time, and stated that the effects of aspartame poisoning are cumulative.

> "Depending on a person's physical state and tolerance level, immediate effects can either be severe (resulting in epileptic seizures, including grand mal, blindness, chest palpitations), or less noticeable (causing blurred vision, bright flashes, tunnel vision, ringing or buzzing in ears, migraine headaches, dizziness, loss of equilibrium, lip and mouth reactions); less noticeable effects may be passed off as temporary or caused by something else." [R17]

Aspartame's promises may be turning sour, as aspartame has received more complaints to the FDA in its short existence than any other 'food' additive in history. Commercial pilots have crashed simulators and even lost licenses due to symptoms that may be attributed to aspartame. Airplane pilots, who frequently consume aspartame, may experience symptoms that include: vertigo, loss of vision, suicidal depression, heart problems, and even grand mal <u>seizures</u>, etc. [R17]

> "An Air Force pilot traced the patterns of tremors and seizures he suffered for two years directly to his patterns of NutraSweet consumption. When he traveled to areas where diet sodas were not available, he was free of the symptoms. But when he resumed intake of the beverages, his tremors resumed, grew more severe and culminated in a grand mal seizure." [R17]

A final warning involves heating aspartame to 85°F, causing its breakdown to toxic substances: methanol (wood alcohol); formaldehyde (embalming fluid); KDP (brain tumor agent); and formic acid (ant sting venom). Mary Nash Stoddard believes this may have happened in 1990, when several soft drink companies shipped many cases of diet soft drinks, some of which may have been expired, to the deserts of Saudi Arabia for US Desert Storm troops during the 'Gulf War' – possibly causing 'Gulf War Syndrome'. The symptoms experienced by Gulf War Syndrome victims are similar to poisonings from the ordinary breakdown and metabolism of aspartame in the body, but, because of the extreme heat and the 'free' sodas that were readily available during the Gulf War, soldiers had the opportunity to consume many, many sodas in a very short time – increasing the severity of all toxic symptoms. [R45-46] Dr. Joseph Mercola of the Optimal Wellness Center also suggests that aspartame in sodas may have had a part in soldiers developing Gulf War Syndrome.

∗ Aspartame may be the most-subtle poison to deliberately be entered into the food chain.

Honey, Honeycomb and Royal Jelly

The natural low water content of honey (about 17%) causes honey to be 'hygroscopic' or water absorbing. Hygroscopicity causes honey to be bactericidal – by virtue of the fact that honey will actually draw water away from the bacteria that the microbes need to live. This bactericidal property of honey will actually kill many human disease-causing germs, including those resulting in typhoid fever, bronchial-pneumonia, dysentery, peritonitis, and pleuritis. [R2D-4C-5A] The highest quality honeys all have a low water content. Naturopaths have understood these therapeutic effects of honey for many years. In fact, the bactericidal properties of honey have made it valuable as a sterilizing agent to cleanse deep skin wounds that might otherwise become infected. In places where modern antibiotic drugs are not available, honey has been used postoperatively on a wound to reduce the risk of infection. Honey has also been used to treat burns with excellent results; when applied directly to burned skin, the skin may not even blister, and it often heals rapidly. [R2E]

Honey and Honeycomb are excellent foods for helping people cope with hay fever, asthma, and allergies caused by air-borne pollens. Honey from local bees contains some local pollen. When bee pollens in honey are eaten in the diet, the body's immune system may become desensitized to these pollen proteins. [R4B-5B] The body may not produce the allergic response to the proteins in pollen that it is accustomed to, and the pollen allergy problem may subside. For the maximum value for allergy relief, the honey or honeycomb should be local. Then, the pollen that is eaten in the honey is the same air-borne pollen, to which people may become allergic.

Royal Jelly is very nourishing, and may contain antimicrobial and antitumor elements. [R13-23] Royal Jelly is extremely perishable and is best eaten fresh. Royal Jelly that is preserved for later is best if processed in a non-freeze-dried manner for all its health benefits to be retained. [R13]

Jacob found honey in a cleft in a rock. In areas with flowering plants, but with limited places for honeybees to make a hive, the cleft of a rock is a common and suitable place for a beehive. [R24]

NIV Deut 32:13 He [the LORD] nourished him [Jacob] with honey from the rock.

Other Sweeteners

Stevia or honey leaf is an herb that is native only to Paraguay and was first cultivated in 1900. In its ancient use, stevia leaves were cut, dried, ground, and added to herbal tea as a sweetener. Stevia's sweetness results from the abundant steviosides and the rare but sweeter rebaudiosides. Stevia contains some protein, calcium, phosphorous and other nutrients, but it is primarily an herb. Most of the best quality stevia still comes from Paraguay, while poorer quality stevia often has a bitter and/or grassy aftertaste. Since Japan banned all artificial sweeteners in the 1960s, they have actively cultivated stevia and they lead the world in its use as a sweetener. Crystalline stevia is nearly 300 times sweeter than cane sugar with no reported side effects from its use. [R41-42] Scientific attention given to stevia as the 'sweetener of the future' include; isolating steviosides and sweeter rebaudiosides, reproducing them in a laboratory, and minimizing the bitter aftertaste. Often to avoid its bitter aftertaste, crystalline powdered stevia is mixed with other sweeteners. Possibly, due to its perceived threat by the sugar and/or aspartame industries, in the US stevia must be labeled as a supplement but never as a sweetener. Possibly due to problems with drug trafficking, pure crystalline steviosides and rebaudiosides aren't even allowed in the US. [R41-42]

Fruit concentrates, when boiled down to syrup, may retain their nutrient value as sweeteners. Molasses is a dark brown nutrient-rich sweet syrup remaining from sugar cane processing after the white sugar crystals are refined away. Light molasses is prized for human use, while thicker blackstrap is molasses that contains more vitamins, minerals and ash is sought for animal feed. Maple trees that are native only to NE Untied States produce a tree sap each fall that can be concentrated into maple syrup, which is a good sweetener, but has a limited nutritional content.

Organic sugar cane may be processed to whole 'evaporated sugar cane juice' or powder in a manner that retains essential nutrients. But, not all products labeled 'evaporated cane juice' were processed equally well, with nutrient retention in mind. If evaporated cane sugar is to retain its full nutritional content, great care is required. All 'white' evaporated cane sugar must be bleached.

Turbinato sugar has no more nutrients than white sugar. Brown sugar is just white sugar with a little molasses added for color and flavor. Brown sugar has no more nutrients than white sugar. Stevia and molasses, maple syrup, evaporated cane juice and fruit concentrates, if processed to retain nutrient value, may be valuable as sweeteners, especially if raw unfiltered honey is scarce.

∗ Honey, in its natural state, is unsurpassed for sweetness and promoting physical health.

---------------------------------- References Ch 15 Honey ---------------------------------

[R1] Magic of Honey\ by Dorothy Perlman; pg 39 honey chart and composition
[R1A] pg 22 invert sugar & quote //R1B] pg 40-41 honey chart & definitions
[R2] Honey and Your Health\ by Bodog Beck, MD; //[R2-2C] pg 17-19 honey content/charts
[R2B] pg 49 granulation of honey //[R2E] pg 123-127 honey in surgery
[R2D] pg 22-23 honey kills bacteria //[R2A] pg 35 sugar addiction //[R2F] pg 44-47 sugar a drug
[R3] Sugar Blues\ by William Dufty; pg 28-31 sugar cane from India – sugar spread by Islam
[R4] Folk Medicine\ by D.C. Jarvis, MD; pg 98-99 vitamins in honey pg 112 Honey charts
[R4A] pg 97 honey & minerals [R4B] pg 111-119 content/chart [R4C] pg 95-96 honey kills germs
[R5] Honey for Health\ by Cecil Tonsley; pg 35-37 bees gather nectar & dry in out to make honey
[R5A-C] pg 38-41 honey content //[R5B] pg 100-103 honey - pollen - hay fever
[R6] Eat, Drink and Be Ready\ by Monte L. Kline, PhD and W.P. Strube Jr.; pg 189
[R6A] pg 189 quote -- Sugar Information Inc. of New York
[R7] Poisons In Your Food\ by William Longgood; pg 3 quote food technologist
[R8] Sweet and Dangerous\ by John Yadkin, MD; pg 3 – 1/5th all calories //[R8A] pg 95-98 sugar – CVD
[R9] Chemical Feast\ by James Turner, atty; health risks from eating aspartame
[R10] The Bitter Truth About Artificial Sweeteners\ by Dennis Remington, MD; pg 80-81 //[R10A] pg 80-100
[R11] Food and Nutrition\ by J. I. Rodale staff; pg 456-457 /[R11A] pg 457
[R12] What the Bible Says About Healthy Living\ by Rex Russell, MD; pg 167-179 honey and health
[R13] Nutrition Made Simple\ by Robert Creyhon, PhD; pg 168-169 royal jelly (Bee Alive 1-800-345-BEES)
[R14] Nutrition and Physical Degeneration\ by Weston Price, DDS diet in relation to physical well-being
[R15] Joy with Honey\ by Doris Mech; honey recipes & w^3.beemaid.com/BeeMaid/Recipes/HoneyCarrotSnackCake.htm
[R16] Sugar Busters\ by Leighton Steward, Morrison Bethea, MD, Sam Anderws, MD, Luis Bulart, MD
[R17] The Deadly Deception\ by Mary Nash Stoddard // Aspartame Safety Net /PO Box 780634 Dallas, TX 75378
[R18] Strong's Concordance\ by James Strong, STD, LLD
pg 490 honey # 1706 H pg 29 ***devash debash*** Gen 43:11
[R19] The ABC to XYZ of Bee Keeping\ by A. I. Root // The Hive and the Honeybee\ (Langstroth) by Roy Grout
[R20] The Great Sugar Scandal (video)\ by Dane & Vicki Griffin {Let's Eat – PO Box 67 – Thompsonville, Ill 62890}
[R21] 700 Club Video\ Infant Baby Formula may encourage Diabetes
[R22] 22 Health Hazards of White Sugar\ by Lynne Melcombe
[R23] Bee Well Bee Wise\ by Bernard Jensen, DC, PhD royal jelly
[R24] The Land and the Bible\ by W.M. Thompson; pg 566 honey in rock
[R25] Proof Positive\ by Neil Nedley, MD; Ch 10 pg 171-191 sugar
[R26] Wiemar Institute – (Reversing Diabetes Seminar) - 1-800-525-9192
[R27] Warning Nutrasweet is a Neurotoxin\ in Flying Safely (magazine); May 92

Aspartame

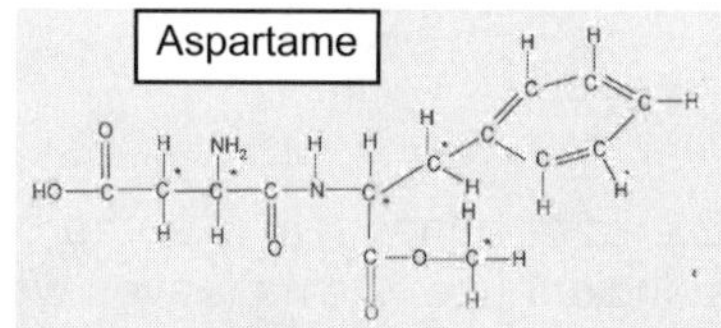

[R28] The 28-Day Antioxidant Diet Program\ by Steven Masley, MD; pg 63-70 glycemic index
[R29] Lick the Sugar Habit\ by Nancy Appleton, PhD; pg 7-11; addictive nature of 'white sugar'
[R30] Molasses\ World Book Encyclopedia 1998 vol 13; pg 689; molasses-syrup from sugar cane
[R31] The Encyclopedia of Nutrition\ by Robert A. Ronzio, PhD; pg 290 Honey contains yeasts that are killed by heat. Bacterial spores in honey are suspected of causing botulism in infants under 1 year old.
pg 300 Blackstrap molasses is the least refined sugar cane – contains minerals Fe, Ch and other micro nutrients.
[R33] Warning Nutrasweet is a Neurotoxin\ from Flying Safely Magazine; May 1992
[R34] Sweet'ner Dearest (book) // [R34A] Is Aspartame Safe? (video) – both – 1-800-814-9800
[R35] Aspartame Disease An Ignored Epidemic\ by H. J. Roberts, MD (Sunshine Sentinel Press)
www.sunsentpress.com J. Roberts, MD // 300 27th Street // West Palm Beach, Florida 33407 // (407) 832-2408
[R36] Bittersweet Aspartame: A Diet Delusion & Nutrasweet - The Bitter Truth; (handout)
Barbara Alexander Mullarey// c/o NutiVoice// PO Box 946// Oak Park, Illinois 60303 // (708) 848-0116
[R37] Worldwide Conference on Aspartame (Internet)\ by Betty Martini
[R38] Exotoxins: The Taste that Kills\ by Dr. Blaylock; Aspartame & MSG (Health Press 1-800-643-2665)
[R39] Honey (Fresno State Library)\ by Eva Crane; pg 264 benefits of honey
[R40] The Honey Book\ by Lucille Recht Penner; pg 19 honey chart
[R41] Life with Stevia: How Sweet It Is! (internet)\ by Daniel Murray, PhD; pg 1-5 stevia as a sweetener
[R42] The Stevia Story\ by Linda Bonvie, Bill Bonvie and Donna Gates; Ch 2 pg 22-30 (1-800-4STEVIA)
[R43] Diabetes (video)\ narrated by Jack Palance; Medical management of Diabetes
[R44] Blood Sugar; Help Yourself to Better Health radio program\ by Monte Kline, PhD (1-800-255-4246)
[R45] The Straight Dope - Did Aspartame cause Gulf War Syndrome?\ by Cecil Adams – Gulf War Syndrome
[R46] Optimal Wellness Center (Internet)\ Dr. Joseph Mercola; Aspartame – overeating – (PKU) Pheylketonuria
[R47] The Maple Sugaring Story (video)\ by David G. and Betty Ann Lockhart – Vermont Maple Syrup
[R48] Devils Candy\ by Susan Kleiner (King 5 TV News 05-18-03) – High Fructose Corn Syrup – 15 yr old sweetener
[R49] Maximum Energy\ by Ted Broer, PhD; Ch 14 pg 156-173 – Aspartame ⇒ a neurotoxin – w^3.TedBroer.com
[R50] Reversing Diabetes\ by Julian Whitaker, MD; healthy food & wise supplements help normalize blood glucose
[R51] Sweetness and Power\ by Sidney W. Mintz; The Place of Sugar in Modern History

∗ Moses likens the Promised Land to milk and honey fifteen times in the *Torah*. Milk and Honey were very nourishing foods in the Hebrew diet, and should be part of a healthy diet today as well.

Chapter 16 Grain and Bread
Whole Grain Bread

Bread (***lechem***) made from complete wheat (***chittah***) and other whole grains has been called the 'staff of life' and a staple of the diet ever since Adam and Eve left the Garden of Eden.

KJV Gen 3:19 In the sweat of thy face shalt thou eat bread (***lechem***), ...

JPS Ex 9:31 And the flax and the barley were smitten; for the barley was in the ear, and the flax was in bloom. vs32 but the wheat (***chittah***) and the spelt were not smitten; for they ripen late.

NIV Num 18:12 I give you all the finest olive oil and all the finest new wine and grain (***dagan***)

Many grains such as: wheat, barley, corn, rice and spelt, as well as flax, were grown in Egypt. Wheat (***dagan***) was often collective in the ***Torah*** for all grains, such as corn, rye, oat and rice. Joseph sent his father ***dagan*** and bread from Egypt. (Gen 45:23) The ease of growing, ease of storage, and vast nutrients are big reasons that grains are an important part of a healthy diet. [R1]

"... three quarters of the people live entirely upon bread or upon that which is made from wheat or barley flour. It [bread] is unquestionably the principle food of the East." [R29]

When the Hebrews lived in Egypt, the grains they ate often came from the Nile River delta. The Nile carried vast mud/mineral deposits. Each autumn the Nile would flood, overflow its bank, and deposit the mineral-rich mud in the Nile delta. This flooding made the Nile delta soil some of the richest and most fertile soil in the world for growing grain. Hearty grains from the Nile delta helped Egyptian armies conquer the world and allowed society time for scholarly pursuits such as astronomy and architecture, yet Egyptian society declined after the Exodus. Later, Greek armies used Egyptian grain to conquer the known world; and later yet, Roman soldiers did the same.

As representative of all grains, complete wheat consists of germ, endosperm, and bran. Wheat germ contains natural oil-soluble vitamins and oils (FAs); bran contains water-soluble vitamins, minerals, fiber and antioxidants; endosperm contains the starch and the gluten. [R10] Wheat germ oil is very valuable for health, but all germ oils are also very susceptible to spoilage. When oils spoil, they become rancid. [R5] Wheat berries (kernels of grain) that are stored intact can keep almost indefinitely without spoilage, as grains found in Egyptian pyramids have proved. Once any grain is cracked or milled, the germ will soon become rancid. Almost all bread, pastry and grain products that are prepared and distributed commercially must be processed to remove the germ before their preparation, to prevent the germ from going rancid on the shelf. Products sold as 'whole wheat' often have had the germ removed, but retain all the rich fiber of the bran. The few commercial grain products that have not removed the germ must be refrigerated or frozen to prevent spoilage. In the days of Moses, grains were ground to flour and used for bread daily, and spoilage wasn't a problem. So important was this grinding of grains to a Hebrew family that the millstone used for this task could not be taken as the payment for a debt. (Deut 24:6) Chaff is a tough husk or outer cover that surrounds the wheat berry. Humans cannot digest chaff. Threshing and winnowing are labor-intensive jobs that separate the wheat-berry from the chaff. Winnowing tosses the grain in the air with a large pitchfork in a very windy area, which allows the lighter chaff to be blown downwind, while the heavier wheat berry remains nearby in a pile.

Jeffrey Bland, PhD in nutrition in an article he wrote for *Let's Live,* discussed the health value of both soluble fiber and insoluble fiber that are found in all whole grains. [R7] (Ch 21 Vegetables)

Today, an ideal way to enjoy fresh complete wheat flour is to buy wheat and other grains in bulk and use a small home grain mill to grind flour fresh as needed for bread and pastries. [R1A]

Melchizedek, the king of peace and priest of God, fellowshipped with Abraham by bringing him bread and wine. Later, Abraham followed this example by serving the three messengers of the LORD a fine 'kosher' meal of bread, and beef, curds and milk. Since the time of Abraham, the breaking of bread with guests has been an invitation of hospitality in Hebrew and Arab culture.

KJV Gen 14:18 ...and Melchizedek, king of Salem brought forth bread and wine: and he was the priest of the most high God.

KJV Gen 18:5 And I will fetch a morsel of bread (***lechem***) and comfort ye your hearts... vs6 and Abraham hastened unto Sarah and said, 'make ready quickly three measures of fine meal, and make cakes [of bread] upon the hearth.' vs8 And he took butter [likely cottage cheese], milk, and the calf which he had dressed, and set it before them; ...

*** For bread to be the 'staff of life' that the LORD intended, bread should be made of complete grain.**

Winnowing and Grinding Grain (i.e. — Wheat)

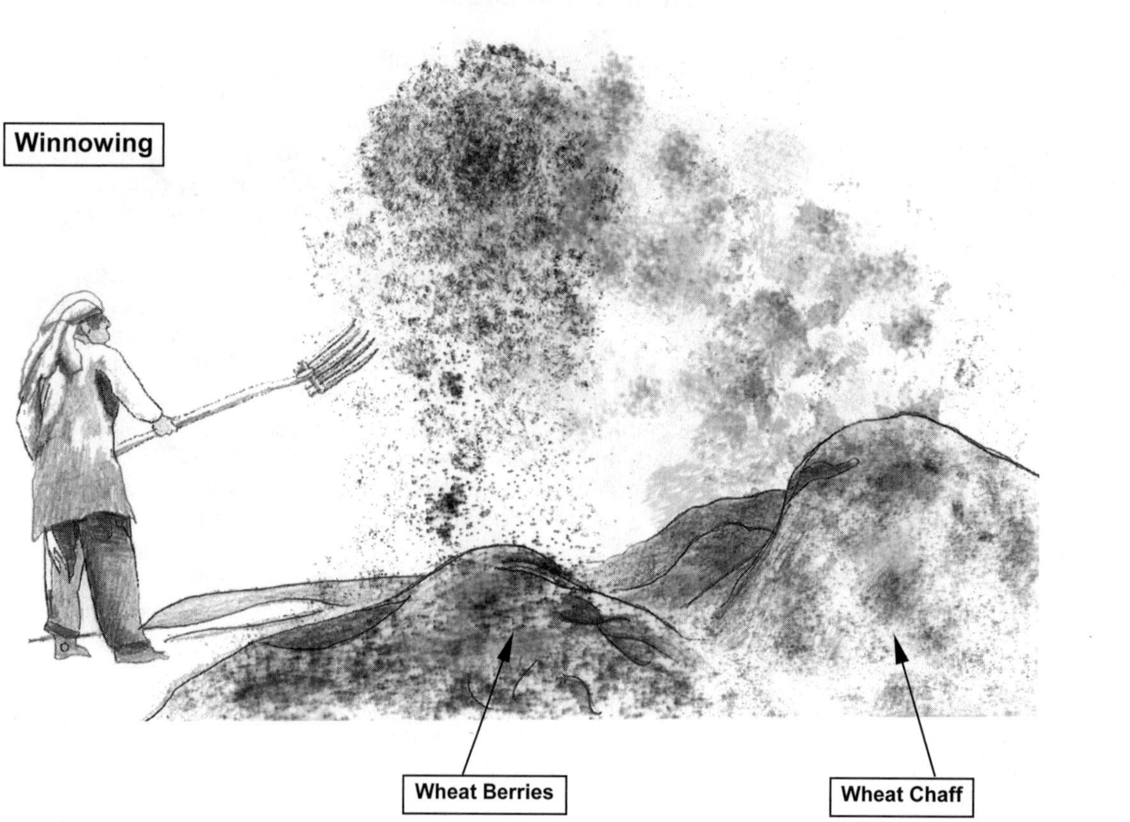

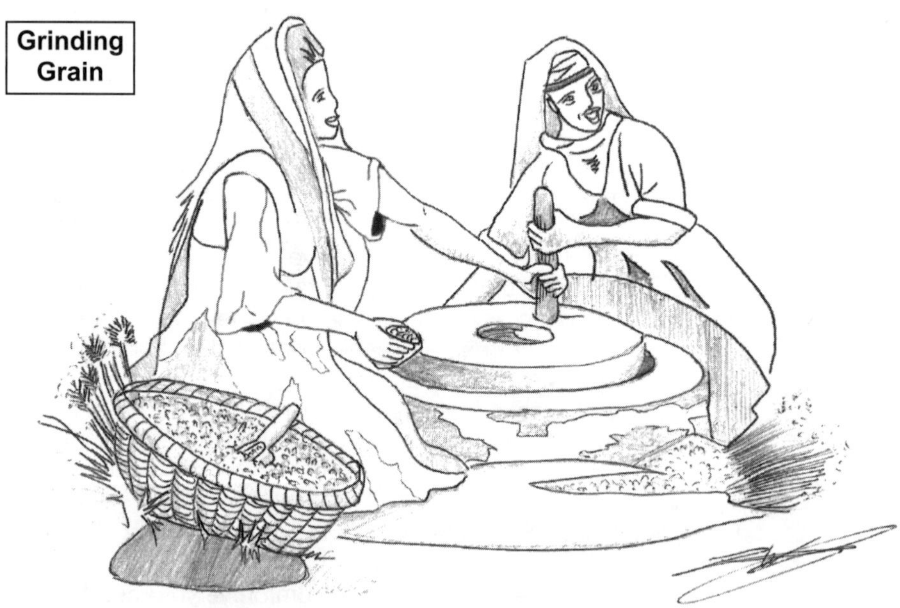

∗ The author is in favor of 'labor saving' advances in grain processing as long as essential nutrients are not lost!

White Flour

In the 1800s, when wheat, rice and other grains were first milled to remove the bran and germ part of the grain, nutritional deficiency diseases such as beriberi soon followed. These nutritional deficiency diseases even caused the death of persons who relied heavily on grains for the bulk of their nutritional intake. Today's laws require the miller of such nutritionally empty flour to make the minimum (possible) necessary restitution of imitation nutrients, so as to prevent the consumer from immediately developing a life-threatening illness. This flour is labeled 'enriched', but by comparison with what God intended, it is really 'nutritionally bankrupt'. While enriching bankrupt white flour does prevent immediate illness, the enriching process does not ensure that consumers will not develop long term deficiencies of vitamins, minerals, enzymes or fiber, which may be causing many of the chronic degenerative diseases plaguing modern society. [R3-4-8-17]

"White flour and sugar supply plenty of calories, but lack the nutrients necessary for the proper utilization of those calories. Vitamin B-6, vitamin E, chromium, manganese, zinc and magnesium, all contained in the 'refuse' left after processing, play a significant role in the body's use of starch and sugar." [R6]

Furthermore, the process of bleaching normally brown wheat flour to white flour involves the use of very harsh chemicals. Agene was the first chemical to be used for this process, before the FDA banned it for use in the United States. Today, the even more powerful chemical nitrogen trichloride is used to bleach the flour white. [R2-3] This counterfeit bankrupt white flour, which is bleached and processed to remove the germ and bran, has one major advantage over freshly milled whole-whole wheat (whole grain) flour: almost unlimited shelf life! This is great for the food processing industry, and very convenient for the baker, but lousy for the consumer. [R2]

Today's removal of nutrients from grains during the milling process to produce white flour, followed by the 'enriching' process of these depleted flours, might be likened to removal of the expert musicians from a symphony orchestra and replacing them with a handful of beginning music students. Once the expert musicians are missing, the music will always be out of harmony. Adding more beginning students to the orchestra will only make the music louder, not more melodious. Only with the original expert musicians, will the symphony be heard in its intended splendor. This is the same issue with any of God's foods: they should be consumed with all their original nutritional elements in their proper place in order to get the full, rich, satisfying nutrition and taste that the LORD intended. As in Moses' era, when the entire wheat berry is used for flour and bread, then all the elements work in concert to provide a well orchestrated, balanced food.

The enriched flour is the product of 'the 'food technologist' who is in the employ of a large corporation that is in business to make a profit. The more profit he can bring about, the greater are his financial rewards. [R2A] His job is to find ways to substitute cheaper ingredients for the more expensive natural ones, to develop money-saving shortcuts, to reduce spoilage, to entice the consumer into buying the company's product. His job is to make stale products appear fresh. The food technologist is not paid to keep people healthy, but to make money for his company.

∗ **The farther removed a food is from its natural state, the less likely it is to be healthy.**

In 1874, in England the first milling of wheat kernels to remove the germ and bran from the endosperm took place. In 1911, the prestigious British medical journal *Lancet* commented: [R3]

"Real bread has been taken out of our mouths by modern methods of impoverishment." [R3]

Dr. Henry Schroeder of Dartmouth Medical College showed that huge percentages of nutrients are **<u>absent</u>** when white (devitalized) flour is produced from the perfect whole wheat kernel. [R3]

Nutrients Lost when Whole Wheat Flour is made into White Flour [R3]

Nutrient	Lost	Nutrient	Lost
Thiamin (B-1)	77.1%	Riboflavin (B-2)	80.0%
Niacin (B-3)	80.8%	Pyridoxine (B-6)	71.8%
Pantothenic Acid	50.0%	Vitamin E	86.3%
Calcium	60.0%	Iron	75.6%
Magnesium	84.7%	Phosphorous	70.9%
Potassium	77.0%	Zinc	77.7%

> " 'the food on your table has had 50% of its nutrients removed.' Countless others echo this leading nutritional researcher's findings: up to 80 percent of the food's value is lost through processing, transportation, freezing, storage, cooking, spraying and chemical additives. Also, most of our foods are grown in soils that are depleted of minerals." [R33]

Kernel of Wheat

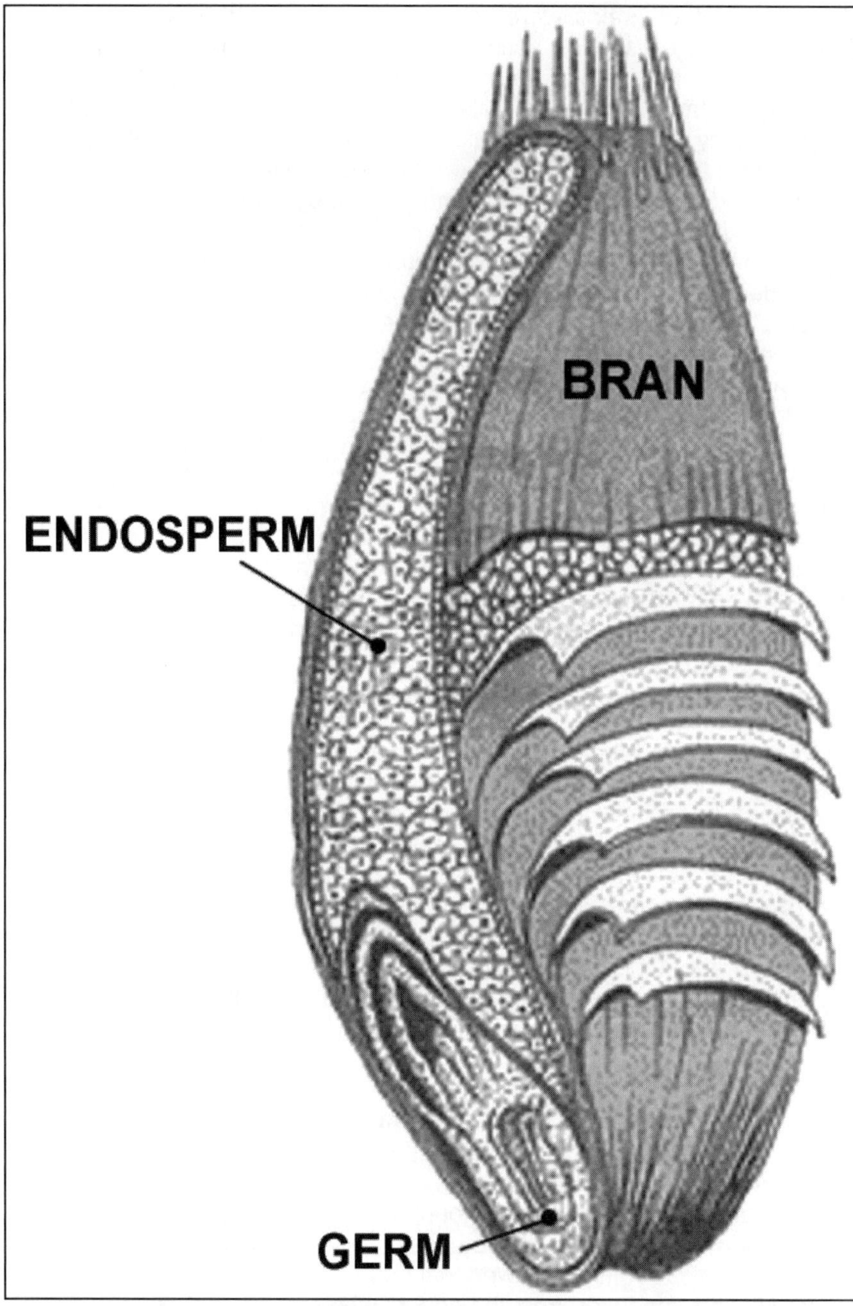

BRAN –
About 14% of the kernel weight. Bran is included in whole wheat flour and is also sold separately. Bran contains a small amount of protein and significant amounts of the 3 major B vitamins, trace minerals and fiber – primarily insoluble.

ENDOSPERM –
About 83% of the kernel by weight and the bulk of white flour. Endosperm contains the greatest share of protein, charbohydrate and iron, as well as the 3 B vitamins – niacin, riboflavin and thiamin. Endosperm contains some – soluble fiber.

GERM –
About 2 ½ to 3% of the kernel by weight. Germ is the embryo or section that sprouts. Germ contains trace minerals, B vitamins, and some protein. Germ contains oils – including vitamin E. Germ is often removed during the milling of flour, as vitamin E and oils spoil very rapidly. Germ is sold separately (is often refrigerated) and is in freshly milled whole whole wheat flour.

Kernel of Wheat reprinted by permission of Kansas Wheat Commission – (also pictured on several Internet websites)

	Whole Wheat Flour Compared with White Flour			Enriched white (still) devitalized flour	
	Whole Wheat Flour	White Flour	% remaining	Enriched White Flour	% remaining
Protein	13.3 grams	10.5 grams	79%	10.5 grams	79%
Calcium	41 mg	16 mg	39%	16 mg	39%
Phosphorous	372 mg	87 mg	23%	87 mg	23%
Iron	3.3 mg	0.8 mg	24%	2.9 mg	88%
Potassium	370 mg	95 mg	26%	95 mg	26%
Sodium	3 mg	2 mg	67%	2 mg	67%
Thiamin	0.55 mg	0.06 mg	11%	0.44 mg	80%
Riboflavin	0.12 mg	0.05 mg	42%	0.26 mg	216%
Niacin	4.3 mg	0.9 mg	21%	3.5 mg	81%

[R4] Diet for a Small Planet

Grain of Wheat

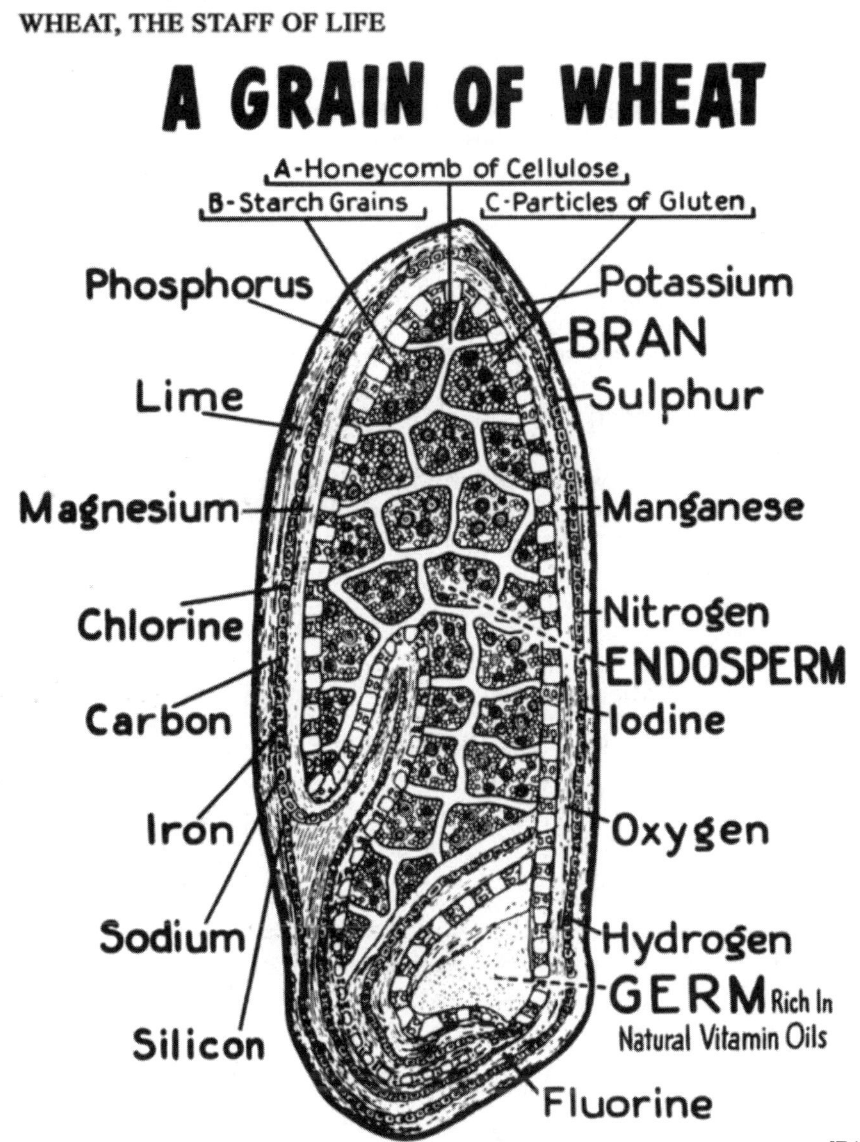

[R1]

Stalk of Wheat

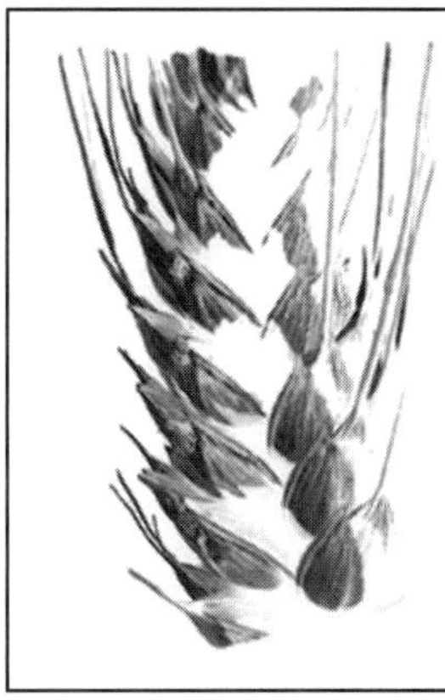

Kernels of Wheat on a stalk are drawn above. Threshing – separates kernels from the stalk when animals (oxen) pull a threahing sled over already cut wheat. Threshing – separates chalf (husk) from the berry (kernal) as well. Winnowing – divides chalf from kernal by tossing both into the air and allowing a wind to blow chalf downwind – kernels remain to be collected and ground into flour for bread.

Grain of Wheat [R1] reprinted from *God's Key to Health and Happiness* – used with permission of Bible Light International

Millstone for Grinding Flour

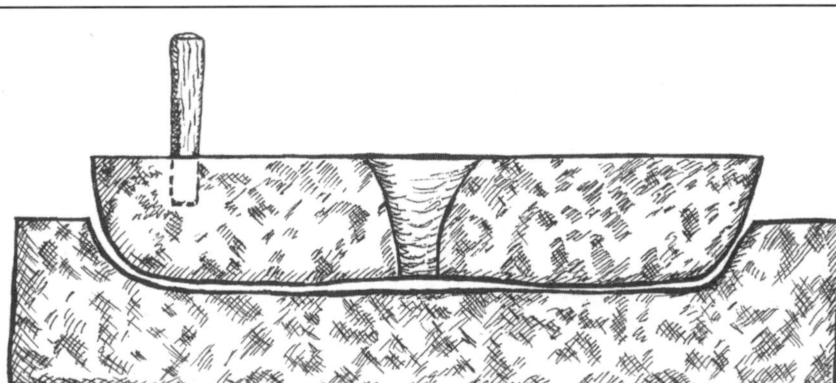

Millstone – for grinding grain (i.e. – wheat) into complete flour. Mornings were the time when women spent 1 to 2 hours per day to grind fresh flour for bread. Whole-whole wheat flour for bread is the 'Staff of Life'.

---------------------------- References Ch 16 Grain and Bread ---------------------------------

[R1] God's Key to Health and Happiness\ by Elmer Josephson; pg 131 Grain of Wheat *sketch*
Grain of Wheat used with permission of Bible Light Int'l PO Box 370 Ottawa, Kansas 66067-0370
[R1A] pg 130-135 whole wheat
[R2] Poisons in Our Food\ by William Longgood; pg 184-185 bleaching flour white
[R2A] pg 47 food technologist
[R3] Eat, Drink and Be Ready\ by Monte L. Kline, PhD and W. P. Strube Jr.; pg 196-197
[R4] Diet for a Small Planet\ by Frances Moore Lappe; pg 66-69 proteins
pg 377 whole Wheat flour compared to white flour chart
[R5] Food and Nutrition\ by J. I. Rodale and staff; pg 66-68 & 82(D)-93 wheat germ & diagram
[R6] Mental and Elemental Nutrients\ by Carl Pfeiffer, MD, PhD; pg 26 white flour & sugar lack
[R7] Let's Live Magazine\ by Jeffrey Bland, PhD; Oct 92: pg 78-79 fiber - Soluble & Insoluble
[R8] Nutrition Against Disease\ by Roger Williams, PhD; pg 206-207 deficient white flour
[R9] Recipes for a Cancer-Free Lifestyle\ by Hanna Kroeger; pg 13 whole wheat vs white flour
[R9A] pg 22 Professor Haupke - mineral quote
[R9B] pg 55 Cancer statement
[R10] The Poisons Around Us\ by Henry Schroeder, MD
[R11] Trace Elements and Man\ by Henry Schroeder, MD
[R12] What the Bible Says About Healthy Living\ by Rex Russell, MD; pg 103-124 grains
pg 109 corn from the KJV is a generic term for grain of all sorts including rice, rye and oats
[R13] From Wheat to Flour\ by Sharon P. Davis; pg 52 wheat kernel picture
[R14] Green Kamut (audio tape)\ by David Sandivold wheat grown in mineral-rich Nile delta
[R15] Whole Grains\ by Sara Pitzer; pg 47 picture of whole grain
[R16] Food in History\ by Reay Tannahill; pg 51-53 bread unleavened and leavened
pg 56-59 kosher - eat no blood - *kashrut* - clean and unclean food
[R17] Supernutrition\ by Richard Passwater, PhD; pg 23 white flour = missing nutrients
[R18] Strong's Concordance\ by James Strong, STD, LLD

pg 1123	wheat	# 2406	H pg 38	***chittah***	Gen 30:14
pg 1123	grain or wheat	# 1715	H pg 29	***dagan***	Num 18:12
pg 141	bread	# 3899	H pg 59	***lechem***	Gen 14:18
pg 219	grain or corn (& wine)	# 1715	H pg 29	***dagan***	Gen 27:28 & Deut 7:13
pg 219	corn	# 1250	H pg 23	***bar***	Gen 42:5 & 25
pg 219	corn	# 7668	H pg 112	***sheber***	Gen 45:23
pg 219	corn	# 7054	H pg 104	***qamah***	Ex 22:6(b)
pg 219	corn	# 1643	H pg 28	***geres***	Lev 2:14(b & c)
pg 98	barley	# 8184	H pg 120	***se'or***	Ex 9:31
pg 356	flax	# 6594	H pg 97	***pishtah***	Ex 9:31
pg 845	rye – (rie)	# 3698	H pg 56	***kuccemeth***	Ex 9:32

[R19] The Wheatgrass Book\ by Ann Wigmore; chlorophyll, enzymes, minerals & vitamins
[R20] Daily Life in Bible Times\ by Albert Bailey; pg 141 picture of winnowing grain
[R21] The New Whole Foods Encyclopedia\ by Rebecca Wood
[R22] Food For Naught\ by Ross Hume Hall, PhD; Ch 1 pg 9-34 lifeless bread
[R23] The Jack LaLane Way to Vibrant Health\ by Jack LaLane
[R24] Your Health Under Siege\ by Jeffrey Bland, PhD
[R25] Proof Positive\ by Neil Nedley, MD; pg 72 fiber chart
[R26] God and Vitamins\ by Marjorie Holmes; pg 288 wheat germ // pg 301 wheat bran
[R27] The Blessings of Bread\ by Adrian Bailey
[R28] The 28-Day Antioxidant Diet Program\ by Steven Masley, MD; pg 86-93 whole grains
pg 86 bran -antioxidants
[R29] Manners and Customs of Bible Lands\ by Fred Wight; pg 44 quote on bread as a staple
pg 182 drawing of threshing pg 47 drawing of bread baking pg 81 drawing of women grinding grain
[R30] Manners and Customs of the Bible\ by James M. Freeman; pg 265 drawing of threshing
pg 375 drawing of hand mill for grinding grain / pg 376 drawing of women grinding grain
[R31] The Laurel's Kitchen Bread Book\ by Laurel Robertson with Carol Flanders, Brian Ruppenthal
[R32] Kernel of Wheat diagram\ by Kansas Wheat Commission 'Kernel of Wheat' diagram
Kansas Wheat Commission / 2670 Claflin Road / Manhatten Kansas / 66502-0255 // 913-539-0255
[R33] The Joy of Health\ by Zoltan Rona, MD; pg 60 – 50 to 80% of nutrients lost in food processing

∗ The author believes that every disease (condition) apart from normal includes a nutritional component.

Chapter 17 Salt
Whole SeaSalt

The Hebrews seasoned their food with salt, as the laws concerning offerings required.

JPS Lev 2:13 And every meal-offering of thine shalt thou season with salt; neither shalt thou suffer the salt of the covenant of thy God to be lacking from thy meal-offering; with all thine offerings thou shalt offer salt (***melach***).

The Hebrews in Israel gathered whole salt from the Mediterranean Sea or the Gulf of Aqaba or the Dead Sea. Salt from the sea or land was then slowly dried by the sun for dietary use. [R4-9] Sodium (Na) and Chloride (Cl) are the most numerous mineral nutrients in salt from the sea, although all minerals necessary for life are also present in whole, unrefined SeaSalt. [R7N-3-5C] ***

Chloride is needed by the stomach in order to efficiently make hydrochloric acid. [R1-2-8-13] Hydrochloric acid, which is produced in the stomach, is a very important part of proper digestion for the glucide of grains, the fiber of vegetables and the protein of any source. [R2] Salting grains, cereals and vegetables is especially important, since these foods, as compared with meat and dairy products, contain only a scant amount of salt. [R10-11] Salting nuts, seeds and beans is also a good idea. The balance of all 71 minerals in whole, unrefined SeaSalt is superior to common, refined table salt for the production of hydrochloric acid. SeaSalt on foods insures the stomach the most efficient production of the hydrochloric acid that is necessary for healthy digestion. [R2]

Sodium in the diet is also valuable for the proper breakdown and absorption of all proteins. [R1-2] Sodium is a component of pancreatic juice and bile. [R8C] The presence of whole, complete SeaSalt in the stomach helps to emulsify fats and oils in order to ensure proper digestion. [R2A] The highest concentration of sodium in the body is found in the stomach. [R20] Whole, unrefined SeaSalt is an ideal source of sodium and the other minerals necessary for this digestion. [R1-2A]

> "Only the wind and the sun serve to dry the ocean brine that is channeled from the open sea into pristine shallow ponds, ... lined with clean food-grade clay. The dazzling white crystals are briskly stimulated by the salt farmer, then hand-gathered from the flowing live salt-water flats. This sea-salt tastes sweet enough to satiate the real hunger for salt that is our instinct." [R2]

Any salt gathered from the sea can be called sea salt. The highest quality SeaSalt retains the sodium and chloride and <u>all</u> the other mineral nutrients as well. *^ [R3] SeaSalt harvested in this manner requires a specially prepared shallow collecting area adjacent to the sea and requires an abundance of sunshine to slowly evaporate the water from the mineral salts. This process is very time consuming, can be very costly, and is quite rare today. [R2A] Today, one of the problems in harvesting SeaSalt this way is finding saltwater that is not contaminated, [R8B] because if the sea-water is contaminated with heavy metals, petrochemicals, industrial pollutants, etc., then the salt may also be contaminated. [R2B] Since ≈1910, most salt from the sea is produced by high heat, vacuum evaporation and suction-drying processes in order to eliminate all unwanted impurities. Modern processes produce the tiny white 'salt crystals' that can be shaken from a saltshaker, but they also cause the loss of most, if not all, of the macro, micro and mini minerals from salt. [R14]

Table for Whole, mineral-rich, SeaSalt [R6]

Minerals (by group)	**Percent by total weight**	**Group**
(1) Sodium and Chloride	84%	Mega
(2) Sulfur, Calcium, Potassium and Magnesium (about ¾ of 1%)	14%	Macro
(3) Carbon, Bromine, Silicon, Nitrogen, Ammonium, Fluorine, Phosphorous, Iodine, Boron, Lithium	1.9997%	Micro
(4) Argon, Rubidium, Copper, Barium, Helium, Bismuth, Tin, Molybdenum, Nickel, Arsenic, Uranium, Manganese, Gold, Vanadium, Aluminum, Cobalt, Antimony, Silver, Zinc, Krypton, Xenon, Chromium, Mercury, Neon, Cadmium, Lead, Germanium, Erbium, Scandium, Gallium, Zirconium, Indium, Niobium, Thulium, Thallium, Lanthanum, Europium, Thulium, Neodymium, Thorium, Cerium, Cesium, Terbium, Beryllium, Ytterbium, Yttrium, Dysprosium, Selenium, Lutetium, Tantalum, Hafnium, Gadolinium, Praseodymium, Samarium, Holmium	0.0003%	Mini (Minerals in groups 1 or 2 may be referred to as 'major minerals'. Any rarer minerals in groups 3 or 4 may be referred to as 'trace minerals'.)
(SeaSalt chart from Jacques de Langre, PhD)	100%	71 Minerals

∗ SeaSalt is the 'gold standard' against which the mineral content of all other salt should be judged.}

∗ Whole, unrefined SeaSalt has an ideal mineral balance to meet human nutritional needs.

Common White 'Table Salt'

According to Jacques de Langre, PhD, founder of the Grain and Salt Society, modern salt refineries remove all of the minerals (of groups 2, 3 & 4) from seawater and brine, leaving pure sodium and chloride. It is the presence of all mega, macro, micro and mini mineral nutrients that renders the SeaSalt so beneficial for health. Taken in larger amounts, not even as a megadose, these same trace minerals may be toxic. Unrefined, hand-harvested ocean SeaSalt carefully and professionally handled will retain all the mega, macro, micro and mini elements originally found in seawater. Every one of the four groups is important for health and must remain, if salt is to perform its role of cellular nutrition, assimilation, [digestion] and regeneration. [R6] Because of the value of salt in digestion (breakdown) and absorption of nutrients from food, the command by the LORD to salt all offerings is perfect to season the food for both taste and nutritional health.

The collection and drying of salt water to produce salt goes on today in Israel in Atlit on the Mediterranean Sea and in Elath on the Gulf of Aqaba. However, salt from Israel today is not the unrefined, still-moist, mineral-rich SeaSalt that the Hebrews initially enjoyed in ***Eretz*** Israel. [R9]

> "The salt used by early mankind was crude, lumpy and wet because the calcium and magnesium it contained attracted water. So salt was 'refined'. The 'impurities' were removed. That is, the things that made it inconvenient to use were taken out. What was finally left was almost pure sodium chloride, which is what we pour from our salt shakers today.... As for the impurities of salt, it was hard to see how such very tiny quantities of extra minerals could make any difference to the human body one way or another." [R5C]

The following quote and chart were provided by the producers of a widely distributed salt, that is sold and labeled as sea salt; but, this devitalized salt is void of most trace minerals. [R6]

> "Our sea salt is derived from sea water and is processed by the solar evaporation method and is pure table salt." [R13]

	Pure 'table salt' that is labeled: sea salt.	
Sodium Chloride		99.990%
Calcium Sulfate		0.005%
Magnesium Chloride		0.003%
Sodium Sulfate		0.002%
Insolubles:		
Heavy Metals	less than 5.0 ppm *	< 0.000005%
Iron	less than 0.5 ppm *	< 0.0000005%
Copper	less than 0.5 ppm *	< 0.0000005%
Average moisture		0.1%
Potassium Iodide added		0.01%

(* ppm is parts per million is converted to decimal 0.00000_%) {chart from Pet Incorporated [R13]}

*^ For purpose of clarity the author will use 'SeaSalt' to refer to whole, full mineral content salt from the sea, while the 99.99% pure NaCl shall be referred to as common mineral-poor refined white-washed 'table salt'.

This fully dried salt is pure sodium and chloride, and is free from environmental contaminates but lacks most of the valuable macro, micro, and mini nutrient minerals found in whole SeaSalt. Calcium sulfate and magnesium chloride are often added to dried, refined table salt to prevent the small, bleached-white salt from clumping and insure the salt can be poured from a shaker.**[R14A]

∗ Ideally, body fluids, such as blood, have an almost identical mineral balance to saltwater.

∗The ideal match of blood with saltwater or SeaSalt, is very rarely found in people today.

SeaSalt provides many minerals that are valuable for nourishing the body and for digestion. All macro, micro and mini minerals in SeaSalt are needed in all biochemical functions of the body. Iodine is among the crucially important trace mineral nutrients in SeaSalt. The thyroid gland is particularly sensitive to a lack of iodine, which may lead to a number of deficiency disorders, including goiter. [R5A-R6-R8] Goiter, which involves a lack of iodine to the thyroid, is one of the oldest known nutrient deficiency diseases. [R8A] In the past, when a goiter was discovered, seafood such as kelp and SeaSalt were recognized as food remedies for this nutrient deficiency disease. [8A-2C-5B] Today, rapidly dried table salt is often 'iodized' by adding potassium iodide in an attempt to meet the body's need for iodine and prevent the development of a goiter. Iodine that is added to pure table salt is not present in the balance with other minerals that is ideal for health. Iodine added to table salt may not be well used by the thyroid, nor by the rest of the body. [R2C-5A]

∗ The ideal mineral balance that is found in SeaSalt may help to prevent or improve common health problems including: thyroid disorder, high blood pressure, chronic fatigue, and digestive disorders.

Whole SeaSalt vs White Table Salt

In centuries past, SeaSalt was valuable to make up for slight mineral deficiencies in foods. "In the past the trace-element deficiencies in our food were not too important because the missing elements were available for the most part in our table salt [SeaSalt]. In recent years, [after about 1910] however, the salt producers have refined their table salt almost to the point of chemical purity in their effort to market a product that will not 'cake' in damp weather. It appears that we still have not profited by past experience with polished rice." {By this, Dr. Hoechstetter is referring to the deficiency disease of beriberi, which became almost an epidemic in rice-eating countries, when brown rice was refined and the vitamin B containing germ [and bran] was removed to make it [rice] white.} [R5A]

The LORD's people have been called 'the salt of the Earth'. Whole SeaSalt or whole salt from mineral-rich land deposits are valuable for seasoning foods and are important for proper nutrition. But, if the healthy SeaSalt has lost its saltiness, or health-giving properties, of what value is it? None, except to be thrown away and trampled under foot! [R10A]

∗ Whole SeaSalt or mineral-rich land salt may be considered the first mineral food supplement ever.

* SeaSalt that retains all 71 minerals should be considered the 'gold standard' against which all other salt should be compared. Many people gathered salt from underground concentrations of salt solutions called 'brine'; as was frequent in colonial times in Virginia or New York. Typically, salt that was collected from salt water was concentrated by solar evaporation, while salt from brine was usually concentrated by boiling over a fire in large cast iron kettles. (Later, as the wood became scarce, solar evaporation was also used for brine salt.) The skill in salt making was in removing impurities as the salt was condensing, while allowing the salt crystals to precipitate, and then gathering the still moist lumps of salt crystals that remained. (It is noteworthy that many times people who were drilling for salt brine ended up finding petroleum, while other people were drilling for petroleum and ended up finding salt brine. Either resource proved highly profitable.) After the industrial revolution of the mid-1800s, many salt brine-rich areas such as Syracuse, NY used the brine as a source of chemicals for manufacturing. This was the age of business trusts and big corporations that began to dominate the economy. In the early days of salt making, the quality of the salt depended upon the source. Salt brine was often contaminated with iron oxide (FeO_2-rust), resulting in a 'red' salt of poor taste, while other salt brine contained excess gypsum. Thus, all salt (including SeaSalt) has needed some processing to remove impurities and collect the salt crystals. Even though all the impurities may not have been removed in the past, the salt of old always contained many essential minerals for health, beside just the sodium and chloride.

The goal of modern salt making is to produce a pure white Na–Cl salt product, regardless of the source, and to have the salt free flowing for convenience of use as 'table salt'. To produce pure table salt all moisture and all minerals except Na and Cl must be eliminated from seawater, rock salt or salt brine. Today, chemists or manufacturers to produce plastics, cosmetics, cleaners, electronics and other convenience items, often use trace minerals that formerly were in SeaSalt and in our bodies encouraging health. 'Leftover' mineral deficient table salt is not ideal for health.

** In areas of the world where salt was lacking or scarce, wars have been fought over salt. Armies have won or lost battles or even wars, depending upon whether their soldiers had salt. Roman soldiers guarding salt were often paid wages of salt. The term 'salary' originated from salt. Soldiers who were incompetent (at guarding salt) were said to be: 'not worth their salt'. [R7G-14G]

*** Salt has had a very important use in Hebrew culture. The term 'salt covenant' is a promise of enduring loyalty and trust, which stems from the nutritional use of salt as a preservative. [R7] Salt preserves foods (especially meats) by absorbing moisture, which prevents bacterial growth. Salt is often contrasted to leaven (yeast), which decays foods (especially grains) until its action is halted, as by heat from baking. Workers were at times paid wages of salt, from whence the term 'he is worth his weight in salt' came. SeaSalt was so valuable for health that a laborer, working in the heat of the day, often carried a small pouch for salt to overcome cramps and/or fatigue.

**** The author cannot over-emphasize the importance of full mineral content SeaSalt or mineral-rich brine or rock salt for balancing mineral and electrolyte needs of the body (blood, lymph, etc.). The minerals that are present in macro, micro and trace amounts in SeaSalt, if taken in higher, unbalanced concentrations, can be very harmful to human health. Healthy salt must be evaluated based on its balanced mineral content; <u>not</u> on convenience of use or taste or looks. [R7A]

(Pepper is an 'irritant' to the digestive system that many people may want to avoid and others must avoid.)

∗ SeaSalt has been the gold standard for quality salt, since before Moses wrote the *Torah*.

------------------------------------ References Ch 17 Salt ------------------------------------

[R1] Are You Confused?\ by Paavo Airola, PhD, ND; pg 190-191; salt
[R2] Seasalts Hidden Powers\ by Jacques deLangre, PhD; pg 1 - the definition of SeaSalt
[R2A] pg 30-31salting vegetables is good
[R2B] pg 52 the Brittany coast of France as an ideal place to hand harvest SeaSalt
[R2C] pg 33-36 balanced Iodine in SeaSalt
[R3] personal correspondence (May 1991)\ with Jacques deLangre sought SeaSalt chart
[R4] personal correspondence (Nov 1991)\ with Jacques deLangre purchased SeaSalt chart
[R5] The Complete Book of Food and Nutrition\ by J.I. Rodale and staff; Section 9 'Salt'; (279-308)
[R5] pg 302 potassium <u>iodide</u> added to processed table salt
[R5A] pg 304-305 (trace minerals =Health) & NE Jour of Medicine; 3 May 1951 quote Dr. Hoechstetter
[R5B] pg 305-308 mix of elements in salt water need also to be in sea salt
[R5C] pg 306-307 quote old lumpy salt with impurities verses modern pure Na–Cl w/out minerals
[R6] The 8 Week Cholesterol Cure\ by Robert E. Kowlowski; pg 88-89 excess sodium & HBP
[R7] Salt Natures Fifth Element\ by John Heinemann, PhD; pg 17 salt covenant
[R7A] pg 9 Hebrews gathered salt form Med. Sea and Dead Sea and land deposits
[R7B] pg 6, 33-34 body fluids an almost perfect match to salt water and SeaSalt
[R7G] pg 22 salary from salt //[R14] pg 13 wages, salary from salt guarding
[R7N] end of book other minerals necessary for life
[R8] Foods and Nutrition Encyclopedia\ pg 1959-1960 Ensminger, Ensminger, Konlande and Robson - 3rd Edition Pegasus Press-648 West Sierra A-Clovis, Calif. 93612 [R8A] pg 1083-1084 /[R8B] pg 1961 /[R8C] pg 1959
[R9] Salt\ from International Standard Bible Encyclopedia (ISBE)
[R10] Rare Earths Forbidden Cures\ by Joel Wallach, DVM, ND and Ma Lan, MD, MS
[R10] pg 355 salt hunger because little salt in grains, fruit and vegetables
[R10A] pg 20 salt traded ounce for ounce for gold
[R10B] pg 279-389 Periodic Table of the Elements
[R11] Food, Nutrition and Diet Therapy\ 7th ed; by Krause and Mahan; pg 184 salt
[R12] What the Bible Says About Healthy Living\ by Rex Russell, MD; pg 203-205 salt
[R13] personal correspondence with Pet Incorporated\ June 1991 table salt chart
[R14] Salt The Fifth Element\ by Garnett Laidlaw Eskew (1948)
[R14] pg 150-151 vacuum, suction salt refining – in 1910, Morton 1st salt that pours
[R14A] pg 172 calcium sulfate and magnesium chloride added to salt
[R14B] pg 13 Roman guard paid in salary of salt or not worth his salt
[R15] Neptune's Gift\ by Robert P. Multhauf
[R16] Folk Medicine\ by D.C. Jarvis, MD; pg 134-137; essential Iodine (I) is replaced by F – Cl – Br
[R17] Salt\ from National Geographic; September 1977; pg 380-401 salt as a resource
[R18] Strong's Concordance\ by James Strong, STD, LLD
pg 873 salt # 4417 H pg 67 ***melach*** Lev 2:13
[R19] The Poisons Around Us\ by Henry Schroeder, MD; balanced minerals ⇒ health
[R20] Trace Elements and Man\ by Henry Schroeder, MD; balanced minerals ⇒ health
[R21] The Hunger for Salt\ by Derek Denton; people crave 'whole' salt
[R22] Lecture at U of W (Oct 1992)\ by Bernard Jensen, DC; balanced minerals ⇒ health
[R23] Help Yourself to Better Health (02-17-2001radio 07-06-2002)\ by Monte Kline, PhD; 'Celtic' SeaSalt
[R24] Help Yourself to Better Health\ by Monte Kline, PhD newsletter update on sea salt
[R25] Proof Positive\ by Neil Nedley, MD; pg 137-141 salt
[R25A] pg 490 mineral chart
[R26] Lick the Sugar Habit\ by Nancy Appleton, PhD; pg 16 mineral wheel by Dr. Paul Eck
[R27] Seaweed Chart\ by Arnold Distributing
[R28] The 28-Day Antioxidant Diet Program\ by Steven Masley, MD; pg 72-73 salt
[R29] Tired or Toxic\ by Sherry A. Rogers, MD
[R30] Living in Divine Health (8 audio cassettes)\ by Ted Broer, PhD; (Tape 7-sBS)
Black Pepper is an intestinal irritant and is similar to 'slivers-of-glass' in the colon – avoid Pepper!

Have you ever seen a child playing on a teeter–totter by himself? That would be pretty silly. It's equally silly to take high doses of isolated minerals to restore health and maintain vitality. A body needs minerals balanced with other minerals, just as a teeter–totter requires balance.

SeaWeed–Kelp chart

Ag	Silver	-47-micro
Al	Aluminum	-13-micro
Au	Gold	-79-micro
B	Boron (5)	micro
Ba	Barium	-56-micro
Be	Beryllium	-4-mini
Bi	Bismuth (83)	mini
Br	Bromine	-34-mini
C	Carbon (6)	massive
Ca	Calcium (20)	macro
Cd	Cadmium	-48-mini
Ce	Cerium	-58-mini
Cl	Chlorine (17)	mega
Co	Cobalt (27)	micro
Cr	Chromium (24)	mini
Cs	Cesium	-55-mini
Cu	Copper (29)	micro
F	Fluorine (9)	micro
Fe	Iron (26)	micro
Ga	Gallium	-31-mini

Ge	Geranium-	32-micro
H	Hydrogen (1)	massive
Hg	Mercury	-49-micro
I	Iodine (53)	micro
In	Indium	-49-mini
Ir	Iridium	-77-mini
K	Potassium (19)	macro
La	Lanthanum	-57-micro
Li	Lithium (3)	micro
Mg	Magnesium (12)	micro
Mn	Manganese (25)	micro
Mo	Molybdenum (42)	micro
N	Nitrogen (7)	mega
Na	Sodium (11)	mega
Nb	Niobium	-41-mini
Ni	Nickel (28)	micro
O	Oxygen (8)	massive
Os	Osmium	-76-mini
P	Phosphorous (15)	micro
Pb	Lead	-82-micro

Pd	Palladium	-46-mini
Pt	Platinum	-78-mini
Ra	Radium	-88-mini
Rb	Rubidium	-37-micro
Rh	Rhodium	-45-mini
S	Sulfur (16)	macro
Se	Selenium (34)	micro
Sb	Antimony	-51-micro
Si	Silicon (14)	micro
Sn	Tin (50)	micro
Sr	Strontium	-38-micro
Te	Tellurium	-52-mini
Th	Thorium	-90-mini
Ti	Titanium	-22-micro
Tl	Thallium	-81-micro
U	Uranium	-92-micro
V	Vanadium (23)	micro
W	Tungsten	-43-micro
Zn	Zinc (30)	micro
Zr	Zirconium	-40-mini

SeaWeed–Kelp Chart above lists the elements in SeaWeed and groups similar concentrations.
Mega, Macro, Micro and Mini mineral groups in Sea Weed relate well to percentages in SeaSalt.
Numbers in ( ) indicate the atomic number of elements that are considered beneficial to health.
Numbers in - - indicate the atomic number of elements that aren't known as beneficial to health.

Elements in SeaSalt that aren't in seaweed include: As - Arsenic #33 / Y - Yttrium #39 / Ti - Titanium #81 & all the Noble gases: He - Helium / Ne - Neon / Ar - Argon / Kr - Krypton / Xe - Xenon / Ra - Radon.

Periodic Table of the Elements

Many important trace minerals for health -V–Cr–Mn–Fe–Co–Ni–Cu–Zn- - - -Se- are found in the same horizontal row # 4.

H 1																H 1	He 2
Li 3	Be 4											B 5	C 6	N 7	O 8	F 9	Ne 10
Na 11	Mg 12											Al 13	Si 14	P 15	S 16	Cl 17	Ar 18
K 19	Ca 20	Sc 21	Ti 22	V 23	Cr 24	Mn 25	Fe 26	Co 27	Ni 28	Cu 29	Zn 30	Ga 31	Ge 32	As 33	Se 34	Br 35	Kr 36
Rb 37	Sr 38	Y 39	Zr 40	Nb 41	Mo 42	Tc 43	Ru 44	Rh 45	Pd 46	Ag 47	Cd 48	In 49	Sn 50	Sb 51	Te 52	I 53	Xe 54
Cs 55	Ba 56	57- -71	Hf 72	Ta 73	W 74	Re 75	Os 76	Ir 77	Pt 78	Au 79	Hg 80	Tl 81	Pb 82	Bi 83	Po 84	At 85	Rn 86
Fr 87	Ra 88	89- -103															

La 57	Ce 58	Pr 59	Nd 60	Pm 61	Sm 62	Eu 63	Gd 64	Tb 65	Dy 66	Ho 67	Er 68	Tm 69	Yb 70	Lu 71
Ac 89	Th 90	Pa 91	U 92	Np 93	Pu 94	Am 95	Cm 96	Bk 97	Cf 98	Es 99	Fm 100	Md 101	No 102	Lr 103

Minerals within the same vertical column often share similar chemical and/or physical properties. The most important mineral interactions often occur between minerals within the same column or row. Elements 89 to 103, such as Plutonium (Pu-94) are often unstable, radioactive and injurious to health.

Chapter 18 Nuts, Seeds and Beans (Legumes)
Nuts and Seeds

----------- **NUTS** ---------------------------------------

Almonds (***shaqed***) and Pistachio nuts (***boten***) are the nuts mentioned in the ***Torah*** by Moses as food, and they are certainly representative of the many fine nuts that the Hebrews ate.

NIV Gen 43:11 Put some of the best products of the land in your bags and take them down to the man as a gift – a little balm and a little honey, some spices and myrrh, some pistachio nuts and almonds.

Nuts and Seeds are concentrated sources of proteins, unsaturated fatty acids (Vitamin F), B-complex vitamins, vitamin E and many trace minerals, including copper and iron. [R1-1A-12-15] Nuts, Seeds and Beans (and grains), due to their natural low water content, may be stored for long periods of time without losing nutritional value. Nuts and Seeds contain oils that are easily damaged by heating, so the most nutritious way to eat them is raw. Almonds are the most nutritious nuts, according to Dr. Jensen. [R6] * Nuts contain few mineral salts for the production of hydrochloric acid; so, adding salt, especially SeaSalt, to nuts often aids in their proper digestion. (Baklava is a tasty desert pastry made from (pistachio) nuts and honey and phyllo dough.) [R31]

---------- **SEEDS** -------------------------------------

The Hebrews certainly included many types of seeds from seed-bearing plants in their diet.

NIV Gen 1:29 Then God said, "I give you every seed-bearing plant on the face of the whole earth and every tree that has fruit with seed in it. They will be yours for food."

NIV Ex 9:31 The flax and barley were destroyed, [by the Plague of Hail] since the barley had headed and the flax was in bloom.

Nuts, Seeds and Beans, as well as grains, are particularly important for their mineral content, and their oil-soluble nutrients, such as essential fatty acids (EFAs) and oil-soluble vitamin E. [R3-24]

Flax seeds are known to be amongst the most nutritious of these seeds.

> '"Flax is an excellent food, because it contains almost a complete diet all by itself. The solid part of the seed is used [by the body to heal] in all of the digestive, eliminative, toxic diseases of the stomach intestines, and colon. Flax is useful in the treatment of constipation. It increases the bulk of the stool, speeds up the movement of the stool out of the body, and thereby prevents the buildup of toxins in the bowel." [R2A]

Nuts, Seeds and Beans, as well as many grains, are excellent sources of many UFAs. [R1C-3] Flax seeds contain the essential fatty acids (EFAs) – Linoleic Acid (LA) and Linolenic Acid (LNA), which may also be called vitamin F. Linolenic Acid is often considered the most important EFA, because only fish oil and flax oil contain the EFA (omega 3) in a substantial concentration. [R1A-2] Flax oil also contains a special phosphorous-containing complex-fat nutrient, lecithin, which is valuable for the digestion of fats and oils and the utilization of cholesterol. [R2B-2C] (see Ch 23) Flax seed is an excellent source of fiber, which helps soften the stool and prevent constipation. Flax seed is mucilaginous and a natural laxative that helps the colon form a slick, mucous layer. Flax seed contains nearly every major and trace mineral. Flax seed contains the oil-soluble vitamins D, E and carotene (pre-vitamin A), and the water-soluble vitamins B1, B2 and C. [R2D] Flax seeds contain complete protein. In his book *Fats that Heal Fats that Kill* Udo Erasmus, PhD promotes flax oil as an alternative source of omega 3 oil, to the more often used fish liver oil.

Canola oil is made from a hybrid (see Ch 7) of the rape seed plant and is being marketed as a healthy alternative to butter and other vegetable oils because the oil is low in saturated fat and like all vegetable oils, contains no cholesterol. Canola oil, however, may also contain some erucic fatty acid that must be eliminated by the body. Erucic fatty acid may scar heart walls and may lead to fatty degeneration of the heart, kidneys, adrenals and thyroid. [R2J] The oil from rape seed was likely never used by people as food before it was altered by hybridization to make canola oil. Canola oil, despite all the hype, is not a perfect or useful oil for health, and is fragile on the shelf. Canola oil, like margarine, is inexpensive to produce, and it requires marketing for sales. [R27]

*note- Nuts and Seeds and Beans are very concentrated sources of nourishment, and some people may have difficulty digesting them. For ease of digestion the author recommends eating nuts, seeds and beans with 'whole SeaSalt' (Ch 17 Salt), and Dr. Jensen recommends eating nuts, seeds and beans with fresh fruit juice, such as pineapple, or with pure water to aid digestion. [R6]

∗ Nuts and Seeds are rich in nutrients, may be difficult to digest, and should be eaten raw.

Beans

----------- **BEANS** – including Legumes ------------

Lentils (***adash***), which are a legume, were the main element of the porridge that Jacob served Esau, and are certainly representative of all the beans that were eaten by the Hebrews. (Esau so lacked insight that he sold his birthright for a bowl of lentil stew and a piece of bread.)

NIV Gen 25:34 Then Jacob gave Esau some bread and some lentil (***adash***) stew.

Legumes are a hearty, versatile bean. Legumes including Pea, Soybean, Lentil and Peanut^^ and are a rich source of proteins, iron, thiamin, riboflavin and niacin. [R1B] Proteins are made from building blocks of molecules called amino acids (AAs). Of the 22 amino acids the body needs, 8 AAs are called essential because the body cannot build them from other amino acids. To efficiently use the protein in food, all 8 essential AAs should be present in the same meal. 'Complete' proteins contain all 8 of the essential amino acids, and include meats, milk and eggs. Foods that are high in 'incomplete' proteins, such as legumes, contain an abundance of certain essential AAs, but a scarcity of other essential AAs. To efficiently utilize the protein from incomplete sources, foods that are high in certain amino acids and deficient in other amino acids are best combined with other foods that have the different abundances and sacristies of AAs. Foods that complete other incomplete proteins are called 'complimentary' to one-another. [R5] Because of their high but incomplete protein content, legumes can be eaten in combination with other incomplete, yet complimentary protein rich foods, so the body can obtain all the required AAs at each meal. Lentils and other legumes, plus whole, grains, such as whole wheat bread, are ideal protein compliments. [R5A] The meal that Jacob served Esau of Lentil stew and whole-grain bread is an excellent example of combining foods to compliment incomplete proteins. Combining several legumes with several whole grains is even better for complementing incomplete proteins. Beans are an excellent source of fiber. When whole grains are processed to white flour, many AAs are lost and their value for complimenting other foods is greatly reduced. [R5B] (Ch 17 Grains)
Beans are ideal to compliment incomplete proteins for protein-rich vegetarian meals. [R5C]
Beans often taste bland without being spiced. Onion, Garlic and SeaSalt are excellent as spices. (Beans are often eaten with pork/ham to add a spicy, toxic, addictive taste to their bland flavor.)

Beans need to be well cooked for easy of digestion. Beans are difficult digest due to sugars that are bound in a manner that makes them difficult for human digestive enzymes to cleave. [R32]
***The digestive system can be trained to digest beans, or any *kosher* food, more efficiently!**
Begin digestive training by eating a small serving of beans at the same time (ie - lunch) every day. To aid efficient digestion, begin a meal with an enzyme-rich fruit or fruit juice, such as pineapple. In time, the digestive system will produce the required enzymes to efficiently digest *kosher* food. Light exercise after lunch (ie - walking or stretching) may aid digestion. SeaSalt often aids digestion. Later, a greater variety and quantity of beans can be eaten on a more flexible time schedule. [R6]

Sprouting greatly potentiates the mineral, protein, vitamin, enzyme and fiber value of Seeds and Beans, as Ann Wigmore quoted Jeffrey Bland, PhD in her book *The Sprouting Book.* [R30A]

> “The germinating seed represents a protein manufacturing machine which is turning out protein... along with the necessary vitamins and minerals for its assimilation and utilization.”

As sprouting potentiates nutrition in nuts, seeds and beans, roasting may damage nutrition. The vitamin C content of a nut, seed or bean is virtually nil, but sprouts readily creates vitamin C. Captain Cook first recognized and used sprouts, for their vitamin C, to prevent scurvy on ships. Sprouts continued to be used for their vitamin C content throughout WWI and WWII in India. [R30] Enzymes in sprouts turn starch and large carbohydrates into simple sugars, fatty acids into fats and complex proteins into simple proteins and individual AAs. Protein and minerals are building blocks for the newly developing plant and are also building blocks for maintaining human health. Minerals are bound in raw seeds and beans (and grains) so they may be difficult to digest, but after sprouting, minerals are naturally chelated with proteins, making them easily absorbed. Sprouts are live food. Sprouts are great with many meals, especially salads or sandwiches. [R30A]
*** Sprouting Seeds and Beans may be thought of as a key that unlocks a treasure chest of nutrients.**
^^ Peanut is technically a legume but is practically considered as a nut, and should be eaten raw. Legumes ‘fix’ nitrogen from the soil, which makes them useful as cover crops and in crop rotation.
*#*note- Carob is a bean routinely eaten by Hebrews, but it isn’t mentioned in the ***Torah/Tanakh***. Carob has a similar taste to chocolate, but carob has no caffeine, much less fat and more protein. Carob is a healthy alternative to chocolate. Carob powder is used like chocolate in desserts. [R23]

*** Beans are nutritious and were eaten often by the Hebrews as part of their healthy diet.**

---------------------- References Ch 18 Nuts, Seeds and Beans ----------------------

[R1] Nutritional Almanac\ pg 191
[R1A] pg 55/ [R1B] pg 188/ [R1C] pg 220-222
[R2] Fats and Oils\ by Udo Erasmus, PhD; pg 34-35/ [R2A] pg 265/
[R2B] pg 263 [R2C] pg 56-57 / [R2D] pg 262-265/ [R2E] pg 86/
[R2F] pg 88/ [R2G] pg 90-95/ [R2H] pg 88 & 95-102/ [R2J] pg 104
[R3] Are You Confused?\ by Paavo Airola, ND; pg 80
[R3A] pg 74
[R4] Unsafe at Any Meal\ by Earl Mindell, PhD; pg 77 &116
[R4A] pg 79-80
[R5] Diet for a Small Planet\ by Francis Moore Lappe; pg 81-82
[R5A] pg 153 /[R5B] pg 377 [R5C] pg 136-137
[R6] Foods That Heal – and – Lecture at UofW\ by Bernard Jensen, DC; 1 Oct 1992
[R7] Eat, Drink and Be Ready\ by Monte L. Kline, PhD and W. P. Strube Jr.; pg 201-203
[R8] The Encyclopedia of Psychoactive Drugs: Caffeine The Most Popular Stimulant \by Richard Gilbert, PhD; pg 19 (&44-45)
[R8A] pg 40-41 /[R8B] pg 44-45 (&19) /[R8C] pg 111-117 &137
[R9] The Coffee Book (Chartwell Books)\ by Jacki Baxter; pg 14-15 early history of coffee
[R10] Coffee (101 Productions, Publishing)\ by Kenneth Davids; pg 21-22
[R11] The Book of Coffee and Tea\ by Joel, David, Karl Schapira; pg 5-9
[R12] What the Bible Says About Healthy Nutrition\ by Rex Russell, MD
[R13] Comptom's Pictured Encyclopedia-1963 Ed. 'Coffee'\ pg 428
[R14] America's Favorite Drug: Coffee and Your Health\ by Bonnie Edwards, RN ∗great booklet (Odonian Press; Box 7776; Berkeley, CA; 94662); pg 24 creosote – gums, tars, resins
[R15] The Book of Coffee and Tea\ by Joel, David & Karl Schapira; pg 5-9 history of coffee
[R16] Coffee and Tea; by Elin Mccoy & Frederick Walker\ pg 9 Islamic prayer - pg10 iron rations pg 9-10 coffee to stay awake at religious services // pg12 soon coffee part of Islamic religious ritual
[R17] Nuts and Seeds – The Natural Snacks\ by Rodale Press – healthy fast food
[R18] Strong's Concordance\ by James Strong, STD, LLD

pg 593	Lentil	# 5742	H pg 86	***adash***	Gen 25:34
pg 49	Almond	# 8247	H pg 120	***shaqed***	Gen 43:11
pg 732	nuts (Pistachio)	# 992	H pg 20	***boten***	Gen 43:11

[R19] Help Yourself to Better Health\ by Monte Kline, PhD; health update on coffee
[R20] 30 Day Health Makeover\ by Marilu Hennen; pg 46 6oz cup coffee = kidneys lose ≈5$^+$ mgs Ca$^+$
[R21] Coffee Plantation (Colombia 1984)\ visit by Jay Nelson Beans may acidify soil ⇒ inhibit plant growth
[R22] Healing Foods from the Bible\ by Bernard Wood; pg 67-70 nuts, seeds and beans
[R23] Carob (Internet Encyclopedic article); healthy alternative to chocolate
[R24] Mental and Elemental Nutrients\ by Carl Pfeiffer, MD, PhD; pg 44
[R25] Proof Positive\ by Neil Nedley, MD; pg 67-69 nuts
[R25A] pg 30-32 acids pg 265-272 coffee
[R26] Creosote - conversation with Travis Shaw -- Army Corp of Engineers – a restricted substance
Creosote byproduct from coal processing and oil refining used for piles for dock piers and for railroad trestles and ties.
------ Creosote is 85% polycyclic aromatic hydrocarbons (PCAH or PAH or PCH) {several hundred PCAHs}
Polychlorinated phenols (PCP) may purposely be added to creosote to increase toxicity to insects.
possibly small amounts of dioxin (a PCP) which is likely carcinogenic – some dioxins from barbequing meat
some dioxins present in burning of any wood product containing Chlorine containing compounds
[R27] New Whole Foods Encyclopedia\ by Rebecca Wood; pg 54 Canola oil is bad news
[R28] The 28-Day Antioxidant Diet Program\ by Steven Masley, MD; pg 107-109 nuts-seeds pg 54, 69, 94-99 legumes or beans
[R29] Sprouting for the New Millennium\ dist by Handy Pantry
[R30] The Sprouting Book\ by Ann Wigmore; pg 2-3 Capt. Cook 1st used sprouts to prevent scurvy.
[R30A] pg 5-6 Dr. Bland quote and nutrition information
[R31] Grains, Rice and Beans\ by Kevin Graham; pg 88 Millet - the 'gruel of endurance' in Old Testament pg 156 Pistachio Nuts with honey and phyllo flour used in baklava.
[R32] The Bean Bible\ by Aliza Green; pg 4-5 digestive problems from beans
[R33] Making the Best of Basics\ by James Talmage Stevens
[R34] The Bible Cure\ by Reginald Cherry, MD
[R35] CBS Sunday Morning (09-07-03); Coffee – Bennet Weinberg wrote 2 books on Coffee Caffeine – one of the fastest acting drugs – blocks the adenosine in the body that causes drowsiness.
[R36] Maximum Energy\ by Ted Broer, PhD; Ch 16 pg 186-196 – avoid Coffee and Caffeine

Coffee

Coffee in History – Coffee plants were originally native only to the high, steeply sloped, mountains of Ethiopia. [R10] Caffeine and acids in coffee beans act as natural insecticides so small insects won't feast on the bright red beans. When a mountain lad saw a wild animal leaping and hopping around after eating coffee beans, he considered them a good source of energy. Possibly, after an Ethiopian invasion of Arabia in ≈525 AD, coffee plants were found in Yemen. [R10] The first method of human consumption of coffee beans was to squash them, combine them with animal fat, and role the mixture into balls called 'iron rations'. [R16] These coffee/fat balls were carried on long treks by warriors and caravan travelers for use as a stimulant. [R9-10-11] Not until ≈1000 AD, did Arabs first boil water and add ground-up coffee beans, to consume coffee as a hot drink. [R9-11] Coffee as a beverage was often used by Moslems to stay awake and alert during their long religious services. [R16A] During the 1200s AD, coffeehouses became part of mainstream Arab life, and they spread throughout the Moslem Arab world. In 1615, many church clergymen first became aware of coffee, and condemned coffee as the 'drink of the devil', however Pope Clement VIII tasted the coffee drink and blessed it. After being blessed by the Pope, coffeehouses and drinking coffee spread throughout Europe and the Christian world. [R9-11] Through the late 1600s AD, almost all coffee came from Arabia, until coffee plants were smuggled throughout the world in the 1700s AD. [R9-10-11] Coffee replaced tea as the most popular drink in America only after 1773, when King George of England continued a tax on tea, which caused the 'Boston Tea Party'. [R8] Today, people of the United States consume 65-75% of all the coffee in the world [R13], and the caffeine in coffee is the world's most popular stimulant drug. [R8]

Amongst the beans that were not consumed by the Hebrews was the coffee bean. [R9-10-11] There is nearly no food value (carbohydrate, protein, fat, vitamin or mineral) in a coffee beverage. Caffeine from any source is a drug. [R8] Caffeine has a chemical structure that is very similar to naturally occurring nicotinic-type neurotransmitters in the human nervous system, which accounts for caffeine's brain stimulating and sleep depressing effects. [R8B] The purine chemical structure of caffeine is also close to the gene structure of DNA, accounting for the fact that caffeine can interfere with the reproduction of cells, which may result in tumors, cancer or genetic defects. [8A]

Natural oils in coffee beans are altered by roasting to become a group of gums, resins and tars including creosote, which are very carcinogenic and become part of the brewed coffee. [R14] The liver's biochemistry isn't designed to biodegrade the gums, tars or resins created in coffee. Similar gums, tars and resins (P{C}AHs) are created in tobacco and marijuana smoke, crude oil refining, and in wood-burning stoves where they collect on the inside of chimneys. Creosote is used to prevent wood (fence posts, railroad ties or pilings) from rotting. No biochemistry in nature easily biodegrades creosote. Creosote is labeled a biological toxin and is no longer public in use.

The author theorizes: Gums, tars or resins in coffee may clog human capillaries, may wall tissues off from their blood supply and may allow a toxic environment to develop. Just as tobacco tars may cause lung cancer; so gums, tars or resins in coffee may promote cancer throughout the body.

Monte Kline, PhD on his Saturday *Help Yourself to Better Health* radio program discussed that caffeine from coffee may inhibit the kidney's ability to eliminate toxins from the blood. [R19]

Acids in coffee are very strong and may upset the digestive system's delicate pH balance, which may encourage stomach disorders and prevent proper digestion of food. Proper digestion is a major problem for the elderly and many people in poor health. (Coffee growers are careful that coffee beans don't drop on the ground and remain to acidify the soil – which may interfere with plant growth.)

Caffeine in coffee, tea, chocolate or soft drinks is a very fast acting drug. Caffeine gives the body a 'lift' by stimulating adrenal glands to produce adrenaline, which causes the liver to convert its storehouse of glycogen to glucose. Glucose is then dumped into the bloodstream, producing a 'coffee high'. The rush from the caffeine high is produced at great expense to the internal organs: the liver is depleted of valuable glycogen; the adrenals are stressed as they produce adrenaline; the pancreas is stressed to stabilize the blood sugar; and the kidneys are stressed, causing many nutrients to be lost or eliminated in the urine. ∗ **Caffeine damages the efficiency of the kidneys.** ∗∗ **Each 6 oz cup of coffee causes the kidneys to lose 5$^+$ mgs of Calcium.** [R20] Like many drugs, caffeine gives the body a quick stimulation but may also produce unwanted side effects, including physical or psychological addictions. [R4-8C] Incidentally, the chemical residues in decaffeinated coffee may be as bad or worse for health than the caffeine that they removed. [R4A]

No matter how you pore it, coffee, latte or espresso does not belong in any healthy diet.
∗ Coffee (with caffeine, acids, gums, tars and resins) is the worst beverage imaginable for health.

Chapter 19 Water
Pure Water

Clean fresh water (***mayim***) is among the most vital needs of the human body. The Hebrews obtained pure drinking water, even while wandering in the desert, as they used unglazed earthen pottery vessels with thin walls for purifying water. Water put into these vessels filtered through the thin earthen walls, within which impurities and contaminants were trapped. Water that filtered through the earthen vessel, as well as water that condensed on the outside would then drip into a glazed collecting vessel below. (Water vapor from condensation collected on the outside of the unglazed vessel only when the vessel contained cold water.) Water vapor that condensed on the unglazed vessel already underwent purification through the 'water cycle' including, evaporation from ground water, vaporization in the atmosphere and re-condensation as water droplets. [R1] (*)

∗ Water free of contaminants and safe to drink was obtained from unglazed earthen vessels.

JPS Lev 15:12 And the earthened vessel, which he that hath an issue toucheth, shall be broken, ...
KJV Lev 15:12 And the vessel of earth, that he toucheth which hath the issue, shall be broken: ...

George Bush in his Leviticus commentary discussed thin-walled, unglazed, earthen vessels. [R1]
"These unglazed earthen vessels were to be broken if they became contaminated. Without glazing as a barrier, any disease causing germs that came into contact with these vessels would permanently be retained within the vessel walls. If this unclean vessel were then used again, any water flowing through it would become contaminated and would be unfit for drinking."

-------- See pictures of how an unglazed vessel may have looked on pages 178 and 179 -------

Today, many effective ways to purify water exist (filters, solar and steam distillation, reverse osmosis or chemical 'ion exchange'). Water purification systems often include additional in-line carbon or cotton filters designed after the Hebrew water-vessel filtration principle. Good filtration systems remove most chlorine, fluorine, chemicals, toxins and microbes from drinking water.

∗ Keeping the cells of the body properly hydrated is essential for continued efficient function. Unfortunately, many of the beverages that are consumed today frequently contain additives that may actually act to draw water out of the cells and thereby may encourage cellular de-hydration. Coffee, tea, soft drinks, diet sodas, sports drinks, meal replacement drinks, packaged mixes and all alcoholic beverages may contribute to cellular de-hydration and decreased cellular function. Hydration is critical in digestion, where water helps digestive enzymes break down food, absorb nutrients and flush away toxins. Dr. Jensen recommended drinking a glass of water during meals. The recommendation of 6 to 8 glasses of pure clean water throughout the day is often proper.

Paul Bragg, PhD, ND in his book *The Shocking Truth About Water* and Allen Banik, OD in his book *The Choice is Clear* and Henry Schroeder, MD in his book *The Trace Elements and Man* discuss inorganic minerals and residues of toxic chemicals that often contaminate public water. Dr. Schroeder states that soft slightly acid water may leach toxic cadmium from the water pipes. Cadmium can replace essential zinc in the vascular system, which may be a major risk factor contributing to atherosclerosis, high blood pressure, and heart or kidney disease. [R13] Dr. Bragg stated that inappropriate, inorganic minerals get into the blood stream and may be deposited on the walls of the arteries. This leads to a general inflexibility of the arteries and a narrowing of the lumen within the artery that can be used for circulation; which is known as arteriolar sclerosis or hardening of the arteries. [R2] Contaminants in drinking water are a huge issue concerning health.

People can only live without clean water for a couple of days. One primary need for water is to flush waste byproducts of human biochemistry and other ingested toxins out of the body. [R12]
"Water is necessary for digestion, assimilation, elimination, circulation, nutrient transport, temperature control, and as a solvent and medium for chemical reactions to take place." [R11]

The LORD God promised His Hebrew followers a good land including abundant clean water.

JPS Deut 8:7 For the LORD thy God bringeth thee into a good land, a land of brooks of water, of fountains and depths, springing forth in valleys and hills.

JPS Deut 11:11 ... a land of hills and valleys, and drinketh water as the rain of heaven cometh down.

* Moses likely had knowledge of desert springs and how to locate them from his years in Midian. Often desert waterways are just below the surface layer of rock formations. Moses may have used this information when he struck off the outer facing of a rock in the desert, which allowed water to flow through the porous limestone at Rephidim (Ex 17) and at Meribah (Num 20). [R10]

∗ Keeping the LORD's lofty standards for pure clean fresh water is essential for ideal health.

Fluoridation

Fluoride is currently added to public drinking water in many USA cities. When fluoridation began in the mid 1940s, many people believed that a 'new and glorious age' had begun for preventative dentistry. George Waldbott, MD wrote in his book *Fluoridation: the Great Dilemma* that the goal of fluoridation was to be a low cost, safe, effective way to reduce dental caries. [R3] The rationale was: that youngsters in an area where fluoride is naturally found in drinking water seemed to have fewer cavities than their peers in towns without high fluoride in the water. [R3A] However, minerals other than fluoride, may have been responsible for reduced cavities. [R8-14] Some early studies seem to support fluoridation of water for the prevention of dental caries. [R3K] The dilemma was, and still is: fluoride is a very toxic substance to the human body, [R5] that can cause sudden acute toxicity (including vomiting, abdominal cramps, diarrhea, shock, or tetany), [R3C- 3B-3N-7] and chronic, slowly developing toxicity including skeletal fluorosis and mottling of teeth and impaired function to most if not all the human glands, tissues and organs. [R3D-3L-7A-15] Sodium Fluoride (NaF) is an enzyme poison with widespread toxic effects throughout the body. [R4]

Leo Spira, MD, PhD in his book *The Drama of Fluoride: Arch Enemy of Mankind* wrote about the toxic chronic effect of exposure to low concentrations of fluoride over a long period of time. [R7] For any chronic poisoning, there is usually a gradual transition from a condition of normality to one of protracted abnormality. Frequently, there is no sharp line of demarcation of symptoms as in acute poisoning; and this fact in itself often makes it difficult to associate a pathological condition with the fundamental causes. Chronic fluoride intoxication's are of greater importance to the public health than are acute toxicities, but in comparison little is known about chronic intoxications as to scope, significance and ultimate tissue and functional changes. [R3D] In his book *Fluoride the Aging Factor* John Yiamouyiannis, PhD wrote that chronic consumption of fluoride both poisons enzymes and decreases the efficient functioning of the immune system. [R4] Since the immune system is responsible for defending the body against disease, decreasing the proper function of the immune system may increase a person's susceptibility to bacterial and viral infections. [R4A] In addition to weakening the body's ability to resist infection, fluoride may also increases the likelihood of the immune system damaging the body's own healthy tissues, as takes place in autoimmune diseases, such as: type 1 diabetes, lupus, fibromyalgia or rheumatoid arthritis. [R4B]

Skeletal fluorosis is a chronic fluoride toxicity, may result in excess calcification of bones, increased bone density, abnormal laying down of the bone, and calcification of ligaments and joints, which frequently leads to rheumatic arthritis and other crippling joint deformities. [R3D]

Tooth mottling is another significant toxic side effect of fluoride toxicity, which disrupts the metabolism of the enamel of teeth. Mottled teeth begin to show white, yellow, or brown spots on their enamels (outer surfaces). Advanced fluoride mottling can cause teeth to appear absolutely black and may cause pitting. [R3E-R3F-3M] The outer portion (¼) of the enamel in fluoride mottled teeth is distinguished by an absence of cementing substance between the enamel rods. Although fluoride mottled teeth may be initially more resistant to decay, when fluoride mottled teeth get caries, the teeth are difficult to fill due to frail tooth enamel. ∗ Thus, fluoride mottled teeth, should they get caries, may need to be crowned, or removed and replaced with bridges or dentures. [R3F]

> "There is ample evidence that mottled teeth, though they be somewhat more resistant to the onset of decay, are structurally weak, and that unfortunately, when decay does set in, the results are often disastrous." [R3F]

The fluoride level at which tooth mottling affects about 10% of the population is about 1.0 ppm in public drinking water. A fluoride level of 0.7 ppm is near the concentration considered optimal for prevention of cavities. [R3G] When fluoride exceeds 2.0 ppm then brownish mottling is seen in many teeth. [R3H] Fluoridation of public water has a very low margin of safety – therapeutic index.

> "No specific biochemical pathway requirement or essential metabolic role for fluoride has yet been discovered in any mammals, including man. The fact that fluoride affects, and is incorporated in the mineralization, of bones and teeth does not demonstrate its indispensability. Although lead, mercury, and cadmium share this property, that fact does not make them essential nutrients." [R3J] If an essential role for fluoride is ever found, an important fact to keep in mind is that many minerals have essential functions at very low concentrations; but, at high concentrations these same minerals can be very toxic. [R3P]

Fluoride is used an insecticide and a rat poison. [R6] Fluoride is a toxic waste by-product of aluminum smelting and manufacturing to be disposed of – or to be sold as 'dental care'. [R16] Fluoride may also replace essential Iodine in the thyroid, risking goiter or thyroid dysfunction. [R21]

∗ When Fluoride is added to water to prevent dental caries, the cure may be worse than the disease.

The Halogens – Fluorine, Chlorine, Bromine and Iodine

Fluorine, Chlorine, Bromine and Iodine are all part of the 'halogen' chemical family. (Ch 17) As a general rule, the lighter molecular weight element in a chemical family is more 'active' and will more easily form compounds than a heavier molecular weight chemical from the same family. Fluorine, as discussed earlier, is the most reactive member of the halogen family, which means it easily forms compounds with other chemicals, and it is the most likely to react with body tissues. Chlorine is added to every public water supply system today to prevent growth of harmful bacteria, which is necessary since public water is stagnant and may sit in reservoirs for months before use. Chlorination of public water is generally effective, however, recent evidence documents that some mutated bacterial spores in the water reservoirs may become resistant to chlorine sanitation. [R11] Cryptosporidium is a microbe that may contaminate public water and is not killed by chlorination. While chlorination of public water usually limits microbial growth, this chlorine is similar to diluted household bleach and is not healthy for drinking water. Chlorine in public water may also be absorbed by the skin during showers, while swimming or in hot tubs. Chlorine in public water may combine with otherwise innocuous organic elements in water to form trihalomethanes (THM) or chloroform. Chloroform and THM are both potent carcinogens and are unhealthy to drink. [R12] Since Chlorine, etc. may be absorbed by the skin, showerhead filters are ideal to remove them. Fluorine and Chlorine toxicity from water, like many other toxicities, may be cumulative over time. Bromine, being a heavier element than Chlorine or Fluorine, is thus less-toxic to human health. Bromine is often a better choice than Chlorine to kill microbes in hot tubs, saunas and Jacuzzis. The best chemical for killing microbes in a swimming pool is ozone. Ozone (O_3) is effective, safe and not toxic. Ozone is created in small amounts in breaking waves and is invigorating to health. Iodine is essential for proper thyroid function. The halogen balance in SeaSalt, sea weed (kelp), and clean saltwater fish is ideal for health and to promote retention of Iodine by the thyroid.

∗ Because Fluorine, Chlorine and Bromine are all lighter than Iodine they can replace essential Iodine from the thyroid, which may interfere with normal thyroid function. [R9]

"It has long been established that fluorides interfere with the action of many [human] enzymes. Not all enzymes are affected, of course, but the action when it occurs is very powerful and takes place at unbelievably low concentrations of fluoride." [R8A]

Today, the most practical scenario is to add Chlorine in the reservoir and to remove it for drinking.

(*Fluorine, Chlorine, Bromine, Iodine are used for elements. – Fluoride, Chloride, Bromide, Iodide are used for compounds.)

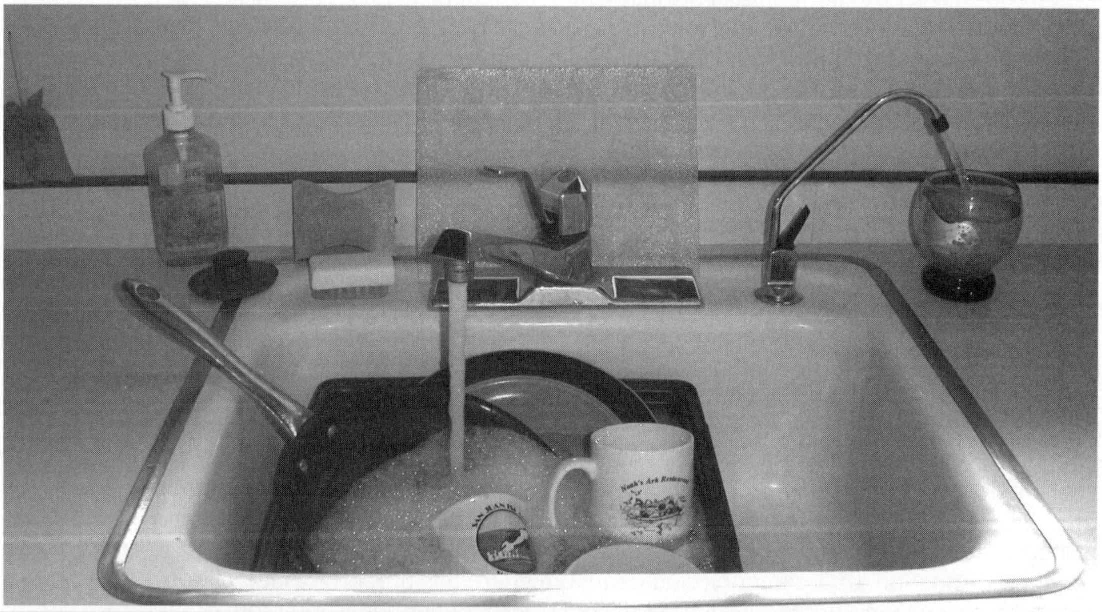

One faucet for tap water for washing dirty dishes – and – a second faucet for clean water for drinking.

Beverages including coffee, many teas, soda pop and those containg alcohol may cause less water to enter cells, resulting in a state of cellular 'dehydration' and decreased cellular efficiency. Water is the medium of exchange by which living organisms conduct the metabolism of life; just as money is the medium of exchange by which people conduct the commerce of free trade.

Photos of one possible, although not yet functional, Hebrew Water Purification Vessel on pages 178 and 179.

---------------------------------- References Ch 19 Water ----------------------------------

[R1] Notes on Leviticus/ by George Bush; pg 138 thin-walled earthened vessel
[R2] The Shocking Truth About Water\ by Paul Bragg, ND; pg 2-4 hard water = hard arteries
[R3] Fluoridation the Great Dilemma\ by George Waldbott, MD pg 23 Fluorides as Industrial Waste
[R3] pg 175 new glorious age [R3A] pg 63 & 64-67 quote on mottled teeth
[R3B] pg 72 &Ch7 &Ch8 the dilemma [R3C] pg 90 acute toxicity
[R3D] pg 98-104 chronic Fluoride toxicity - skeletal fluorosis
[R3E] pg 62 effects of Fluoride mottling [R3F] pg 176 weakened mottled tooth enamel
[R3G] pg 66 Key 1.0 ppm Fluoride [R3H] pg 67 mottling exceeding 2.0 ppm
[R3J] pg 82 quote no essential biochemical need for Fluoride
[R3K] pg 67-71 preliminary studies on Fluoride reducing dental caries
[R3L] pg 148-168 Fluoride – enzyme poison [R3M] pg 66-69 advanced tooth mottling
[R3N] pg 120 chronic Fluoride toxicity [R3P] pg 76-77 debate on essential Fluoride
[R4] Fluoride the Aging Factor\ by John Yiamouyiannis, PhD
[R4] pg 26-33 Fluoride decreases WBC – increases susceptibility to infection
[R4A] pg 24 Fluoride increases likelihood of autoimmune disease
[R4B] pg Ch 1 & 26 Fluoride accelerates aging
[R5] Fluoridation and the Truth Decay\ by Gladys Caldwell and Philip E. Zanfagna, MD; pg 5-8
Top-Ecol Press 18416 Van Owen//Reseda, Calif 91335
[R6] Compton's Pictured Encyclopedia (vol3-1963 Edition)\ pg 423 cockroach NaFl as insecticide
[R7] The Drama of Fluoride Arch Enemy of Mankind\ by Leo Spira, MD, PhD; pg 42-46 chronic toxicity
[R7A] pg 93-104 tetany (Lee Foundation for Nutritional Research; Milwaukee 3 Wisconsin - Dr. Leo Spira)
[R8] The American Fluoridation Experiment\ by F. B. Exner, MD and G. L. Waldbott, MD; (Devlin-Adair, NY 61)
pg 5 Origins of US Fluoridation in Hereford, Texas from Feb 1943 Readers Digest – Town Without a Toothache
[R8A] pg 36 Fluoride as an enzyme poison // Stannous (Tin) Fluoride = SnF_2
[R9] Folk Medicine\ by D.C. Jarvis, MD; pg 134-137 essential Iodine (I) may be replaced by F - Cl - Br
[R10] Encyclopedia of Bible Life\ pg 417 subject - high water table in desert
[R11] Come Alive\ by Bernard Jensen, DC, PhD; pg 62 water quote
[R12] What the Bible Says About Healthy Living\ by Rex Russell, MD; pg 208-209 water
[R13] Drinking Water Fluoridation & Ingested Fluoride\ by International Academy of Oral Medicine & Toxicology
[R14] Help Yourself to Better Health\ by Monte Kline, PhD Fluoride and Water updates (1-800-255-4246)
[R15] HYtBH Radio (09-20-99)(04-17-99)(11-20-99)\ by Monte Kline, PhD and Paul Genung, DDS; Fluoride
[R16] HYtBH Radio (04-20-02) (04-27-02)\ by Monte Kline, PhD and Paul Genung, DDS; Fluoride in drinking water
[R16] Uninformed Consent\ by Hal Huggins, DDS and Thomas Levi, MD, JsD; 'what you don't know'
[R17] The Water Book\ by Halloway & Joiner-Bey, ND + Water Myth and Magic (tape/CD) – www.pentawater.com
[R18] Strong's Concordance/ by James Strong, STD, LLD (***mayim*** – a dual noun used as a singular)
pg 1108 water # 4325 H pg 65 ***mayim*** Deut 8:7
[R19] Trace Minerals and Man\ by Henry Schroeder, MD; fluoridation controversy
[R20] Food Nutrition and Diet Therapy (7th Ed)\ by Krause and Mahan; pg 706-707 starvation
[R4A] pg 180 up to 10 days maximum survival w/out water
[R4B] pf 181 water loss and death or disorder
[R21] The Fluoride Question\ by Anne-Lise Gotzche; pg 104-105 Fluoride is the lightest halogen and can displace essential Iodine from the thyroid - may cause a goiter – (back pg Body Pollution/ by Gary Null)
[R22] Your Body's Many Cries for Water (audio+book)\ by Fereydoon Batmanghelid; age↑⇒ cellular hydration↓
[R23] The Coming Water Crisis (US News Aug 12, 2002) \ by Lavelle and Kurlantzick
[R24] Is Our Water Safe to Drink?\ by Gordon Millichap, MD
[R25] Proof Positive\ by Neil Nedley, MD
[R26] Your Health Under Siege\ by Jeffrey Bland, PhD
[R27] Body Pollution\ by Gary Null, PhD
[R28] The 28-Day Antioxidant Diet \ by Steven Masley, MD
[R29] Eating by the Book\ by David Meinz
[R30] The Bible Cure\ by Reginald Cherry, MD

All food is balanced between Toxins and Nutrients.

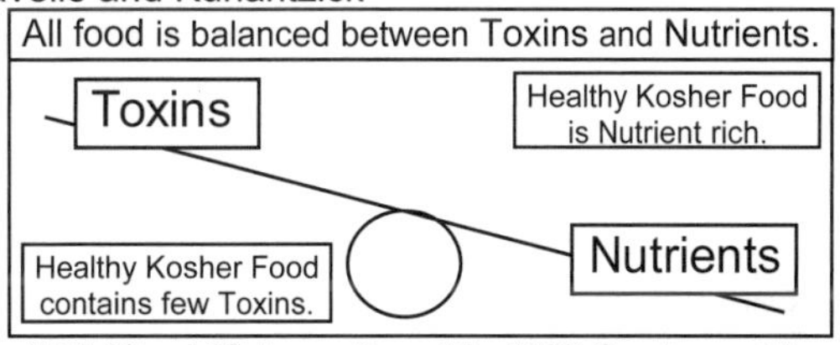

[R29] Milwaukee Fights Crypto with Ozone Retrofit; Civil Engineering (NY) 98 vol 68; issue 9; pg 13 - 1993 Cryptosporidium
[R32] Brunning Pottery/ 2908 6th Ave S / Seattle, Wash 98134 / (206)-623-1007 water purification vessels
[R33] Sacred Balance (video -#2)\ on PBS (1-800-543-3764) /Penta-water /PCBs /Bali – water & agriculture
[R34] Consider Jesus (radio-05-24-04)\ by Wayne Taylor; (In ≈1200 AD, the ArchBishop of Canterbury 1st added chapters to the Scripture. – At 9,200 ft, Mt. Herman is the primary source of water for the Sea of Galilee + Jordan River + Dead Sea.)
[R35] The Town Without a Toothache (Feb 1943)\ in Reader's Digest – Hereford, Tx + fluoride in the water {[R8]}
[R36] Fluoridation of Public Water Supplies\ by Louis J. Ronsivalli

Fluorine in salt-water is ≈1.3 ppm (parts per million). Fluoridation (NaF) of the public water is ≈ 0.7 ppm.
What's the problem? Fluoride advocates may argue that fluoridation (NaF) of public water at ≈ 0.7 ppm is less than the 2.0 ppm that's known to be toxic, or the 1.3 ppm Fluorine in sea food and/or in SeaSalt.
∗ Fluoride (NaF) added to water/ toothpaste at 0.7 ppm is an isolate, not balanced by any other minerals.
NaF is a rat poison, an insecticide and a toxic byproduct of aluminum smelting and fertilizer production.

Chapter 20 Fruit and Fruit Juice (Wine)
Vitamin C and Enzymes

The LORD gave mankind every fruit for food in the Garden of Eden (***Gan Eden***). (Gen 3:23) Fruit contains fat, protein and carbohydrate. Fruit can meet all nutritional needs in an ideal world. In the Garden, the environment was great, and fruit was likely the only food that man required. Man's nutritional needs were greater after leaving Eden, and a greater variety of food was needed.

NIV Gen 1:29 'Then God said, "I give you every seed bearing plant (vegetable) on the face of the whole Earth and every tree that has fruit with seed in it. They shall be yours for food."

Moses listed several fruits (***periy***) from the Promised Land and Egypt that the Hebrews ate.

NKJV Num 11:5 We remember the fish which we ate freely in Egypt, the cucumbers, the melons, the leeks, the onions, and the garlic;

NKJV Num 13:23 'They ... cut down a branch with one cluster of grapes; they carried it between two of them on a pole. They also brought some of the pomegranates and figs."

All fruit has a maturity date, or ripe date, which means that there is a time to pick the fruit when it is completely vine ripened. This is the time that all the nourishment from the sun and the soil are passed from the plant to the fruit. Ripe fruit contains all the protein, fat, fiber, enzymes, vitamins, minerals and mature fruit sugar (carbohydrate) that the fruit is intended to provide. Today, most fruit is picked when it is still 'green' – before it is ripe. Green fruit keeps much longer at the market or on the shelf but is much lower in nutritional value than vine ripened fruit. Bernard Jensen, DC says many people get stomach cramps or indigestion from eating poor quality 'green' fruit. [R5]

∗ Fruit of modern hybrid varieties that is picked while still 'green' may rot before ripening.

When autumn's apples are kept in storage until spring or summer many vitamins/minerals have lost their nutritional value or potency. The best way to eat one-season fruit all year round is to pick fruit ripe and freeze or dry it quickly without adding sugar. Fortunately, fresh flash-frozen fruit, and fruit dried without sugar, such as raisins, figs, dates and prunes are found in most markets today.

∗ Fruit that is fresh, ripe, in season and from non-hybrids is of the highest nutritional value.

Fresh vine-ripened fruit is bursting with vitamin C. Abundant vitamin C is essential to health. Vitamin C in quantities needed to prevent scurvy is far below what is needed for optimum health. Vitamin C from fresh fruit or raw milk is also superior in quality to vitamin C made by a chemist. Fruit also contains rutin, hesperidins and bioflavonoids (carotenoids and flavonoids) – antioxidant pigments that are part of a food-based vitamin C complex. Food-based vitamin C complex may be stored in the body and used as intended by the LORD for building and maintaining good health.

Norman Cousins in his book *Anatomy of an Illness* discussed the critical role of vitamin C in restoring and maintaining collagen connective tissue, and in his recovery from crippling arthritis.

Linus Pauling, PhD in chemistry and Nobel Prize winner believed man lost the biochemistry to produce vitamin C as part of evolution. The author believes that primates (humans) may have lost the biochemistry for producing vitamin C as a result of sin and the curse in Eden. (Gen 3:17)

"... where as most species of animals can synthesize ascorbic acid [vitamin C], man and other primates ... are unable to synthesize the substance, and require it as a vitamin." [R11]

Fruit, of course, isn't the only food with enzymatic value, but fruit may be the most important. Enzymes are necessary for every body process to function efficiently. Enzymes in digestion work to split proteins. Stomach enzymes and acids begin protein digestion. Ripe fruit contains more enzymes than green fruit. Pineapple contains papain as well as acids that augment digestion. Papaya contains bromelain that augments digestion. Citrus contains pectinase and acids that augment digestion. Apple, avocado, fig, grape, guava, kiwi, mango and tomato are other fruits that also contain enzymes that have been identified. Prune and plum contain yet unidentified enzymes that are very effective in promoting regular bowel movements and keeping the colon clean. Other fruits certainly contain valuable enzymes that haven't yet been identified. Flavonoids and minerals are often required as co-enzymes to enhance an enzyme's activity. Digestion without enzymes working efficiently may result in unwanted residues of fecal matter in the colon; and is like running a track meet in heavy work boots, you'll feel slow, sluggish and worn-out at the end. Enzymes whether produced by the body or from food need a proper pH (acidity) in the digestive system to work. Fruit acids promote an environment that activates enzymes and the absorption of nutrients by maintaining the required digestive pH, while the acids in coffee/tea may hinder digestion. [R27]

∗ The nutritional needs of the body for vitamin C and enzymes make plenty of ripe fresh fruit a must.

Fruit Juice and Wine

Wine was an important part of the Hebrew diet and vineyards were central to land use.

NKJV Num 18:12 "All the best of the oil, all the best of the new wine {***tiyrosh***} and the grain, their first fruits which they offer to the LORD, I have given them to you."

Grapes were often squeezed into fresh juice (***tiyrosh***) or allowed to ferment to wine (***yayin***). [R14] ***Yayin*** was usually mixed with water for drinking. ***Yayin*** also refers to a fruit syrup paste that remained after the liquid from fruit juice was heated away. ***Yayin*** paste could be spread on bread as jam/jelly or ***yayin*** could be reconstituted with water and/or honey and herbs into a drink. ***Yayin*** paste was often preserved in skins, which is an ancient equivalent of canning. Reconstituted ***yayin*** was often mixed with 2 to 20 parts water before it was drunk. Reconstituted ***yayin*** would not easily ferment and was often non-alcoholic. The mixed water and fermented ***yayin*** in Moses' time likely had an alcohol content of less than 3%. Wine must have more than 3.2% alcohol today to be labeled alcoholic. Today, most wine is made by adding white sugar and yeast to fruit (grape) juice to produce an alcohol content of 10-13%. Fermentation of most fruit without added sugar produces a 6% alcohol cider. Drinking ***tiyrosh*** before fermentation took place was the way to enjoy all the nutritional value of the fruit juice. Heating ***tiyrosh*** to produce ***yayin*** inactivates many microbes, enzymes and vitamin C. Fortunately, fresh fruit juices can be refrigerated today for a short time to delay fermentation, preserving enzymes and vitamins. Fresh fruit juices are often recommended as a nutritional aid to digestion for the enzymes and vitamins they contain, and to maintain or promote a healthy digestive pH. [R27] The value of wine with meals as an aid to digestion and to balance pH cannot be overemphasized. If new wine (***tiyrosh***) sits, then yeast on grape skins and in fruit juice may ferment fruit sugars into a alcoholic wine. Alcoholic wine in large amounts and undiluted is strong drink (***shekar***), while ***yayin*** was always diluted with water. If wine fermentation proceeds unabated, *actetobacter* bacteria may turn alcohol into vinegar and the wine is spoiled. Vinegar in French means 'sour wine'. [R39] In the 1800s, the French and all other nations had this problem with wine until Louis Pasteur showed that heating wine to 145°F for 30 minutes halted all fermentation, killed bacteria and left the wine with the desired flavor and alcohol content. [R31-32]

(Pasteurization is named for Louis Pasteur, who, in 1864, first pasteurized beer and wine, but never milk.)

*** (The ***Torah*** used ***tiyrosh, yayin*** and ***shekar*** to refer to the fruit of the vine (i.e. - wine), which may cause confusion.)

NIV Deut 18:4 You are to give them the firstfruits of your grain, new wine {***tiyrosh***} and oil, ...

JPS Gen 14:18 And Melchizedek brought forth bread and wine {***yayin***}, ...

Fermentation of fruit sugar in grapes into alcoholic wine (***yayin***) is first mentioned in the ***Torah*** after Noah left the Ark. (Gen 9:21) Many ***Torah*** students conclude that alcoholic wine did not exist before the Flood, due to the radically different atmosphere/environment of the pre-Flood Earth.

Overeating and drinking strong alcoholic wine is a sin against God and His commandments. A youth may drink to excess as an act of rebellion against his parents or God. Overindulgence of alcohol and alcoholism is still a sin against the LORD by adults and is usually an act of rebellion against God; just as youth may rebel against parents. The impaired judgment that comes from drinking alcohol {***shekar***} may cause consequences that are worse than the original drunkenness. Noah was a righteous man of God, but Noah's drunkenness after the Flood lead to a terrible incident with his son Ham, which caused Noah to curse Ham's son Canaan. (Gen 9:20-24) Lot was a righteous man, but his drunkenness precipitated his incest with his two daughters. (Gen 19)

KJV Gen 9:21 And he [Noah] drank of the wine {***yayin***} and was drunken {***cobe***}; ...

KJV Gen 19:32 Come, let us [Lot's daughters] make our father [Lot] drink wine {***yayin***}, ...

KJV Deut 21:20 And they [the parents] shall say unto the elders of his city.
This our son is stubborn and rebellious, he will not obey our voice, he is a glutton, and a drunkard {***cobe***}.

KJV Deut 29:6 ... neither have ye drunk wine {***yayin***} or strong drink {***shekar***} ...

Impaired judgment due to drunkenness often causes people to sin against their neighbors: as the death toll on US highways indicates that 50% of all deaths are alcohol related. [R29]

Shekar was never spoken of well by Moses. Brews such as beer (5% alcohol) from grain may have begun in a bakery, when yeast for bread making contaminated barley soaking in water. [R50] Many of the oldest known and be preserved recipes for beer are found on clay tablets from Egypt.

The health valve of wine for the heart results from proanthrocyanidines and other nutrients in grapes that remain in the wine, and not from any alcohol in wine. [R7] Grape skins make wine red. Red wine may be more nutritious than white wine. Today, (***shekar***) wine is often 10 to 13% alcohol.

∗ Fresh is the best way to enjoy all the nutritional value and flavor of the 'fruit of the vine'.

Olive Oil

Olive oil is prominent in the Hebrew diet, but olives were never recorded as being eaten. Olives are excruciatingly bitter straight from a tree and are never eaten fresh. Olives are cured in salt brine for a month or more to remove water-soluble oleuropein, before being eaten. [R40-41]

JPS Ex 23:11(b) In like manner thou shalt deal with thy vineyard, and with thy oliveyard.
KJV Deut 6:11 ...wells digged that thou diggest not, vineyards and olive trees ...
NIV Deut 24:20 When you beat the olives from your trees, ...
KJV Deut 28:40 Thou shalt have olive (***zayith***) trees throughout all thy coasts, ...

Olives are a fruit that is rich in monounsaturated oil (Oleic fatty acid) and other UFAs. [R2] Linoleic fatty acid (LA) is an EFA that is vital in large amounts for ideal healthy body function. Olives that are allowed to ripen on the tree contain more linoleic acid and are therefore more valuable for health than olives that are picked green. [R3-4] This ripening of olives is important: **since all fruit contains more nutrients when the fruit is allowed to fully ripen on the vine.** Dr. Elliot Berry discusses that olive oil and other monounsaturated oils like almond or avocado may reduce blood cholesterol and protect the body from cholesterol oxidative artery disease. [R10]

"During infancy, olive oil helps growth, bone formation and the delicate process of 'brain myelinization'; and aids the body to resist infection. In adults, olive oil is effective in preventing diseases of the arteries and heart. Rich in vitamin E, it slows down the aging process in the skin and the bones, and protects the bones from decalcification, osteoporosis and fractures. [R21]

Steven Masley, MD in his book *The 28-Day Antioxidant Diet* discusses the antioxidant value of olive oil and the antioxidant value of other monounsaturated fats and oils from plants.

"Monounsaturated fats provide an excellent source of Vitamin E. They also contain a vast array of antioxidants that remain essential to your health. Monounsaturated fats have been proven to decrease the oxidation of cholesterol in your blood stream." [R28]

Olives were frequently pressed into pulp by the Hebrews to extract olive oil. Olive pulp was usually pressed for olive oil and repressed several times, which produced several 'grades' of oil. The highest grades of the 1st pressed olive oil were used as food and for sacrifice to the LORD. Lower grades of later pressed olive oil were burned in lamp stands and used for making soap. [R42]

"Oil extracted from olives by mechanical or other methods which do not modify its basic properties, results in a completely natural product which maintains the taste plus chemical and biological values of the olive oil. Within the Virgin grade, there are three recognized quality levels:" [R19]

Extra (*Extra*): Oil of the best taste characteristics, and with an acidity not exceeding 1%.
Average (*Coriente*): Oil with a good taste, and acidity levels not exceeding 3.3%.
Strong (*Lampante*): Inadequate taste and/or acidity levels above 3.3%. [R19]

"It [E. V. Olive oil] should taste fruity on the tip of the tongue and feel spicy on the back of the throat. It's the bite in the back of the throat that means the oil [Extra Virgin Olive oil] is full of the antioxidants and polyphenols that keep your body healthy." [R45]

Olive oil must be consumed without being heated excessively to retain its healthy properties.

"For centuries olive oil has been used to maintain the suppleness of skin and muscle, to heal abrasions, to give body and sheen to hair and soothe the drying effects of sun and wind." [R19]

"People on high blood pressure medications may be able to reduce the amount of medicine they take if they substitute extra virgin olive oil for other types of fat in their diet..." [R19] [R20]

Olive oil, like fresh fruits and fresh vegetables, is valuable for preventing colon cancer. [R35]

Today, 'cold-pressed' refers to a low heat oil extraction that retains high nutritive value.

Extra Virgin Olive oil stimulates the gall bladder to release its stored, enzyme-rich, bile salts. Bile salts are made by the liver, stored in the gall bladder and are crucial for proper digestion and fat absorption [R41], promoting easy stool eliminations, and preventing fecal deposition in the colon.

∗ High quality Extra Virgin Olive oil, fresh Lemon juice and fresh Apple juice have a healthy effect on the gall bladder that promotes bile to be released and may be important to prevent gall stones. [R43]

Olive oil soap cleanses, softens, moisturizes and keeps skin elastic and keeps pours open. [R42]

Clean water, fertile soil and a climate suitable to grow/raise healthy foods, including fruit, are what the LORD promised to the Hebrews. As promised, the Promised Land delivered the 'goods'. But, even the best resources of ***Eretz*** Israel still must be used wisely, if good health is to follow.

KJV Deut 8:8 A land of wheat, and barley, and vines and fig trees, and pomegranates; a land of olive oil and honey.

∗ The author encourages everyone to rountinely include Extra Virgin Olive Oil in their diet.

-------------------------- References Ch 20 Fruit and Wine --------------------------------

[R1] The Genesis Diet\ by Gordon Tessler, PhD fruit as the ideal food for man

[R2] Encyclopedia of Fruits Vegetables Nuts and Seeds for Healthful Living
\by Joseph M. Kadans, ND, PhD: pg 132-133 /(Parker Publishing Co. Inc.; West Nyack, New York)

[R3] Nabali Olive Oil Ripening and Oil Properties, Nutrition and Health (Journal 1991 Vol 7)
\by Muhammad Attumeid, Hamed R. H. Takruri, Rafat F. Daqqaq; (Faculty of Agriculture, University of Jordan)
pg 151-154 Olives picked 'green' had lower nutritional content than 'vine ripened' olives.

[R4] What You Should Know About Olive Oil (Let's Live - Aug 1992) \ Betty Kamen, PhD; pg 34-37

[R5] Nutrition Lectures (1984 Hidden Valley Ranch)\ by Bernard Jensen, DC; fruit enzymes aid digestion

[R6] Body Pollution\ by Gary Null, PhD; pg 12 Olive oil

[R7] The Complete Book of Juicing\ by Michael Murray, ND; pg 9 fresh juices have antiviral activity
pg 12 no weight loss if the body not fed; the body feels like it is starving
pg 13 metabolism ↓ – energy ↓ – no weight loss – no fat burned
pg 15 oxidants (produce free-radicals) smoking //pg 21 proteins
** pg 26 vitamins and enzymes like catalysts -//- collagen – Vitamin C needed for production
pg 39 Enzymes 1) Synthatases - build up complex body molecules - anabolism
2) Hydrolases - add H_2O - break down complex foods - digestive enzymes
digestion requires enzymes - costs the body a great deal of energy -//- law of adaptive secretion
pg 80 anthrocyanidines = color pigments ⇒ health benefits
bilberry = a variety of blueberry ⇒ better light and dark adaptation by the eyes
pg 88 cranberry inhibits bacteria like E. coli from adhering to mucus membrane of bladder
thereby cranberry prevents/treats bladder infections
pg 91 grapes contain flavanoids called procyanolic oligomers

[R8] Poisons in Your Food\ by William Longgood; Ch IV pg 61 acute verses chronic poisons
[R8A] Ch IV pg 55-56 & 59 DDT and other pesticides are cumulative poisons

[R9] Fresh Vegetable and Fruit Juices\ by Norman Walker, DSc more nutrients in fresh juices

[R10] Olive Oil\ in Dispatch from Jerusalem Vol 19 No 5 Sept/Oct 94; pg 12 quote Elliot Berry

[R11] Vitamin C and the Common Cold\ by Linus Pauling, PhD, pg 58 Vitamin C & evolution

[R12] What the Bible Says About Healthy Living\ by Rex Russell, MD; pg 139 white oil

[R13] The Art of Making Wine\ by Stanley F. Anderson and Raymond Hill

[R14] Alcohol (radio 04-28-2000 audio)\ by John MacArthur – wine – ***yayin*** – boiled to be a thick paste or fruit concentrate syrup like jelly – difficult to ferment after reconstituted – mixed with water: 2-3% alcohol

[R15] Wine Drinking (06-20-1975)\ by Robert Stein; Christianity Today

[R16] Jewish Encyclopedia (1901) vol 12\ pg 533 ***yayin*** as fruit paste, often mixed with water

[R17] Olive Leaf Extract (Internet)\ by James R. Privitera, MD - olive oil (leaf) as a medicine

[R18] Strong's Concordance\ by James Strong, STD, LLD

pg 372	fruit	# 6529	H pg 96	***periy***	Gen 1:29
pg 376	Garden	# 1588	H pg 28	***Gan***	Gen 3:23
pg 296	Eden	# 5731	H pg 85	***Eden***	Gen 3:23
pg 1174	new wine	# 8492	H pg 124	***tiyrosh***	Gen 27:25
pg 1174	old wine (paste)	# 3196	H pg 49	***yayin***	Gen 9:6
pg 1174	strong drink	# 7941	H pg 116	***shekar***	Num 28:7
pg 285	drunk	# 7937	H pg 116	***shakar***	Deut 29:6
pg 285	drunkard	# 5435	H pg 81	***cobe***	Deut 21:20
pg 740-41	oil	# 8081	H pg 118	***shemen***	Deut 8:8
pg 742	olive	# 2132	H pg 35	***zayith***	Deut 28:40

*** ***Tiyrosh***, ***Yayin*** and ***Shekar*** are all beverages from the fruit of the vine (wine), which may cause confusion.
Tiyrosh is fresh non-fermented fruit juice and is best translated – new wine.
Yayin is fruit syrup or fruit syrup reconstituted with water to a low alcoholic beverage and is translated – wine.
Shekar *is a strong undiluted alcoholic beverage usually drunk by barbarians and is translated – strong drink.*
Today's '80 Proof' whisky – 40% alcohol ñ has a much higher alcoholic content than any ***Shekar*** in the ***Torah***.

[R19] Olive Oil from Spain (Internet Article-2000)

[R20] Journal of the Archives of Internal Medicine (March 27, 2000)\ by L. Aldo Ferrarra, MD

[R21] Olive Oil\ by Silvana Bevilacqua Calzolari; pg 12 quote on healthy aspects Olive oil
pg 13 health reference // Olive oil expert Professor Ancel Keys
pg 18 oldest Olive oil press found in Palestine
pg 39-43 Olive oil production

[R22] The Feast of the Olive\ by Maggie Blyth Klein

-------------------- References continued Ch 20 Fruit and Wine ----------------------------

[R23] Bible Wines\ by William Patton; pg 27 Grapes 1st for grape juice (i.e.- wine) – 2nd eaten
[R24] The Grape Cure\ by Johanna Brandt; Grape juice as an aid to digestion and health
[R25] Proof Positive\ by Neil Nedley, MD; pg 164-166 fruit
pg 186 Olive oil and other oils
[R26] Wine in the Bible\ by Samuele Bacchiocchi (SDA)
[R27] The Complete Book of Enzyme Therapy\ by Anthony Cichoke, DC
pg 46 bromelain pineapple
pg 47 cellulose avocado
pg 49 ficain or ficin fig
pg 49 lactase tomatoes, persimmons, apples, peaches
pg 49 lipase avocado
pg 50-51 papain papaya
Pg 51 pectin's citrus fruits
Pg 51 peroxides apple, grape, mango and other fruit
Pg 52 protease pineapple, papaya, fig, guava, kiwi
[R28] The 28-Day Antioxidant Diet Program\ by Steven Mosley, MD;
pg 54 red wine
[R28A] pg 56 olive oil // [R28B] pg 78-80 fruits

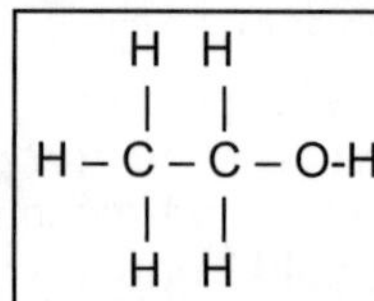
Ethyl Alcohol is a byproduct of (fruit) sugar fermentation by yeasts.
CH_3CH_2OH or C_2OH_6 or Ethyl Alcohol

Ethyl Alcohol is an intoxicant. Methyl Alcohol is very toxic and may cause blindness in alcohol from inept home distilleries.

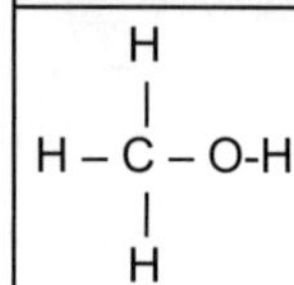
Methyl Alcohol or wood alcohol is poisonous and is part of Aspartame.
CH_3OH or COH_4 or Methyl Alcohol

[R29] The Coming Plague\ by Laurie Garrett; pg 506 alcohol abuse quote
[R30] Anatomy of an Illness\ by Norman Cousins Vitamin C is required by collagen tissue.
[R31] Pasteurization\ in Encyclopedia Americana 2000; Vol 21; pg 518 1864 Wine & Beer
[R32] Pasteurization\ in Britannica Micropedia 1997; Vol 9; pg 190 1860s Wine & Beer
[R33] California study shows levels of unhealthy pesticide residues increased in foods in 1980s
[R34] Wine\ by Robert Teachout – wine as a beverage in biblical times
[R35] California Olive Oil Council (Internet-2000) Olive oil and colon cancer
[R36] Olive Oil from Trees to Table\ by Peggy Knickerbocker and Laurie Smith
[R37] Nutrition for Health\ by Alice Chase, DO, PhD
[R38] tape by GNLD on pro-anthrocyanidines in wine
[R39] Encyclopedia Britannica 1997\
Vinegar; – Micropedia Vol 12 pg 380 vinegar in French = sour wine
Beverages; (Wine) – Macropedia Vol 14 pg (884-890) pg 885 bacterial spoilage of wine

Fruit juice that is labeled 'from concentrate' allows a food technologist to concentrate the juice and then reconstitute the juice by adding water. Reconstituted fruit juice from concentrate has lost most, if not all, of it nutritive properties.
These processes are often convenient for companies and the food technologist but are often poor for the consumer.

[R40] Olives The Life and Lore of the Noble Fruit\ by Mort Rosenblum
pg 12 healthful properties of Olive oil
pg 13 don't eat straight from a tree // Olive oil graded by acidity
pg 14 black pitted canned olives far removed from being a nutritionally healthy food
pg 59-60 Olives cured in salt brine to remove bitter water soluble element – oleuropein
pg 62 picking to milling to oil
pg 64 fresh oil – more antioxidants -//- grades of oil
pg 65 Olive oil soap in Israel
pg 70 old oil press found from Promised Land
pg 77 make oil quickly - before fermentation
pg 88 Olive trees produce fruit well only every other year.
[R41] Medical Physiology (5th Ed)\ by Arthur Guyton, MD; pg 838-839 bile salts – liver + gall bladder
[R42] The Natural Soap Book\ by Susan Miller Cavitch; pg 22-24 Olive oil soap
[R43] Dr. Christopher's 3 Day Cleansing Program\ by John R. Christopher, ND, MH
Olive oil, Lemon juice and Apple juice cleanse the gall bladder
[R44] e-mail correspondence concerning Olives from an Olive distributor
[R45] Virtuosity, Extra Virgin Olive Oil is Divine (Better Nutrition Feb 03)\ by Kimberley Lord Stewart; pg 47-51
[R46] The UnCook Book & The Gourmet UnCook Book \ by Elizabeth Baker; raw fruit & vegetables
[R47] A Good Cook Book … Ten Talents\ by Frank K. Hurd, DC, MD and Rosalie Hurd, BS
[R49] The Book of Jewish Foods\ by Claudia Roden
[R49] The New Complete Joy of Home Brewing\ by Charlie Papazian; pg 5 beer = barley + yeast
[R50] Egypt and the Age of the Pharaohs\ by Guillemette Andreu; pg 95-96 Beer and bread are made from the same ingredients of grains, barley and starchy wheat. Beer was the common drink of Egyptian meals. Egyptians also drank milk and ate dairy products at meals, but beer was likely the adult beverage of choice.

Chapter 21 Vegetables and Herbs
Antioxidants

Plants are important every diet for the minerals, phytonutrients and antioxidants they contain.
NIV Gen 3:18 ... and you will eat the plants [vegetables and herbs] of the field.
NIV Num 11:5 ... the fish we ate ... also the cucumbers, melons, leeks, onions and garlic.

Vegetables (***eseb***) are an important source of minerals for human health. The quality of the vegetables as determined by the quantity of minerals, vitamins, proteins, enzymes, and oils they contain, which is directly tied to principles of 'sustainable agriculture' used to grow them. (Sec 3) Vegetables have no mature date like fruits; eaten earlier vegetables are young and tender, eaten later vegetables are bigger and tougher. Minerals, in combination with proteins and EFAs, build all body tissues and enhance enzymes/vitamins. Enzymes and vitamins are catalysts that increase the efficiency of all body functions and help regulate the body's metabolism. [R6-8] Green leafy vegetables are rich in chlorophyll. Vegetables naturally chelate minerals, which makes minerals easier to assimilate. Chlorophyll is the green plant protein that plants use via photosynthesis to convert sunlight, CO_2 and minerals from the soil into new tissue that man/animals use as food. Bernard Jensen, DC said the body can absorb chlorophyll more easily than any other food. [R1]

A variety of vegetables are healthy for many reasons, including the antioxidants they contain, as discussed by my friend, Steven Masley, MD in his book *The 28-Day Antioxidant Diet Program*.
"Antioxidants play a critical role in guarding our cell walls from free radical attack.
On a cellular level, free radicals start chain reactions within our tissues, damaging
one compound after another until the cell's functional capacity is destroyed."
∗ "Antioxidants block this process by neutralizing free radicals." [R28]

Oxygen is vital for health, including to help efficiently burn carbohydrates as fuel for energy. But oxygen and UV light can also encourage free-radical formation, which are destructive to tissues. Antioxidants that neutralize free radicals include vitamin C, vitamin E, certain enzymes, carotenoids, flavonoids, as well as many trace minerals. Carotenoids and flavonoids are both antioxidant pigments found in colorful fruits and vegetables, which protect plants against the damaging effects of UV sunlight. [R28-28A] Garlic is also a valuable antioxidant food herb. [R28B] Beta-carotene is a carotinoid in carrots that the liver can convert into vitamin A for use in the eye. Pesticides, waste products of manufacturing, UV-b, coffee and tobacco products act as unwanted toxic 'oxidants' that may cause damage to tissues that are not well stocked with antioxidants.

Phytonutrients are chemicals in plants and the nutritional research topic of the 1990s. New phytonutrients including antioxidants, some of which are essential to normal health, are being discovered yearly. Phytonutrients are often linked to preventing/treating illnesses, such as cancer.

Andrew Weil, MD in his book *Spontaneous Healing* discusses the process of reductionism: which analyzes foods to find chemical(s) made by plants that produce health-promoting effects. Reductionism reproduces these 'phytochemicals' in a laboratory as 'isolated' chemicals, apart from the plants in which they were originally identified. Reductionism isolated the broad spectrum and very potent antimicrobial agent, allicin, from garlic, and then turned it into the chemical, kyolic. [R36] In 1897, reductionism isolated acetoacylic acid in willow tree bark, and, in 1899, produced it as aspirin. Willow tree bark is only valued as a drug for pain or fever relief – there is no food value to lose. Reductionism is important in many antioxidant, vitamin, mineral and phytochemical supplements. In 1929, vitamin C was found in food, such as fruit, vegetable and milk, and then produced in a lab. Reductionism allows people to take a much higher 'quantity' of the phytochemicals than they could get from eating plants, but in the process the food 'quality' of the plant is lost. Practically speaking: 'Reductionism often turns a food into a drug.' Lutein is a carotenoid found in vegetables, such as kale. Lutein is also found in the macula of the eye. Lutein cannot be made by the body. Lutein is scarce in eyes with macular degeneration. Lutein may help to prevent or treat ARMD. (Ch 51) Reductionism may turn a phytochemical in kale into a pharmaceutical lutein in ARMD formulations. Isolated vitamins, minerals and other phytochemicals taken in proper amounts may be valuable for treating degenerative disease, such as ARMD, but they shouldn't be thought of as replacements for the nutrient value of fresh whole foods from whence they came. The quantity and quality of phytonutrients in a plant may depend upon the health of the soil in which the plant is grown. (Sec 3)

The LORD made man from dust (minerals) of the earth and He instructed man to eat mineral-rich plant foods for health. (Gen 3:18) A variety of vegetables provide minerals, antioxidants and phytonutrients in the balance that is proper for maintaining a healthy metabolism and long life.

∗ Antioxidants, phytonutrients and minerals in whole food are critical to maintaining health.

Fiber

Fiber is a big component of vegetables and is very important for the health of the colon. [R4-7]

"Fiber is a special kind of carbohydrate. One common definition [of fiber] – a physiologic understanding that focuses on the functioning of the intestines and other bodily organs and tissues during digestion – is that fiber is a natural component of plant food which cannot be broken down by the enzymes in the human digestive tract." [R5]

All food from plants (Section 3) contains some fiber: either insoluble or soluble. [R5-R6]

"Insoluble fiber gets its name from the fact that it does not dissolve in water, as well as in the liquid environment of the stomach and intestines." [R5A]

"Soluble fiber does dissolve in water, as well as in the gastro-intestinal tract." [R5A]

Insoluble fiber is the 'roughage' part of food that works like a brush to keep intestines clean. Insoluble fiber includes parts of the plant cells and walls, which is also known as cellulose. [R5]

"The most important function of the insoluble fiber is to absorb water in the large intestine and thus increase the size and softness of the stool. The cellulose in insoluble fiber cannot be digested, but it can take in water like a sponge. This process helps prevent constipation."

If insoluble fiber works like a brush to sweep the intestinal tract clean, then conversely an absence of or less-than-optimal insoluble fiber contributes to the poor colon heath of constipation (difficult or infrequent bowel movements) or diverticulitis (inflammation of bowel pockets). [R5G-5H] High fiber diets increase the speed or 'transit time' for food to move through the digestive system. The normal food transit time of 24 to 30 hours for a high fiber diet reduces the risk of slow moving feces contributing to disease. [R9A] Autopsies reveal that colon pockets often contain several pounds of impacted food waste (i.e. - feces) that may contribute to cancer and other ill health. [R17-10] A fiber brush may account for the lower incidence of certain diseases in people who eat a proper amount of insoluble fiber. [R5J] Prominent sources of insoluble fiber include cereal grain bran (especially wheat bran), barley and raw mature vegetables (especially raw cabbage). [R5A-5C-6]

'Soluble' fiber includes pectins, gums and mucilages, which are found within plant cells. [R5-5D] Soluble fiber helps regulate the absorption of starches, thereby normalizing blood sugar, and helps carry excess cholesterol through the colon, and normalize blood cholesterol. [R5E-7] The important soluble and insoluble fiber value of fruits and vegetables tends to be greatly reduced by cooking, while the important soluble fiber value of cooked or sprouted grains and beans may be potentiated (increased), as cooking or sprouting these foods may improve their digestibility and bio-availability. [R6] Prominent sources of soluble fiber include oat bran, legumes, fruits and vegetables. [R5A-D-F/6]

Insoluble fiber passes through the colon, brushing it clean. One item eliminated by soluble fiber is cholesterol that is dumped into intestines with bile salts. A high fiber diet may reduce the blood level of bad LDL-cholesterol, thereby reducing the risk of cardiovascular disease. [R1-R4]

Since cooking vegetables helps make some vegetable minerals more bio-available to the body, but also results in the loss of important fiber and enzymes, Dr. Bernard Jensen advised eating 40% of vegetables cooked, but the 60% majority of vegetables should be eaten raw. [R1]

David Reuben, MD in his book *The Save Your Life Diet* warned of low fiber diet cancer risks;

"... lifetime low-roughage diets are probably converting their own bile acids into awesome cancer-producing compounds within the confines of their own large intestines." [R9A]

Colon cancer is one disease that everyone recognizes may be directly related to too little fiber in the diet, as toxic fecal matter builds up in pockets within the colon. The American Cancer Association recommends several servings of raw fiber-rich vegetables per day for colon health. Fiber may help to dissolve wastes and toxins from the colon and eliminate them in the stool. Some studies recommend as much as 25 grams of total fiber per day to keep the colon clean, yet this amount of fiber is very difficult to get by diet alone. Supplements may help provide required fiber. Mineral-rich food, grown on healthy soil, may provide the highest quality soluble and insoluble fiber.

∗ Dietary fiber is essential to colon health and to prevent chronic degenerative disease.

Mushrooms

Mushrooms aren't mentioned in the ***Torah***. Mushrooms are not green and leafy, do not bare seed that reproduce and may need to be excluded as a food. (Gen 1:29) Mushrooms contain very little starch, protein, enzymes, vitamins and minerals. Some mushrooms are deadly poisonous. People with digestive disorders and especially *candida* yeast infections must avoid mushrooms (cooked or uncooked), since mushrooms are fungi that will encourage the overgrowth of yeast.

∗ If in doubt, leave Mushrooms out, as they may be more harmful than beneficial to health.

Herbs – Aloes – Garlic – Oregano – Olive Leaf

Herbs are nature's medicine chest (i.e. – naturally occurring drugs). Herbs may also be food. All food contains calories in the form of carbohydrate, protein or fat. Food provides the body with building blocks for developing and repairing healthy tissues or as fuel to be burned for energy. Drugs often cause the body to mobilize nutrients that were stored from foods previously eaten. Drugs do not nourish the body, but they may cause nourishment stored in tissues to be used up. Herbs may have drug-like properties. For an illness, the right herb or drug may have a valuable effect on health by helping the body to mobilize the nutritional elements needed for recovery. Plants, such as garlic, are both herb and food. Herbs, like an herbal tea, should not be consumed as if they were food, nor should herbs be eaten in place of food. The indiscriminate use of drugs and some herbs may cause stored nutrients to be mobilized and lost, and may leave the body in a weakened and vulnerable condition. Used wisely, as in an acute illness, herbs can be very valuable for health, but used improperly or indiscriminately, herbs may do more harm than good.

The gel that comes from the leaves of the aloe plant has marvelous healing properties. Aloe Vera is great as a burn ointment, including sunburns. Aloe Vera also helps heal skin rashes and other skin ailments. [R22] Aloe plants, however, are not listed in the Nutritional Almanac as food.

"...incredible non-toxic potency. ...(Aloe) gel is an ingenious mixture of antibiotic, antistringent, coagulating agents, while also being a pain and scar inhibitor and a growth stimulator." [R22]

Aloes grow readily in Israel and other Mediterranean lands. Only since ≈1960, have Aloes been stabilized in a bottle, so their non-toxic, therapeutic value can remain potent as a gel or juice. [R17]

KJV Num 24:6 ... as the trees of lign aloes (***ahaliym***) which the LORD has planted, ...

When visiting Cali, Colombia, in 1984, the author got food poisoning, and my entire digestive system felt like it was on fire. I had a bottle of Aloe Vera gel with me for such an occasion. After I swallowed the Aloe, I felt the gel slowly travel through the digestive system. The burning in the digestive system was relieved from top to bottom, inch by inch. I used Aloe Vera as a drug with an excellent result. The next morning I felt fine, but I don't use Aloe Vera internally on a regular basis. The author recommends that aloes may be used internally as natural medicine, but not as food.

Garlic is from the onion family, and is used as food for flavor and nutrition, and as an herb. Garlic as an herb is discussed by many authors, including Joan and Lydia Wilen in their book *Garlic: Nature's Super Healer* and by Robert Creyhon, PhD in his book *Nutrition Made Simple*.

"Garlic has been found to have antibiotic and antifungal properties. Garlic has been found to be an important stimulator of the body's defense system known as the immune system." [R15]

In addition to it's stimulating taste, garlic also helps the body improve circulation; manage high blood pressure, high cholesterol and high triglycerides; and reduce *candida* yeast, bacterial and parasitic infections. Garlic promotes the growth of friendly bacteria. Garlic may help remediate or prevent some cancer. Garlic's selenium makes it a valuable antioxidant. [R15] Garlic is an herb with remarkable health-promoting properties that can be used in disease therapy or in prevention.

Cass Ingram, MD in his book *The Cure is in the Cupboard* discusses oregano as a food and the herbal value of oregano oil. Oregano herb in the ***Torah*** is called Hyssop. The common spice oregano is often just wild sage, which is fine to flavor food but has no therapeutic value. [R24B] Dr. Ingram discusses oregano's incredibly high mineral content and oregano oil's antiimicrobial value that can be used both externally and internally. [R24A-24] Oregano oil is a potent herb. [R35]

"Wild oregano is a veritable mineral treasure-house, containing a density of minerals that would rival virtually any food." "Oil of oregano is the premier antiseptic and posses a wide range of microbial killing powers. Uniquely, there is no tendency for microbial resistance." [R24]

"Hyssop's volatile oil produces a camphor-like odor that is also responsible for its health benefits." [R35]

Hyssop or Oregano was used for its therapeutic properties as part of a cleansing for leprosy.

JPS Lev 14:4 then shall the priest command to take for him that is to be cleansed two living clean birds, and cedar-wood, and scarlet, and hyssop.

Various resigns and gums were used as spices and for worship of the LORD. (Ex 30:34) [R31]

Olive leaf was the plant brought to Noah that indicated life returned the land after the Flood. Olive leaf is used as an herb for its potent antibacterial, antiviral and antifungal properties. [R23]

KJV Gen 8:11 And the dove came in to him [Noah] in the evening; and, lo, in her mouth was an olive leaf plucked off; so Noah knew that the waters were abated from off the earth.

∗ The herbs in the *Torah* are representative of all herbs used as food or as drug for health.

------------------------ References Ch 21 Vegetables and Herbs ----------------------------------

[R1] Lecture at Hidden Valley Health Ranch (1984)\ by Bernard Jensen, DC

[R2] Poisons in Your Food\ by William Longgood; pg 61 chronic toxicity

[R2A] pg 59 AMA quote //[R2B] pg 56 Warburg – cumulative effects of toxicity

[R2C] pg 55 poisons not easily washed off foods

[R2D] pg 57 insecticides like war nerve gas ⇒ very toxic

[R3] The Chemical Deception\ by Marc Lappe, PhD

[R4] Come Alive\ by Bernard Jensen, DC, PhD

R5] The Fiber Prescription\ by Myron Winick, MD; pg 11 definition of fiber

[R5A] pg 4 soluble vs insoluble fiber //[R5B] pg 45 insoluble fiber absorbs water

[R5C] pg 107 insoluble fiber foods //[R5D] pg 106 soluble fiber foods

[R5E] pg 28 soluble fiber eliminates unwanted LDL-cholesterol

[R5F] pg 27 soluble fiber dissolves in water //[R5G] pg 44 insoluble fiber limits constipation

[R5H] pg 52-56 diverticulosis and colon health

[R5J] pg 7 colon cancer = (bad) fats↑ + insoluble fiber↓

[R6] Foods and Nutrition Coarse\ by Jeffrey Bland, PhD

[R7] Let's Live Magazine\ by Jeffrey Bland, PhD; Oct 92: pg 78-79 Fiber - Soluble + Insoluble

[R8] Mental and Elemental Nutrients\ by Carl Pfeiffer, PhD, MD; pg 212-307 all minerals

[R8D] pg 266 selenium deadly yet essential //[R8E] pg 212-213 essential minerals

[R9] Save Your Life Diet\ by David Reuben, MD; pg 3-36 poor diet - chronic disease

[R9A] pg 30-31 quote / low fiber - cancer risks

[R10] The Poisons Around Us\ by Henry Schroeder, MD

[R11] Trace Elements and Man\ by Henry Schroeder, MD

[R12] What the Bible Says about Healthy Living\ by Rex Russell, MD

[R13] Bakersfield Newspaper; Sept 89 despite best efforts California food contains more pesticide residues

[R14] Green Kamut (audio tape)\ by David Sandivold (1-800-362-8482) minerals for colon health

[R15] Nutrition Made Simple\ by Robert Creyhon, PhD; pg 137-141 garlic for health

[R16] Garlic The Miracle Nutrient\ by Earl Mindell, PhD; garlic for health

[R17] Garlic Natures Super Healer\ by Joan and Lydia Wilen; garlic for health

[R18] Strong's Concordance\ by James Strong, STD, LLD

pg 479	herb	# 6212	H pg 92	***eseb***	Gen 3:18
pg 228	cucumbers	# 7180	H pg 105	***qishshu***	Num 11:5
pg 591	leeks	# 2682	H pg 42	***chatsiyr***	Num 11:5
pg 754	onions	# 1211	H pg 23	***betsel***	Num 11:5
pg 377	garlic(k)	# 7762	H pg 113	***shuwm***	Num 11:5
pg 49	aloes	# 174	H pg 09	***ahaliym***	Num 24:6
pg 506	hyssop	# 231	H pg 10	***ezowb***	Num 19:6
pg 742	olive (leaf)	# 2132	H pg 35	***zayith***	Gen 8:11
pg 589	leaf (olive)	# 5929	H pg 88	***aleh***	Gen 8:11

[R19] Minerals: Kill or Cure\ by Ruth Adams and Frank Murray, ND

[R20] Rare Earths Forbidden Cures\ by Joel Wallach, BS, DVM, ND and Ma Lan, MD, MS

[R21] Aloe Vera Natures Soothing Healer\ by Diane Gage; pg 6 Aloe Vera gel –stable as of 1960s

[R22] The Aloe Vera Handbook\ by Max Skousen; pg 7-8 Aloes heal skin disorders + quote

[R23] Olive Leaf Extract (Internet)\ by James R. Privitera, MD

[R24] The Cure is in the Cupboard\ by Cass Ingram, MD; pg 6 quote // [R24A] pg 24 mineral value

[R25] Proof Positive\ by Neil Nedley, MD; pg 489-490 minerals // pg 490 – mineral chart

[R25A] pg 39-41 phytochemicals

[R26] Lick the Sugar Habit\ by Nancy Appleton, PhD; pg 16 mineral wheel chart

[R27] Spontaneous Healing\ by Andrew Weil, MD; pg 171-173 garlic

[R27A] pg 151 reductionism (aspirin – 1st synthesized 1899)

[R28] The 28-Day Antioxidant Diet Program\ by Steven Masley, MD; pg 6-8 antioxidants //pg 6 - quote

//[R28A] pg 100-102 garlic // [R28B] pg 81-85 vitamins

[R29] Antioxidant Revolution (audio)\ by Kenneth Cooper, MD; (tape2–side1) deadly quartet of blood chemistry {High Blood Pressure – High Blood Glucose – Low HDL Cholesterol – High Triglycerides (fat)} + Low Antioxidants

[R30] The World of Herbs (video)\ by Leslie Bremness; many herbs ⇒ health

[R31] Miracle Foods from the Bible\ by Reese Dubin; pg 274-275 cloves

[R32] Comeback Carotenoids\ by Jack Challem; pg 192 (Nutrition and Science News) vol 3, No 4 Apl 98

[R33] Shinzen Green\ (1-866-438-4733) Japan's barley green – rich in fiber & help friendly bacteria grow

[R34] Supreme Greens\ by Dr. Alex Guerrero; (1-800-672-9328) acidic food ⇒ disease green food ⇒ alkaline

[R35] Hyssop (pamphlet)\ by Natures Way Herbs; hyssop oil ⇒ healthy properties of Hyssop (Oragano)

[R36] What Would Jesus Eat?\ by Don Colbert, MD; pg 90 allicin antimicrobial in garlic ⇒ kyolic

[R37] Tired or Toxic\ by Sherry A. Rogers, MD ch 6 – mineral deficiencies compromise the immune system

[R38] Answers to Questions (audio)\ by Dr. Richard Schultz; Herbs to cleanse the colon (1-877-823-2463)

[R39] The Green Pharmacy\ by James A. Duke, PhD

[R40] The New Whole Foods Encyclopedia\ by Rebecca Wood

Minerals

Minerals that are required for life/health are called 'essential'. Some essential minerals are needed by the healthy body in large amounts, while other minerals are needed in small amounts. Calcium is needed in large amounts. Trace minerals, such as Cobalt, that are essential in small amounts are often toxic in large amounts. Heavy metals, such as Lead, are often toxic, even in trace amounts. The chemical state of the mineral is also critical for health. Chlorine in SeaSalt is essential in large amounts. Chloride in household bleach is very toxic, even in small amounts.

"Selenium ... is among the most poisonest elements in the universe;
and yet in pure form, it is an essential trace mineral for animals and man." [R8D]

There are currently ≈20 minerals listed as essential for human life. As more scientific research into biochemistry has been done, the list of minerals known as 'essential' for health has increased.

2 Mega: Chloride, Sodium 4 Macro: Calcium, Magnesium, Potassium, Sulfur
3 Micro: Iodine, Phosphorous, Silicon 11 Mini: Boron, Cobalt, Copper, Chromium, Iron,
(Mini) Manganese, Molybdenum, Selenium, Vanadium, Zinc, Fluorine* {*some people question Fluorine}

Nickel and Tin are currently under investigation to determine whether they are essential, while Lithium is used to treat emotional disorders, and Bismuth is used to treat stomach disorders.

Carbon, Hydrogen, Oxygen and Nitrogen are fundamental building blocks of all body tissues.

∗ The easiest way to get all the minerals necessary for health is by eating mineral-rich food.

Plants grown on mineral-rich soil were the only foods necessary for health in antediluvian times. After the Flood the environment became less hospitable, plants became more scarce and meats from animals as well as plants became valuable for health. (Ch 43) Clean animals, fish and birds eating a mineral-rich diet are themselves mineral-rich, making them ideal as mineral-rich foods. Today, mineral-rich soils are rare, and mineral-rich crops, animals and people are also very rare. Whole, mineral-rich SeaSalt was the first mineral supplement used by the Hebrews for health.

∗ Minerals are needed in ratios with other minerals for homeostasis or 'balanced equilibrium'. Cells, organs and tissues ideally require more than the minimum necessary quantity of minerals, and in the most bio-absorbable state (from food), so cells can take in the minerals that are needed and allow excess minerals to pass on. Healthy cells transport minerals across cell membranes to concentrate minerals in specific ratios for ideal function. Mineral balances in neural cells create membrane potentials or electrical gradients. Minerals are used to: build strong bones, teeth and tissues; produce hormones and enzymes; eliminate toxins; and control the biochemistry of life. Mineral intake can range from – absent; deficient; sufficient (RDAs); optimal; to excess (toxic). Minerals are key parts of all antioxidant systems that minimize free-radical damage to tissues. Mineral-rich cells/organs are ready to go to work, while mineral-poor cells are tired and worn out.

∗ Magnesium, as found in chlorophyll, activates 67 human enzymes that help produce energy.

Many mineral deficiency diseases have now been identified, including goiters of the thyroid. Goiters have been successfully treated for centuries with foods from the sea that contains Iodine. Thyroids need Iodine balanced by other minerals. A concentrated pill of pure Iodine can be toxic. Kelp is an Iodine-rich seafood that is ideal to prevent or treat Iodine-deficiency goiters. Goiters don't often develop quickly, and tired thyroids must slowly build up mineral balances to restore health.

Pica is a condition in which people crave missing minerals. Children eat paint, pencils or dirt while pregnant women are famous for craving unusual foods, trying to obtain missing minerals.

Minerals in concentrations higher than optimal are often toxic and upset ideal ratios. (Ch 51) Fluorine may be essential in minute amounts, is often considered safe in moderate amounts, yet is known to be toxic when exceeding 2.0 ppm. (pg 156) ∗ **Mercury is very toxic in minute amounts.**

Supplements can add minerals to the diet and make up for foods that are mineral deficient. ∗ Many mineral supplements aren't well absorbed, and what is absorbed may not be well used. Calcium of the wrong type may not be used to build strong bones, and may form painful Calcium deposits in joint spaces. Whey or bone meal powders as Calcium supplements help avoid this risk. Knowing how to keep minerals in proper balances/ratios with other minerals may seem to be an overwhelming task, but is made simpler by understanding that foods naturally balance minerals. If people eat an over abundance of mineral-rich foods or food supplement powders, tissues will just build up mineral reserves, while extra minerals will easily pass through the colon or kidneys. Chelated mineral supplements are in a form that closely mimics minerals in plants. Low quality multi-minerals are often little different from ground-up rock (limestone), such as in calcium -----ate. Colloidal mineral aggregates may be contaminated with dirt or contain excess (toxic) Aluminum.

Coffee damages the kidney's efficiency to balance electrolytes, causing a great loss of minerals.

∗ Powdered mineral-rich food is one safe effective way to supplement for human mineral needs.

Chapter 22 Eggs and Oils
Nutrition in Eggs

Moses records eggs from a wild 'game' bird's nest as being part of the Hebrew diet.

JPS Deut 22:6 If a bird's nest chance to be before thee in the way, in a tree or on the ground, with young one or eggs, and the dam [hen] sitting upon the young, or upon the eggs (***beytsah***), thou shalt not take the dam with the young;

Eggs were used as food, provided they were from clean fowl. (Lev 11 and Deut 14) [R15-19] Most eggs eaten in the time of Moses were probably from wild game birds, since hens were kept by the Hebrews in Israel to lay eggs only after the Babylonian captivity. [R15-19]

The egg yolk is very high in protein and egg white is almost pure protein. [R1] Egg protein has the highest biological value for man of any food, because the balance of amino acids in eggs is in the best ratio for digestion, absorption and utilization to build or rebuild healthy tissue. [R2-24-11]

Egg yolks are a rich source of protein, EFAs, fat-soluble vitamins, water-soluble vitamins and minerals. [R1] Today, due to their fat and cholesterol content, eggs are questioned as to their place in the diet, often without consideration of the valuable nutrients eggs also contain.

Bernard Jensen, DC in his book *Food Nutrition for Man* stated that egg yolks are very high in cholesterol, but are also one of the foods that is highest in lecithin in nature. Dr. Jensen also described egg yolk as a perfect source of protein. [R13] Dr. Jensen encouraged eating eggs, but warned that overcooking eggs destroys much of the nutritional value of lecithin. [R13]

"God put lecithin right next to cholesterol so you could get the balance,
God didn't make mistakes but we do." [R13]

"The overwhelming evidence of recent years is that eggs belong in a well-balanced diet. We should eat plenty of fresh fruits and vegetables, 60% of them raw, and whole grain cereals as well. But of the basic protein foods, eggs are second only to mother's milk in total nutritional value. The nutrients from eggs feed every cell in the body, brain and nerves, bones and ligaments, muscles and membranes, organs and glands." [R13A]

Lecithin is a very important and complex molecule that gets its name from the Greek word for egg yolk. Lecithin's critical biochemical function is determined by its chemical structure. Lecithin is made of <u>two</u> parts: 1) choline, which is soluble (dissolves) in water and is a vital component of nerve tissue; and 2) glycerol and fatty acids, this part of Lecithin is soluble in fats. The highest quality lecithin has an essential fatty acid (Linoleic - LA /or Linolenic - LNA) in the middle position on the glycerol backbone. Lecithin's structure not only allows it to be soluble in both fat and water; but it also acts in a similar manner to detergents, in the respect that lecithin can hold other molecules that by themselves are not water-soluble in suspension in water. [R5-9A] Lecithin is a complex molecule, and its ability to hold other fat-soluble molecules in suspension within a water medium is what makes lecithin so very valuable for health. [R5A-5B] (Chart 09 Fat)

∗ Lecithin can act as a fat emulsifier within the blood stream by keeping fat-soluble triglycerides and cholesterol in suspension within the water based liquid of human blood.

Paavo Airolo, PhD, ND wrote about lecithin in his book *Are You Confused?* [R7]

"Lecithin is a natural emulsifier of fat and it prevents cholesterol (which is fat) from collecting in chunks and attaching to the walls of the blood vessels, causing arteriosclerosis. ... lecithin is a good preventative of hardening of the arteries by its emulsifying effect on cholesterol."

Lecithin is included in foods products containing fat and water-soluble ingredients to insure uniform mixing of water and fat elements. Lecithin, beside its emulsifying property, is also an important food for building healthy body tissues: 80% of the human sexual fluid is lecithin; 20% of the white matter that surrounds the brain and the myelin sheath that surrounds the nerves is lecithin (also 13% of this is cholesterol); and 30% of the dry weight of the brain is lecithin. [R14]

Linus Pauling, PhD in his book *Vitamin C and the Common Cold* wrote about eggs: [All 3-R9]

"We must educate people away from the dangerous idea that you can control heart disease by not eating foods such as eggs, butter, and milk. This oversimplified idea is totally wrong."

Dr. C. W. Carlson, professor of animal sciences at South Dakota State University, wrote:

"The egg contains many beneficial and essential nutrients-protein (globulins), lecithins, polyunsaturated fatty acids, vitamins, and minerals (iron as well as sulfur, and many others). It is a great disservice to the consuming public to deprive them of these plus nutritive factors for no substantiated reason." [R9]

∗ Eggs and Milk contain many nutrients, such as lecithin, that are needed for life and health.

Eggs and Cholesterol

Zoltan Rona, MD in his book *The Joy of Health* discusses that eating eggs does not elevate blood cholesterol, as 85% of blood cholesterol is manufactured in the liver and intestines. [R22] Cholesterol is a nutrient! Cholesterol is essential for health. The human body can manufacture the cholesterol it needs in the liver or get the cholesterol it needs from food sources. [R5A-5B-9]

Dr. C. W. Carlson of South Dakota State University also wrote about cholesterol:

"A person in caloric equilibrium synthesizes approximately 800 mg of cholesterol per day if none is consumed in the diet. Dietary intakes are compensated for by reduced synthesis. With increased caloric intake, the blood cholesterol levels immediately rise." [R9]

Cholesterol is not soluble in water-based blood and must be transported in the blood stream as a complex of elements (<u>including Lecithin</u>) called a 'lipoprotein'. Medicine and science have documented that fat and cholesterol can become deposited on artery walls forming plaques. Plaque can lead to cardiovascular disease, high blood pressure, stroke and heart attack. [R5A] High blood triglycerides and/or LDL blood cholesterol are associated with increased risk of CVD. However, 40% of people have a heart attack with normal cholesterol. [R30] The Framington study documented the health of over 5,000 men and women who were all initially free from circulatory disease by giving them physical examinations every two years over a time period of 25 years. In the 30 to 49 year age group, persons with serum cholesterol levels of 260 or higher were found to have four times the numbers of cardiovascular events (CVD) as those with cholesterol levels at or below 220. [R9C] ∗ **Elevated (LDL) cholesterol adds a risk for CVD accidents, such as stroke and heart attack, however <u>LDL blood cholesterol has no relationship to dietary cholesterol</u>.**

Roger J. Williams, PhD wrote about cholesterol in his book *Nutrition Against Disease*.

"The cholesterol-rich foods that many people are trying to avoid also contain lecithin, which tends to dissolve dangerous cholesterol deposits. The lecithin helps the body to handle cholesterol and prevent it from accumulating in arteries." [R9-10]

Carl Pfeiffer, PhD, MD in his book *Mental and Elemental Nutrients* also discussed eggs. [R3]

"Egg eating does not explain or cause heart disease. Instead of blaming eggs, it would seem wiser to concentrate on correcting an otherwise poor diet. As we have seen, nutrients such as vitamin C, niacin, magnesium, zinc and chromium, possibly lecithin, and other factors such as natural carbohydrates and regular exercise produce and maintain lowered cholesterol levels, which are negatively associated with atherosclerosis. High cholesterol levels are promoted when the diet is mainly refined junk foods without trace elements."

Like the 'quality' of all foods, the nutritional value of eggs are sensitive to the manner in which eggs are produced. [R5-20] Eggs with the highest nutritional value come from hens that are kept by the 'free-range' method; from hens that live out-of-doors in fresh air and sunlight and are free to eat their normal diet of bugs, worms, grains and other vegetable material. These eggs are also 'fertile'; from females (hens) that were free to have sexual relations with the male rooster. [R27]

Eggs in supermarkets may not compare favorably, from the aspect of nutritional content, to the eggs in the time of Moses. Modern 'factory chicken' eggs may be laid by chickens that are cooped up in tiny cubicles under artificial light all their life and are fed a highly artificial diet including: hormones, antibiotics and a chemical mush. [R5C-7A-R13A] By comparison to 'factory chicken' eggs, fertile eggs from 'free-range' hens that are fed a better diet, including: more grains, lecithin, minerals, vitamins and EFAs, results in more of these micro-nutrients in the yolk.** [R4-5-7A-27]

Udo Erasmus, PhD states in his book *Fats and Oils*: [R5]

"The result of the change in the composition of chicken feed is eggs high in OA [oleic acid], but low in the essential fatty acids (LA and LNA), eggs with the same amount of cholesterol, but less of the essential fatty acids required to metabolize and transport it [cholesterol] properly in the human body. ... plant sterols, which are found naturally in all vegetables and which reduce the cholesterol content of eggs by up to 35%, were removed from the chicken's diet. Commercial eggs therefore contain more cholesterol than home grown barn yard eggs."

One approach to prevent plaque developing on artery walls is to eliminate or limit dietary cholesterol and in extreme cases to prescribe medications that prevent the liver from making cholesterol. The nutritional approach discusses that dietary and/or liver-made cholesterol is <u>not</u> the problem, rather the problem is a lack of lecithin, EFAs, and/or other micro-nutrients, which are needed to utilize cholesterol and allow human cholesterol transporting carriers work properly. [R10] If this approach is correct, the best preventative measures against CVD may come from eating free-range, fertile eggs, raw milk dairy products and other food with high micronutrient contents.

∗ **Lecithin, EFAs, vitamins and minerals increase HDL cholesterol and reduce risk of CVD.**

Oils

Fats and oil soluble nutrients are found in many foods. Milk, whole-germ grains, nuts, seeds, beans, fruits, vegetables and eggs all contain some oil or fat nutrients. Meat fats are terrible for health, containing few nutrients and many toxins. Partially hydrogenated trans-fatty acids are more cause related to heart attacks than the long-chain saturated fatty acids in meat fat. [R21] One very healthy fat is fish liver oil; which is the highest food source of vitamin A. Vitamin A is also found in raw milk and nuts and seeds oils. Vitamin D, which is technically a hormone, is found primarily in raw milk. Vitamin E is found in the germ of whole grains, such as wheat. Lecithin is found in the highest amount in raw milk, soy oil and egg yolks. Olive oil is rich essential fatty acids. * Kosher foods contain these known and other unknown oil-soluble essential nutrients for health.

The naturally occurring oils in foods or properly produced 'cold pressed' oils from foods, such as: olive oil, grain germ oils, nut oils or seed oils and cod liver oil along with sunlight, provide the body the raw materials to make it's own hormones. Polyunsaturated oils from plants sources are very stable in the unbroken complete food, but very subject to spoilage and rancidity after being removed and isolated from the outer protective food layers. Even the best 'cold processing' procedure may remove some protein, essential fat, vitamins and minerals from the finished oil. Unfortunately, the commonly used methods to produce most oils today leave the finished oil completely void of vitamins, minerals, essential fatty acids, essential amino acids, fiber, lecithin, phytosterols as well as leaving residues of unwanted solvents. Rex Russell, MD calls the refined 'white oils' that lack all essential nutrients, a hazard to health. Dr. Russell labels these oils 'white' due their similarity to white sugar and white flour, and their lack of essential fat-soluble nutrients found in natural oils of foods or in cold pressed oils. [R12] Full nutrient oils are frequently especially important for women to balance their monthly hormones or transition comfortably to menopause.

Neil Nedley, MD in his book *Proof Positive* warns against extreme very low fat diets. [R25]

"Intake of total fat per se, independent of the relative content of the different types of fatty acids, is not associated with high blood cholesterol and coronary heart disease."

"We now know that we can have a healthful diet that includes moderate levels of fat if we are using the best [quality] types of fat."

Steven Masley, MD in his book *The 28-Day Antioxidant Diet Program* discusses how oxidant free-radicals contribute to arterial plaque formation and how antioxidants prevent the problem.

"Oxidants, like tobacco, convert cholesterol into plaque, a hardened substance that forms inside the lining of our arteries and blocks blood flow. Antioxidants prevent fat from being oxidized and can slow or reverse this plaque forming process." [R28B]

Olestra is a new oil designed to be too-big to be absorbed in the intestines, so people can eat it without gaining weight, but olestra also blocks the absorption of needed nutrients. Avoid olestra. [28C]

Dr. Rex Russell recommends following three basic principles to choose a healthy diet. [R12]

1) Eat only what God created for food. 2) Eat what God created for food before the food is processed to become nutrient deficient or toxic products are added. 3) Avoid all addictions.

"Over the past few years consumption of seed oil [corn, maize and sunflower] has increased in Italy; these oils are purchased above all because they cost less than olive oil. Nutritionally these oils are actually inferior to olive oil, even if they do contain a high percentage of unsaturated fats." [R31]

[Seed oil is marketed to create an illusion of health and youth, even though seed oil is known to be inferior to Olive oil.]

Lecithin, essential fatty acids (EFAs), protein, fat and water-soluble vitamins, minerals and fiber are nutritional elements that are vital to health. When these nutrients are present in their proper balance in the diet, then digesting and utilizing fats and cholesterol from nutrient-rich foods, such as eggs and milk is no problem. However, when these nutrients are absent/deficient in the diet; then metabolism and transportation in the blood of fats and cholesterol may become faulty, which often leads to an increased risk of cardiovascular disease (CVD). Today, many people are <u>overfed</u> with 'empty' high calorie foods, and yet <u>undernourished</u> due to a shortage of: water and oil-soluble vitamins, minerals, protein, enzymes, EFAs, fiber and other micronutrients. Micronutrients that are missing appear to contribute to cardiovascular disease and other chronic degenerative disease.

** 'Fertile Eggs' result from a rooster's sperm penetrating an egg yolk, which substantially changes the biochemistry of an egg. 'Fertile Eggs' develop into new life; while non-fertile eggs don't develop into new life. Lecithin and male hormones from sperm add to the nutritional content of an egg yolk. Eggs that are 'fertile' are nutritionally superior to ordinary, non-fertile, supermarket eggs. [R27]

Free-range, fertile eggs and raw milk dairy products in the diet do not raise LDL cholesterol and do not elevate triglycerides and do not cause an increased risk of CVD or stroke or heart attack. Raw milk and fertile, free-range eggs may provide key micronutrients that prevent CVD events.

---------------------------- References Ch 22 Eggs and Oil --------------------------------

[R1] Nutrition Almanac 1979 Edition\ pg 206-207 nutritional value of eggs
[R2] Nutrition and Your Body; by Benjamin Colimore, MA and Sarah Stewart Colimore, LPT; pg 12-17; nutrients in eggs
[R3] Mental and Elemental Nutrients\ by Carl Pfeiffer, MD, PhD; pg 85-86 nutrients in eggs
[R4] Making Fats and Oils Work for You\ by Lewis Harrison; pg 117 nutrients in egg yolks
[R5] Fats and Oils\ by Udo Erasmus, PhD; 226-229 (pg 227 quote) commercial egg production
[R5A] pg 56-57 lecithin & 58-65 cholesterol
[R6] Know Your Nutrition\ by Linda Clark
[R7] Are You Confused?\ by Paavo Airolo, PhD, ND; pg 80 lecithin
[R7A] pg 62 free-range verses factory eggs
[R8] Fats that Heal Fats that Kill\ by Udo Erasmus, PhD
[R9] Supernutrition\ by Richard Passwater, PhD; pg 100-101 nutrients in eggs
[R9A] pg 131-135 lecithin, diet and cardiovascular disease (CVD)
[R9B] pg 77-80, 94, 127-128 autopsies of soldier & CVD – cholesterol doesn't count
[R10] Nutrition Against Disease\ by Roger Williams, PhD; pg 75-76 cholesterol is vital for health
[R11] Your Health Under Siege\ by Jeffrey Bland, PhD; pg 70 eggs and cholesterol
[R12] What the Bible Says About Healthy Living\ by Rex Russell, MD; pg 139 white oils
[R12A] pg 55 3 principles of healthy food choices
[R13] Food Healing for Man\ by Bernard Jensen, DC; pg 16 lecithin quote
[R13A] pg 286- also 'free-range' statement
[R14] Sex and Nutrition\ by Bernard Jensen, DC essential nutrition for healthy sex
[R15] Eating in Jerusalem Exhibit of King David Museum\ in Jerusalem Israel
[R16] Egg Science and Technology\ by Powrie and Nakai; pg 116
[R17] Nutrition and the Chicken\ by Scott Nesheim Young; pg 230
[R18] Strong's Concordance\ by James Strong, STD, LLD

pg 297	egg(s)	# 1000	H pg 20	***beytsah***	Deut 22:6
pg 740-41	oil	# 8081	H pg 118	***shemen***	Deut 8:8
pg 742	olive	# 2132	H pg 35	***zayith***	Deut 28:40

[R19] Harpers Encyclopedia of Bible Life; eggs a common Hebrew food after Babylonian captivity
[R20] Answers to Question Frequently Asked About Eggs; (Egg-land's Best; PO Box 370; Rochester, Wash 98579-0370) — more nutritious chicken feed results in higher quality nutrition in the eggs
[R21] Health\ (magazine) March 98; pg 17 nutritious eggs
[R22] The Joy of Health\ by Zoltan Rona, MD; pg 54 eggs are nutritious & don't raise cholesterol
[R23] Food for Nought\ by Ross Hume Hall; pg 100 (more protein)
pg 242 cholesterol is necessary for every cell in the body – including hormone formation
[R24] Good Fat Bad Fat\ by William P. Castelli, MD and Glen C. Griffin, MD
[R25] Proof Positive\ by Neil Nedley, MD; pg 69 quote low fat theory
[R26] Low Fat Lies\ by Mary Flynn and Kevin Vigilante
[R27] Fit and Free\ by Rick Kasper; pg 110-111 fertile eggs
[R28] The 28-Day Antioxidant Diet Program\ by Steven Masley, MD; pg 149 avoid Olestra
[R28A] pg 50-62 fats + cholesterol diagram //[R28B] pg 60 quote plaque formation
[R29] Medicinal Fatty Acids in Inflammation\ by Joel M. Kremer, MD
[R30] Help Yourself to Better Health (March 31, 2001)\ by Monte Kline, PhD heart attacks
[R31] Olive Oil\ by Silvia Bevilacqua Calzolari; pg 74-75 olive oil being replaced by corn oil
[R32] Olives\ by Mort Rosenblum
[R33] Miracle Foods of the Bible\ on TV from the Food Network (04-06-03) 1 lb Olive ≈1 oz Olive oil – Olive Oil (Elliot Berry) – Omega 3 Essential Fatty Acids from fish oils – Wine – Honey – Manna –
[R34] Diet for a New America\ by John Robbins – health risks from modern 'factory chicken eggs'
[R35] Diet for a New America (video)\ by John Robbins – modern factory chicken egg production – also discusses challenges to human health and the environmental risks from modern animal husbandry
[R36] Fit or Fat for the 90s (PBS video)\ by Covert Bailey; cholesterol is wax-like – HDL vs LDL – exercise
[R37] Train Up Your Children in the Way They Should Eat\ by Sharon Broer (1-800-592-HEAL)
[R38] Eating to the Glory of God\ by Ted Broer, PhD and Sharon Broer (1-800-592-4325)
[R39] Fit at Forty\ by Ted Broer, PhD www.TedBroer.com
[R40] The Right Fat Diet (CD)\ by Udo Erasmus, PhD; Flax oil – $w3$ EFA www.UdoErasmus.com

Maintaining homeostasis – balanced biochemistry – prevents health problems; while restoring homeostasis often helps to remediate many health problems.

Chapter 23 Manna
What Was It?

Manna! What was it? Everyone has heard of manna, but nobody really knows what it was. Since ***manna*** means: 'What is it?' obviously the Hebrews did not know what manna was. [R18] Manna is also called 'angels food'. (Ps 78:25) No ***Torah*** translator knows what ***manna*** means, since they all transliterate manna into every language. [R18] The LORD only provided ***manna***, the 'bread from heaven', to the Hebrews that wandered in the wilderness for 40 years. (Josh 5:12)

NKJV Ex 16:4 Then the LORD said unto Moses, "Behold, I will rain bread from heaven for you. And the people shall go out and gather a certain quota every day, that I might test them, whether they will walk in My law or not."

KJV Ex 16:15 And when the children of Israel saw it, they said one to another, It is manna: for they wist [knew] not what it was. And Moses said unto them, this is bread which the LORD has given you to eat.

We know that Moses maintained perfect health during the 40 years of wilderness wandering, because, at the end of his life, his eyesight was not dim nor was his strength gone. (Deut 34:7) Since ***manna*** was his only source of nutrition for ≈40 years, ***manna*** must have supplied all essential nutritional needs: complete protein, including all 8 essential amino acids for building the muscles and organs of the body; carbohydrates for fuel and energy; all essential fatty acids; all the oil-soluble vitamins, including A, D, E, F, and K; all the water-soluble vitamins, including B complex and C complex; and soluble and insoluble fiber for bulk to keep the colon clean and maintain the health of the digestive system; as well as all other undetermined essential nutrients. There is <u>no single food</u> that meets all nutritional requirements for optimal health and longevity.

<u>∗ Manna could have been either: a combination of several common, naturally occurring foods; or one unique, very special food that is not available today.</u>

If ***manna*** was a single, unique food that was provided by God for only 40 years, then any knowledge of ***manna*** will have to wait until God explains it in heaven. (Deut 29:29) However, if ***manna*** was a combination of foods that are available today, then the best place to search and discover what ***manna*** was, is from within the text of the ***Torah***, as well as the text of all Scripture.

Fifteen times in the ***Torah***, Moses likens the future home of the Hebrews to the 'land of milk and honey'. The Hebrew word for land (***eretz***) is also the place the on which the ***manna*** fell. [R18]

KJV Ex 16:14 There lay a small round thing {***manna***) as a hoar frost on the ground (***eretz***).

JPS Ex 16:31 And the house of Israel called the name thereof Manna: and it was like coriander seed, white; and the taste of it was like wafers made with honey.

NIV Num 11:7-9 The manna was like coriander seed and looked like resin. vs8 They cooked it in a pot or made it into cakes. And it tasted like something made with olive oil. vs9 When the dew settled on the camp at night, the manna also came down.

The LORD used giving of manna for six days, but not on the Sabbath, as a means of finding out whether His people would be faithful to Him and faithful to His commandments. (Ex 16:4)

Milk is the most complete food there is. (Ch 16 Milk) [R2] As nutritionally perfect as milk is, it does not contain large amounts of certain vital trace minerals. Dr. Jarvis emphasized that honey contains all the vitamins and many minerals that nutritionists consider necessary to health. [R1] Milk is teeming with nutrients that honey doesn't contain. Milk, when powdered, is small white roundish granules that could fit the description of ***manna***. (Ex 16) A.I. Root lived for many days with vigor, energy and health on a diet of just milk and honey along with a little orange juice. [R3] Milk and honey together are a perfect combination, and the hallmark of the *kashrut* Hebrew diet.

∗ Everyone is subject to the 'Laws of Health' from the LORD that Moses wrote in the *Torah*.

∗ People who obey Moses reap a benefit, while people who disobey the LORD pay a price.

∗ Perhaps <u>concentrates</u> of all clean Meats, Fish, Fowl, Milk, Honey, Grains, SeaSalt, Nuts, Seeds, Beans, Fruits, Vegetables, Olive oil, and Eggs may have been what comprised ***manna***. Concentrated powders or resins, each in the ideal form to retain nutritive values, of all foods that Moses wrote about in the ***Torah*** could have been ***manna***! Whatever ***manna*** was; ***manna*** was perfect nutrition. ***Manna*** plus other instruction in the ***Torah***, led to perfect health for ***Moshe***.

∗ Food dense in nutrients and low in toxicity comprised the *kosher* Hebrew diet of Moses.

∗ *Manna* may have been concentrates of all the foods that Moses discussed in the *Torah*.

Manna as Perfect Nutrition

Society, today, doesn't enjoy the health of Moses. Perhaps one reason for the poor health today can be traced to the fact that today's foods don't always contain all the nutrition in ***manna***. Moses was not the only Hebrew to enjoy the benefit of perfect nutrition that ***manna*** provided. As the Hebrews wandered in the wilderness, the LORD provided and no one's feet were swollen.

JPS Deut 8:4 Thy raiment waxed not old [did not wear out] upon thee,
neither did thy foot swell, these forty years.

Swollen feet are often a sign of a nutritional deficiency disease, such as pellagra or beriberi. Deficiency of a single isolated vitamin or mineral usually resulted in a specific set of symptoms. During the day of Moses, when someone developed a nutritional deficiency, often more than one vitamin or mineral shortage was experienced and symptoms were from more than one deficiency. Beriberi is a thiamin B_1 deficiency causing muscular weakness and loss of feeling in hands–feet. Pellagra is a niacin B_3 deficiency causing (4 Ds) diarrhea, dementia, dermatitis and finally death. Scurvy is a vitamin C deficiency resulting in loss of appetite, bleeding gums, swollen ankles, etc. Osteoporosis (Calcium deficiency) and Rickets in children (vitamin D deficiency) weaken the bones. Eating a restricted or mono-food (category) diet risks developing a vitamin or mineral deficiency. The major mode of transportation during Moses' day was walking and swollen feet were common and incapacitating. No one experienced a vitamin or mineral deficiency by eating only ***manna***. ***Manna*** was nutritionally perfect and it could also be prepared, fixed and eaten in a variety of ways.

KJV Num 11:8 And the people went about, and gathered it [***manna***], and ground it in mills,
or beat it in a mortar, and baked it in pans, and made cakes of it: ...

Variety is important in any diet. Even though the Hebrews ate a mono-food diet of ***manna*** for forty years, they found a variety of ways to prepare ***manna*** and feature ***manna's*** different tastes. Gathering ***manna*** was not without controversy, as instructions by Moses were very specific.

NKJV Ex 16:16 "This is the thing which the LORD hath commanded; 'Let every man gather it [***manna***] according to each one's need, one omer for each person, according to the number of persons; let every man take for those who are in his tent.' " vs17 And the children of Israel did so and gathered, some more, some less..vs19 And Moses said, "Let no one leave any of it till morning." vs20 Notwithstanding they did not heed Moses. But some of them left part of it until morning, and it bred worms and stank. And Moses was angry with them. vs21 So they gathered it every morning, every man according to his own need. And when the sun became hot, it melted.

{An *omer* is the 10th part of an *ephah*. (Ex 16:36) – An *ephah* is ≈15 cups or ≈1¾ quarts or ≈1¾ liters.}

Manna as a Hebrew Test

Manna lasted overnight only on the eve of the Sabbath and through the Sabbath day.

NIV Ex16:22 On the sixth day, they gathered twice as much—two omers for each person— vs23 He said to them "This is what the LORD commanded: tomorrow is to be a day of rest, a holy Sabbath to the LORD. So bake what you want to bake and boil what you want to boil. Save whatever is left and keep it until morning.' " vs24 So they saved it until morning, as Moses commanded, and it did not stink or get maggots in it. vs26 Six days you are to gather it, but on the seventh day, the Sabbath, there will not be any." vs30 So the people rested on the seventh day.

It is likely there was nothing inherent in ***manna*** that would always cause it to spoil overnight, since on the 7th day ***manna*** lasted for two days. It is likely that the LORD arranged overnight variables of temperature, humidity, wind, etc. to be ideal for maggots to flourish and ***manna*** to spoil for 6 evenings, while on the 7th evening conditions were ideal for ***manna*** to be preserved. Hebrews that tested the LORD found out that the instructions of Moses were given to be obeyed.

∗ Forty years of wilderness wanderings was interactive history between the LORD and the Hebrews. ***Manna*** had a three-fold purpose: 1st as perfect nutrition; 2nd as a Hebrew obedience test; and 3rd, as a witness to the Hebrews who crossed the Jordan River and inherited the Promised Land, a sample was put in a jar and was placed in the Ark of the Covenant along with Aaron's rod and the two original tablets of stone, upon which the LORD wrote the Ten Commandments. (Ex 16:33) ***Manna*** provides testimony to the wisdom of the LORD for all generations: past, present and future. {The author does not know how the LORD provided ***manna*** for the Hebrews in the wilderness.}

∗ *Manna* was everything that the LORD designed it to be, and everything the Hebrews needed it to be.

Manna as Food Concentrates

Zoltan Rona, MD in his book *The Joy of Health* discusses the value of food concentrates. [R8] "Live whole food concentrates might well be the most logical and convenient answer to the deteriorated quality of foods available from supermarkets today. Whenever possible, use whole food concentrates rather than single nutrient tablets or capsules. That's because when one isolates a single component from a given food, a lot of the benefits of the complete food are lost. Supplemental vitamins and minerals cannot duplicate the mixture of nutrients and many yet to be identified substances of value to health found in natural foods. Whole foods contain what are called 'phytochemicals' which are linked to both the prevention and treatment of such major degenerative diseases as heart disease, strokes, high blood pressure, and cancer. The only way to get these phytochemicals is by eating whole foods or live whole food concentrates." "Under emergency survival conditions, when people do not have access to live whole foods, the only option may be live whole food concentrates. Live whole food concentrates are processed and converted from live whole food at temperatures less than 100°F, thereby maintaining the 'life' within the food. Temperature during the conversion process is the crucial deciding factor distinguishing 'live' from 'dead' food." [R8]

Udo Erasmus, PhD discusses nutritional deficiency diseases in his books, such as *Fats and Oils*: "The deficiency theory suggests that the cause of degenerative disease is a deficiency of vitamins, minerals, fiber, and essential fatty acids which are necessary for metabolism of cholesterol and fats in the body, but which have been systematically refined out of our foods by processing methods which came into widespread use since just before 1900. Refined sugars, refined oils, and refined starches are all deficient in minerals and vitamins. The finding that increasing the vitamin and mineral intake lowers cholesterol and triglyceride levels in the blood lends weight to the deficiency theory. The fact that just cutting down our consumption of refined sugars and fats stops many degenerative conditions and increases vigor and longevity lends weight to the deficiency theory." [R4]

Understanding the devastating nature of nutritional deficiency disease is further complicated by the fact that there is often a 'gradation' of symptoms from the well-nourished, ideal state of optimal health to a gross deficiency of clinical disease such as diabetes, heart disease or scurvy. Myron Brin, PhD suggests that the first noticeable signs or symptoms of nutritional deficiency disease may be adverse behavioral or personality effects that are caused by subtle physiological changes, followed by more recognizable physiological dysfunction that leads to an obvious, observable clinical illness, ending in terminal tissue pathology and disease (such as cancer). [R5]

Bernard Jensen, DC, PhD candidly discussed the cause of all disease, when he said: [R22] "The fact is there is only one major disease, and that is malnutrition. All ailments and afflictions to which we may become heirs are directly traceable to this major disease."

Hebrew sage Maimonides (1135 to 1204 AD) recognized the value of food to health when he said; "Most diseases that man is afflicted with are due to bad foods." [R30]

To malnutrition, the author adds acute and/or chronic toxicity as an important risk for disease.

Moses indicated that ***manna*** is ideal physical nourishment; just as ***Torah*** instructions are food for thought. Joshua followed the advise of Moses to make his path prosperous. (Josh 1:8)

KJV Deut 8:3 And he [the LORD] humbled thee, and suffered thee to hunger, and fed thee with manna, which thou knewest not, neither did thy fathers know; that he [the LORD] might make thee know that man doth not live by bread only, but by every word that proceedeth out of the mouth of the LORD doth man live.

All the instruction in righteousness from the mouth of the LORD that is found in the ***Torah*** is as important, if not more important, to total health as any instruction by Moses on diet and food.

∗ 1st, recognize the health principles taught by Moses in the *Torah* — 2nd, practice obedience!

If proteins, essential fatty acids and minerals are analogous to the materials to build a house: then vitamins (water- and oil-soluble) and enzymes are analogous to workers who build the house. Vitamins and enzymes are necessary to speed up biochemical reactions that are required for life. Without efficiently functioning vitamins/enzymes, the biochemistry of life will slowly grind to a halt. A body without vitamins/enzymes is like a work slow-down, which results in an unfinished house. Workers are essential to build a house, but without construction materials, workers are helpless. Workers, like enzymes, are not part of the raw materials, nor are they part of the finished product; but the best quality raw materials and the best workers together result in the best, finished house.

∗ For the healthiest diet, the author eats food that is nutrient dense and also low in toxins.

---------------------------------- References Ch 23 Manna ----------------------------------

[R1] Folk Medicine\ by D. C. Jarvis, MD; pg 98 minerals in honey
[R2] The Milk Book\ by William C. Douglass, MD; pg 66-67 nutrition in milk
[R3] The ABC to XYZ of Beekeeping\ by A. I. Root; pg 421 milk and honey fast
[R4] Fats and Oils\ by Udo Erasmus, PhD; pg 312 micronutrient deficiency leads to disease
[R5] Food and Nutrition Coarse\ by Jeffrey Bland, PhD; references the work of Myron Brin, PhD
pg 55 progression of symptoms in nutritional deficiency disease
[R6] Surviving into the 21st Century (audio tape)\ by David Sandivold { w^{3}.GreenKamut.com }
[R7] The Healing Miracle of Green Food (audio tape)\ by David Sandivold {1-800-452-6884}
[R8] Making the Best of Basics\ by James Talmage Stevens;
pg 169 quote from Zoltan Rona, MD on food concentrates
[R9] The Joy of Health\ by Zoltan Rona, MD; pg 60 up to 80% of all nutrients lost by processing
[R10] Diet for a Small Planet\ by Francis Moore Lappe'
[R11] Honey and Health\ by Bodog Beck, MD
[R12] What the Bible Says About Healthy Living\ by Rex Russell, MD; pg 55 three principles
[R13] Back to Protein\ by Barbara Doyen
[R14] Food is the Best Medicine\ Henry Bieler, MD; treats illness as a nutritional deficiency
[R15] The True Cost of a Failed Agricultural System (Acres 1999 audio)\ by Arden Andersen DO, PhD
[R16] Food in History\ by Reay Tannahill; pg 55-56 kosher - eat no blood - *kashrut* -
[R17] Foods and Nutrition\ by Rodale Press
[R18] Strong's Concordance\ by James Strong, STD, LLD

pg 658	manna	# 4478	H pg 67	***manna***	Ex 16:15
pg 141	bread	# 3899	H pg 59	***lechem***	Ex 16:4
pg 474	heaven	# 8064	H pg 118	***shameh***	Ex 16:4
pg 581-3	land (ground)	# 776	H pg 17	***eretz* – *erets***	Ex 16:16
pg 846	right	# 3787	H pg 58	***kasher*** – (*kashrut*)	Esther 8:5

Kosher is an Americanized transliteration of *kashrut* or ***kasher***, which is accurately translated – 'right'.
Kosher or *kashrut* can also mean clean, fit or proper, as it is commonly used to describe Hebrew food.
Kosher also properly discusses – meats from an animal, fish or fowl on the clean lists and meats that are trimmed of fat, and slaughtered so the blood from the meat is drained by the still-beating heart.
Kosher has also come to mean – not eating milk products and herbivore meat at the same meal. (Ch 14)
Since fish and fowl do not produce milk, it is felt they are permitted as *kashrut* with dairy products.
In 1992, the author had a kosher pizza in Israel with cheese and tuna fish, but no beef was allowed.
To the author, kosher best describes healthy Hebrew food, rather than restricted dairy/meat combinations.
[R19] Poisons in Your Food\ by William Longgood; food toxins and nutrient deficient food
[R20] Spontaneous Healing (audio)\ by Andrew Weil, MD; (sd 2) reductionism
[R21] Foods That Heal\ by Bernard Jensen, DC, PhD All healthy foods contain healing nutrients.
[R22] Lecture at Hidden Valley Ranch\ by Bernard Jensen, DC All disease is from malnutrition.
[R23] Goat Milk Magic\ by Bernard Jensen, DC, PhD; benefits of raw Goat's milk
[R24] Notes on Exodus\ by George Bush; a good ***Torah*** Commentary
[R25] Proof Positive\ by Neil Nedley, MD; pg 489-490 vitamin/mineral wheels
[R25A] pg 56-57 progression of coronary artery disease atherosclerosis diagram
[R25B] pg 93-95 the fate of many clogged artery charts
[R26] Lick the Sugar Habit\ by Nancy Appleton, PhD; pg 15-16 mineral chart and deficiency/toxicity
[R27] Orthomolecular Nutrition\ by Abram Hoffer, MD poor nutrition ⇒ poor biochemistry ⇒ poor health
[R28] The 28-Day Antioxidant Diet Program\ by Steven Masley, MD Free-radical 'oxidant' chemicals are 'terrorist chemicals' to be destroyed with anti-oxidants before the free-radicals harm human health.
[R29] Protein Power\ by Michael R. Eades, MD and Mary Dan Eades, MD
[R30] 1995 San Diego Leadership Conference (Enrich audio tape)\ by Julian Whittaker, MD {1-800-300-0219}
[R31] Dr. Whitaker's Guide to Natural Healing\ by Julian Whittaker, MD
[R32] Encyclopedia of Nutritional Supplements\ by Michael Murray, ND vitamins - minerals – RDAs
[R33] Environmental Poisons in Our Food\ by J. Gordon Millichap, MD; pg 133 Rabbi Maimonides
[R34] Oasis Clinic w^{3}.oasisofhope.com / Ralph Moss w^{3}.ralphmoss.com / alternative cancer therapy
[R35] Toxemia Explained\ by John Tilden, MD; pg 31 No fool is a bigger fool than the fool who fools himself.
[R36] Great Minds of Medicine (audio)\ by William Castelli, MD; (tp1) poor food ⇒ heart disease & osteoporosis

∗ If Osama Bin Laden eats no pork and President Bush eats pork, who would be more likely to get trichinosis?
President Bush, whom I respect greatly, said; We can't allow terrorists to strike and then just repair damages, we must seek and identify terrorists before they strike, and then we must prevent them from acting against us. So it is with health: we must seek and identify people and circumstances that cause emotional harm and/or prevent growth and avoid them; we must minimize conditions that promote plague; and we must identify and avoid nutritionally deficient food and food contaminated by toxins, if we are to enjoy the same health as Moses.

Minerals, Vitamins and RDAs

Mineral	RDA	Optimal (adult male)	Main Functions in the Body	Best Food Sources
Calcium	1,000 mg	1,000 to 2,000 mg	bones, teeth, muscles, nerves	milk & dairy
Magnesium	400 mg	500 to 1,000 mg	bones, teeth, muscles, nerves	grains - greens
Sodium	none	deficiencies unknown	nerve transmission (w/Potassium)	SeaSalt
Potassium	none	1.9 to 5.6 g (gram)	heart – balance pH & Blood pressure	fruit-vegetable
Chlorine	none	deficiencies unknown	stomach – hydrochloric acid	SeaSalt
Phosphorous	1 gm	200 to 400 mg	bones, teeth & energy release	meat-dairy-bean
Sulfur	------	deficiencies unknown	used in all protein building	all proteins
Boron	none	1.5 to 3^+ to 5 mg	modulates Calcium absorption	fruit-vegetable
Chromium	none	200 to 600 mcg	utilizing glucose - enzymes	whole grain
Cobalt	none	perhaps 3 mcg	absorbed/used as part of vit B_{12}	meats - liver
Copper	2 mg	0.5 to 2 mg	hemoglobin formation	many foods
Fluorine	? 3.8 mg ?	? 1.5 to 4 mg ?	(incorporated into teeth and bones)	0.7% added to water
Iodine	150 mcg	150-200 mcg	thyroid function & metabolism	kelp & SeaSalt
Iron	10 mg	15 to 30 mg	hemoglobin & energy production	grains-beans
Manganese	none	2.5 to 5 mg	enzymes – blood sugar & thyroid	nut-grain-green
Molybdenum	none	75 to 250 mcg	enzymes – uric acid & detoxification	bean-grain-green
Selenium	70 mg	100 to 400 mcg	antioxidant & immune function	grain-nut-onion
Silicon	none	20 to 40^+ mg	collagen in bone & connective tissue	grain-vegetable
Vanadium	none	10 to 60 mcg	glucose metabolism	grain-bean-green
Zinc	15 mg	30 to 100 mg	digestion, insulin, growth, prostate	beans - meat
g = gram / mg = milligram / mcg = µg = microgram / IU = International Unit / tbs = tablespoon / grain = whole grain				
vitamin A	5,000 IU	5,000 IU	vision – eye tear film – immunity	liver - fish liver oil
vitamin D	200 IU	200 to 400 IU	bone structure	–sunlight-fish oil-butter
vitamin E	15 IU	400^+ IU	antioxidant – immunity – heart	wheat germ
vitamin F (LA & LNA)	none	1 to 2 tbs	cell membrane – essential hormones	olive-flax-fish oils
vitamin K	80 mcg	150 to 500 mg	blood clotting	greens
B_1 -Thiamine	1.5 mg	50 to 100 mg	digestion–enzymes (def=beriberi)	rice–been–seed
B_2 -Riboflavin	1.7 mg	5 to 10 mg	energy – vision – mucus membranes	meat–nut–grain
B_3 -Niacin	20 mg	100 to 300 mg	energy–blood sugar (def =pellagra)	meat–nut
-Biotin	30 mg	30 to 300 mg	metabolism – synthesis fat & AA	meat–bean–cheese
B_5 -Pantothine	4 to 7 mg	250 to 300 mg	RedBloodCell (RBC)–hormones–energy	meat-grain-bean
-Folic Acid	200 mcg	400 to 1,000 mcg	DNA synthesis – works with B_{12}	green-bean-grain
B_6 -Pyridoxine	2.0 mg	50 to 100 mg	synthesis protein &hormones–immunity	grain–nut–seed
B_{12} -Cobalamin	6 mcg	50 to 500 mg	synthesis RBC – DNA & metabolism	meats - liver
Inositol	100 to 500 mg	12 grams	liver & brain & nerve & muscle function	citrus-grain-n-s-b
Choline	350 to 500 mg	15 to 25 grams	in lecithin – brain & liver function	egg–soy–beef
vitamin C	60 mg	1 to 5^+ g (gram)	immunity – collagen – antioxidant	fresh fruit & milk
vitamin P (Bioflavonoids)	none	150 to 1,000 mg	antioxidants – help vitamin C work	plant pigments in
Bioflavonoids – Rutin, Hesperidin, Citrin, Flavones & Flavonals – function with vitamin C				fruit & vegetables
Carotenoids	none	≈15 mg	vision & antioxidant – pre-vitamin A	plant pigments

Balances and ratios between minerals may be more important than the quantity of any mineral. Minerals–Vitamins work well only in relation to concentrations of nutrients with which they interact. The ideal balance for Calcium to Magnesium is ≈2 to 1 and for Calcium to Phosphorous is ≈3 to 1. If 100 mg of Calcium is optimal for health, then ≈50 mg of Magnesium and ≈33 mg of Phosphorus are also needed to use the Calcium. If Magnesium and Phosphorous aren't present in optimal amounts, then Calcium is underutilized, causing a Calcium deficiency; while taking more isolated Calcium supplements will only lead to a buildup of excess Calcium that will become toxic. ∗ **Paradoxically, someone may have both a Calcium deficiency and a Calcium toxicity at the same time!** ∗ Under utilization of Calcium may result in osteoporosis; while excess Calcium may result in toxic arthritis. [R26] Ratios may explain why one person initially does well on a mineral–vitamin formula, but over a period of time benefits decrease; while for another person a mineral–vitamin formula may quickly be toxic. Toxicity is only a problem with high-potency mineral–vitamin supplements. Ranges exist for ratios that promote health, but today deficiencies and/or excesses are common. Using high potency vitamin/minerals supplements to maintain proper balances is a job for a professional, such as Michael Murray, ND, who wrote the *Encyclopedia of Nutritional Supplements*, or Monte Kline, PhD who wrote the *Help Yourself to Better Health* manual. Nutrient deficiencies allow/invite diseases and excesses cause toxicities. Foods grown organically on nutrient-rich soils balance all minerals–vitamins, minimizing the risk of deficiencies while avoiding the risk of toxicities.

∗ Powdered food is a safe way to supplement for ideal balances and for avoiding toxicity.

Mineral and Vitamin Interaction Chart

Minerals are needed in ideal ratios and Minerals interact with one another for proper function. Vitamins and Minerals often interact with one another to enable Enzymes to function efficiently.

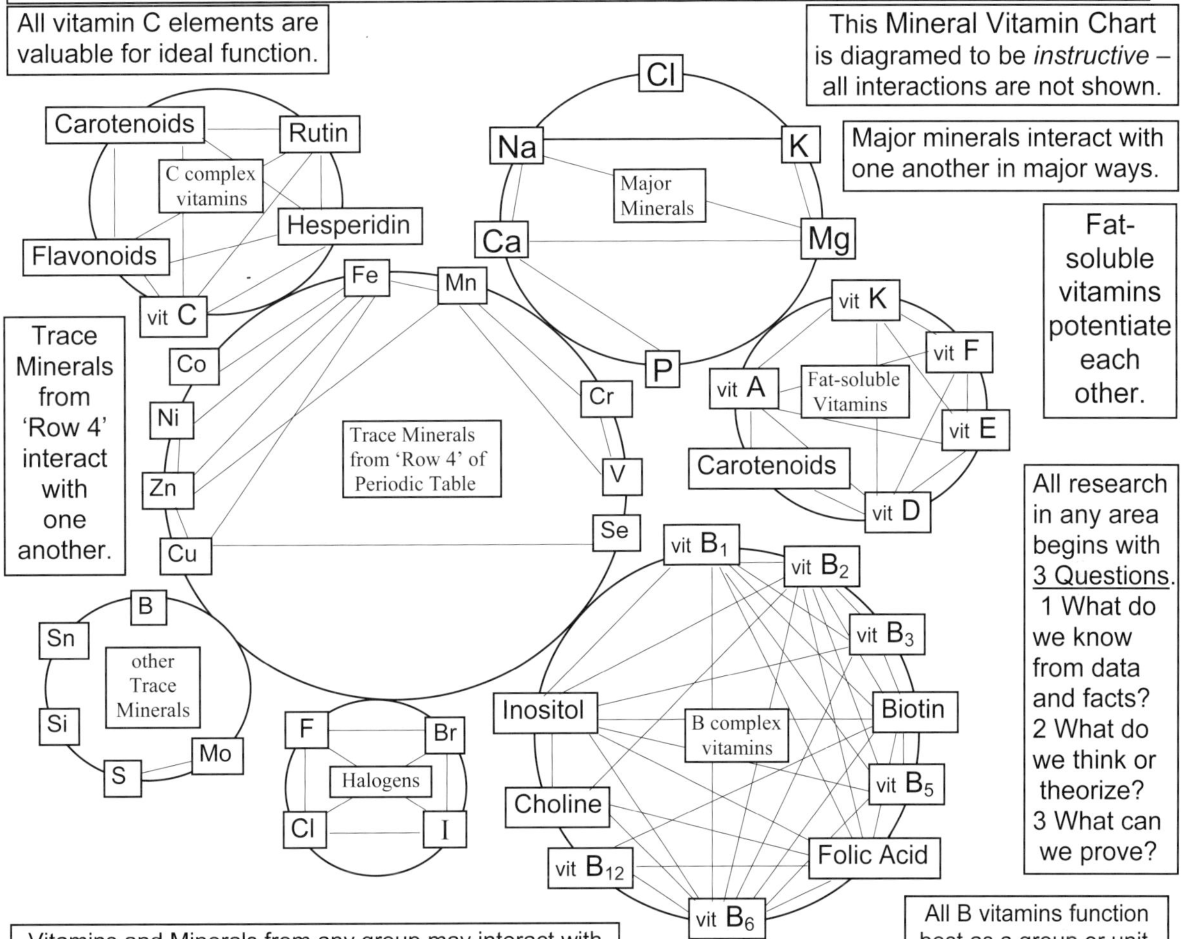

Vitamins and Minerals from any group may interact with one another — as vit B_{12} interacts with vit C and vit E.

∗ Fluorine, Chlorine, Bromine and Iodine are in the 'Halide' column and they all interact with one another.

The author imagines: All vitamins–minerals are primarily part of groups that need one another for proper function, like notches on a gear wheel need all other notches for the gear to function. Individual vitamins–minerals also interact with other vitamins–minerals from outside their group. Finally, nutrient groups must also interact with other groups to form fully-functioning life, in the same way that gears of a fine clock or watch all interact with one another to keep accurate time.

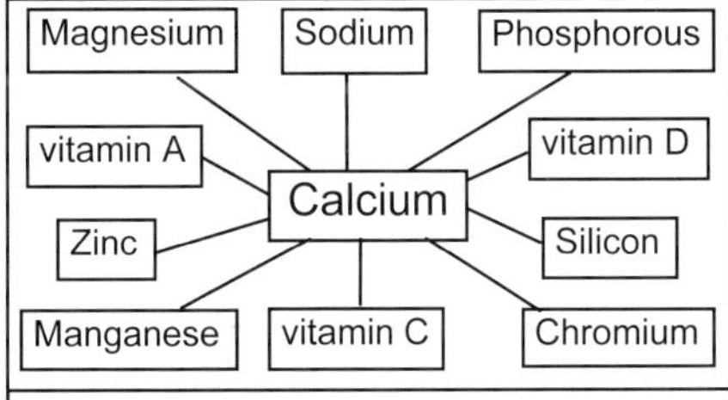

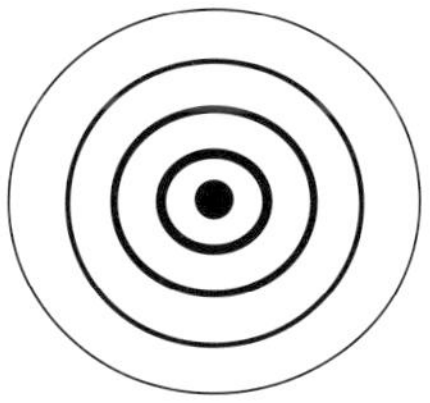

Hierarchies of nutritional needs may be similar to other health hierarchies. – As Always: First Things Must Be First – Make certain that all essential nutritional needs are meet, digestion is functioning efficiently, the colon and the skin are flushing away all wastes, before losing pounds–inches from unwanted places.

Calcium is known to interact with each of the above nutrients for its proper absorption and utilization. Fully functional Calcium requires ratios with other vitamins/minerals that may vary with stress–activity.

Whole, organically grown *kosher* foods are always helpful for maintaining proper balance-ratios of essential nutrients. Drugs and non-kosher foods frequently inhibit the kidneys' ability to the maintain the nutrient levels required for health.

Non-kosher food and drugs that stress glands may result in worn out organs that encourage disease and/or defy healing.

Unglazed Thin-walled Earthen Vessel – for Water Purification

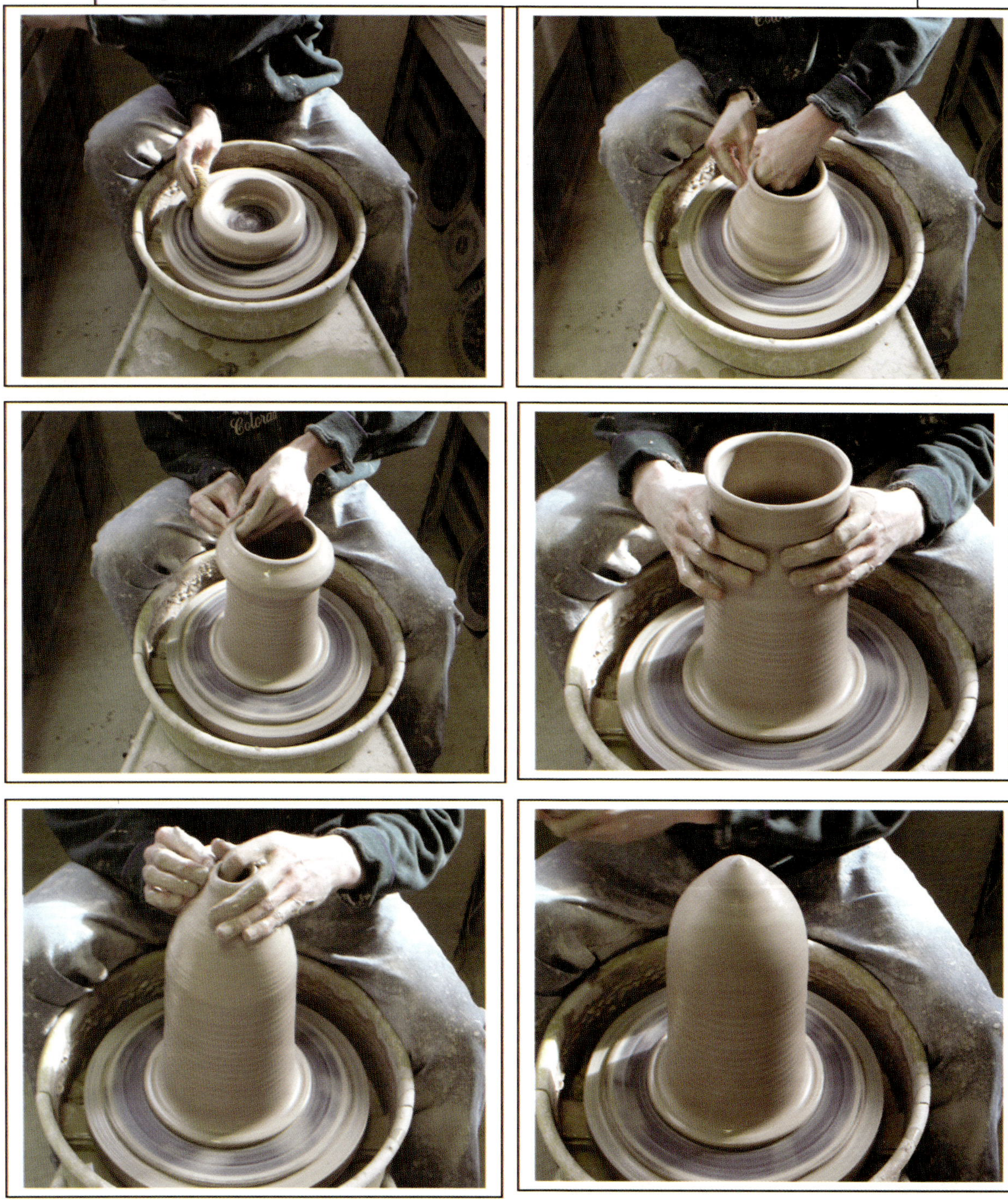

Kai Brunning of Brunning Pottery made several thin-walled vessels for the author.

The author had several clay vessels made for water purification as discussed by George Bush. So far, no vessel has been sufficiently porous enough to profuse water for water purification. Larry Brunning suggested including aggregate material, such as sand, with clay to produce a clay–aggregate combination for the vessel wall that is porous enough to easily profuse water. A friend suggested adding straw to the clay in a similar manner to making bricks in Egypt, and after firing the straw will burn away, leaving sufficient porosity for the vessel to profuse water. The author hasn't yet mixed various clays and various aggregates to find a good combination. If anyone, especially with pottery experience, wants to offer advise on which clays and which aggregates to mix in which amounts, please send e-mail to: Moses5in1Torah@msn.com .

Water Filtration Vessel as it may have been used – suspended from a wooden tripod.

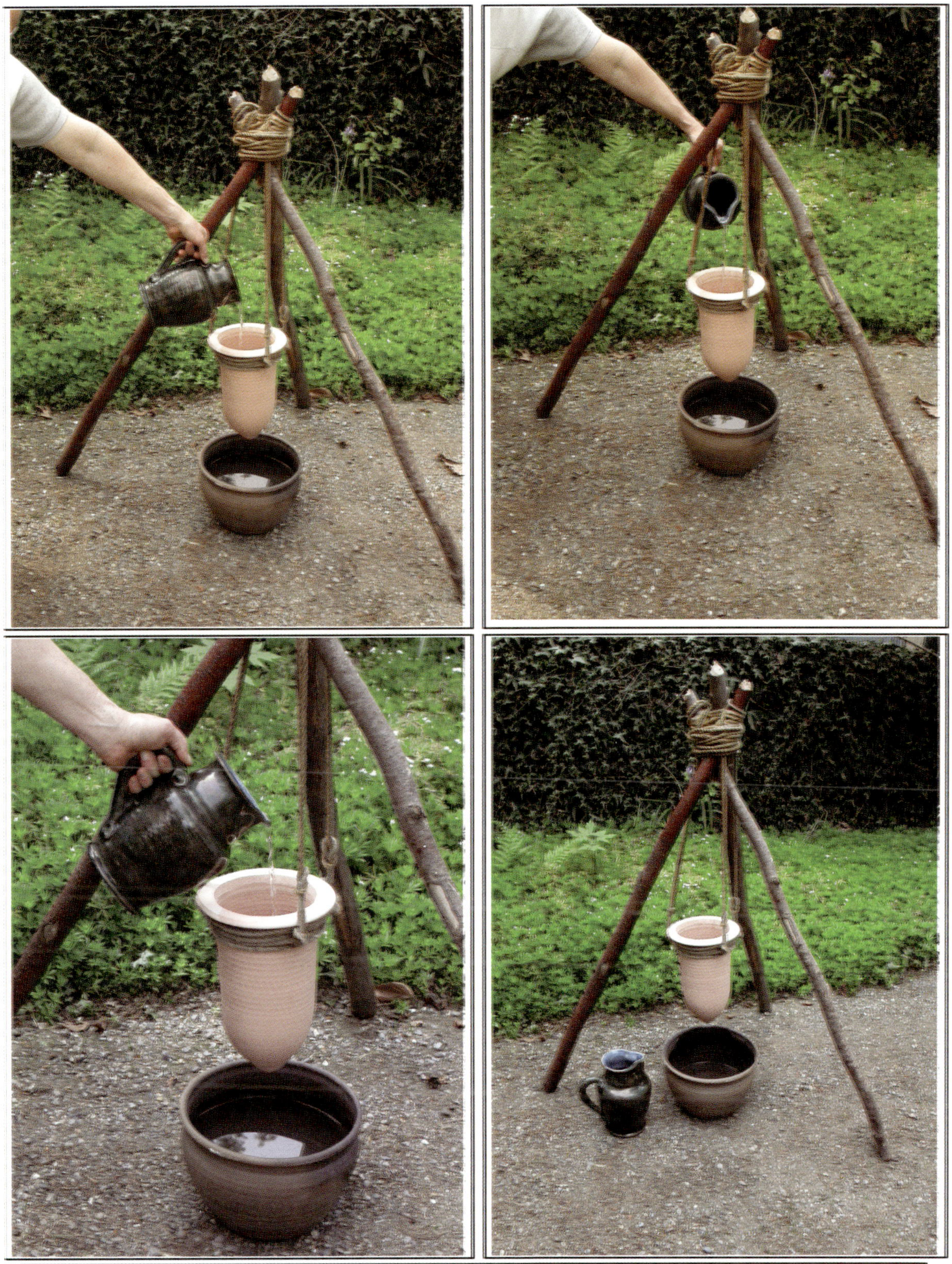

Water inside a unglazed water purification vessel must be relatively cool/cold compared with the outside desert air temperature, to promote condensation on the outside of the vessel. This type of condensation also happens when a cool glass of liquid, especially with ice cubes, is taken out-of-doors on a warm afternoon. Even in relatively warm dry climates, there is usually enough water vapor in the air to cause considerable condensation on the outside of the cool/cold glass.

Passover Foods and the Seder

The Passover Feast commemorates and celebrates the 'Exodus' of the Hebrews from Egypt. Each year the sequence of the Exodus events is re-told on the anniversary of the original Passover. The Passover, causing the death of the firstborn of Egypt, is the last of Ten Plagues that the LORD brought upon Pharaoh and the nation of Egypt to force Pharaoh to allow the Hebrews to leave Egypt. (The Hebrews were slaves for many of the ≈210 yrs that they spent in Egypt from the Famine to the Exodus.) The Exodus events including the Passover are delineated in a holiday booklet, called a '***Haggadah***'. The ***Haggadah*** orchestrates the order of observances during the Passover meal, called the '***Seder***'. ***Seder***, which means the 'order of service', includes seven foods, which are symbolically important. The ***Seder*** is designed to help each Hebrew generation to personally experience the Exodus events. (All foods, details and observances of the Seder, as it exists today, may not have been finalized until the ***Mishnah*** of ≈220 AD.)

Matzah is a ≈6 inch square flat bread that is made without leaven. Leaven is yeast that is added to bread dough. Leaven (yeast), under warm moist conditions for several hours begins to digest the carbohydrates (starch) in the dough. A byproduct of this leavening process is CO_2, which is what causes the dough to rise and makes bread soft, light and fluffy. The Hebrews didn't have time to allow leaven to lighten to dough, because they were to leave Egypt quickly and the had to make enough ***matzah*** to last for a six day trek to the Red Sea and the one day to cross the Red Sea. Later, Moses required the Hebrews to commemorate the series of Exodus events with a series of feasts, including the Feast of Unleavened Bread or ***Hag HaMatzot***. ***Hag HaMatzot*** requires the Hebrews to remove all leaven from their house. The ***Bedikot CHametz*** is a ceremony where the head of each household inspects the house for leaven and removes any leaven that is found. Today, most leaven is removed before the ***Bedikot CHametz*** search, except for a token amount that is hidden and is left to be found. During the ***Bedikot CHametz*** ceremony the leaven that was found is taken out of the house and is buried in the ground. Leaven is used consistently throughout Scripture as a symbol to represent sin. The ***Bedikot CHametz*** ceremony cleanses the house of sin and helps to prepare all members of the household to be in the proper frame of mind to appreciate all the events of the Passover and Exodus.

CHaroset is a sweet mixture of crushed nuts, apples, raisins (or wine), cinnamon and honey. ***CHaroset*** is often eaten with ***matzah***. When ***charoset*** is eaten between two pieces of ***matzah*** it is symbolic of the mortar between bricks that the Hebrews slaves used to build the cities for Pharaoh.

Egg (hardboiled) is symbolic of life. Eggs were likely added to the ***Seder*** after the Babylonian exile.

Karpas is the green parsley that is symbolic of spring and the renewal of life.

Salt water is symbolic of the tears shed by the Hebrews, during their slavery in Egypt.

Maror is the bitter horseradish herb that symbolizes the bitterness of Egyptian bondage.

Lamb was eaten for the Passover. Lamb is symbolized on the Passover plate by a small bone. The Passover lamb was required to be a lamb without spot or blemish. The Passover lamb was to be roasted and eaten in one meal, without breaking any of its bones and without any meat left uneaten. Several households likely shared a single Passover lamb. As Moses wrote of the Passover lamb, he always used lamb as a singular, rather than a plural, even though thousands of families ate a lamb. Moses also began general language of 'a lamb', followed by the more specific term 'the lamb', and finally the most personal term 'your lamb' to describe the Passover lamb. The linguistic style of Moses helped later readers to become personally cognizant of the events that transpired during the Exodus. After the destruction of the Jerusalem Temple in 70 AD, chicken has often been substituted for lamb.

Wine is drunk four times during a ***Seder***. Wine is consistently symbolic of joy throughout the Bible. The four glasses of wine represent the four-fold promise of Hebrew deliverance by the LORD. (Ex 6:6-7)
The ***Seder*** begins by drinking of the 1st cup of Wine, the Cup of Sanctification.
Next the parsley is dipped in the salt water and eaten.
The ***Seder*** continues by drinking of the 2nd cup of Wine, the Cup of Praise.
Three ***matzah*** are found in a three-pocketed linen napkin called a ***matzahtosh***. The middle ***matzah*** is taken from the ***matzahtosh*** and is broken in half. Half of the broken middle ***matzah*** is called the *afikomen* (Greek - that which comes after) and is wrapped in a napkin and is hidden until after dinner is over.
The remaining 2½ ***matzah*** are eaten during the ***Seder*** service with ***charoset*** and/or ***maror***.
The ***Seder*** leader is required to explain to the children the symbolism of the Passover foods/events.
Diner is eaten. After dinner the *afikomen* (desert - comes after) is found and eaten as the desert.
The ***Seder*** continues by drinking of the 3rd cup of Wine, the Cup of Redemption.
Scripture related to the Exodus, the Passover, the hope of celebrating future Passovers in Jerusalem, and the expectation of the prophet Elijah appearing to herald the advent of the Messiah are read.
The ***Seder*** concludes by drinking of the 4th cup of Wine, the Cup of Acceptance.

The ***Seder*** is a spiritually rewarding experience to help everyone appreciate the Passover/Exodus events.

Passover Food Pictures

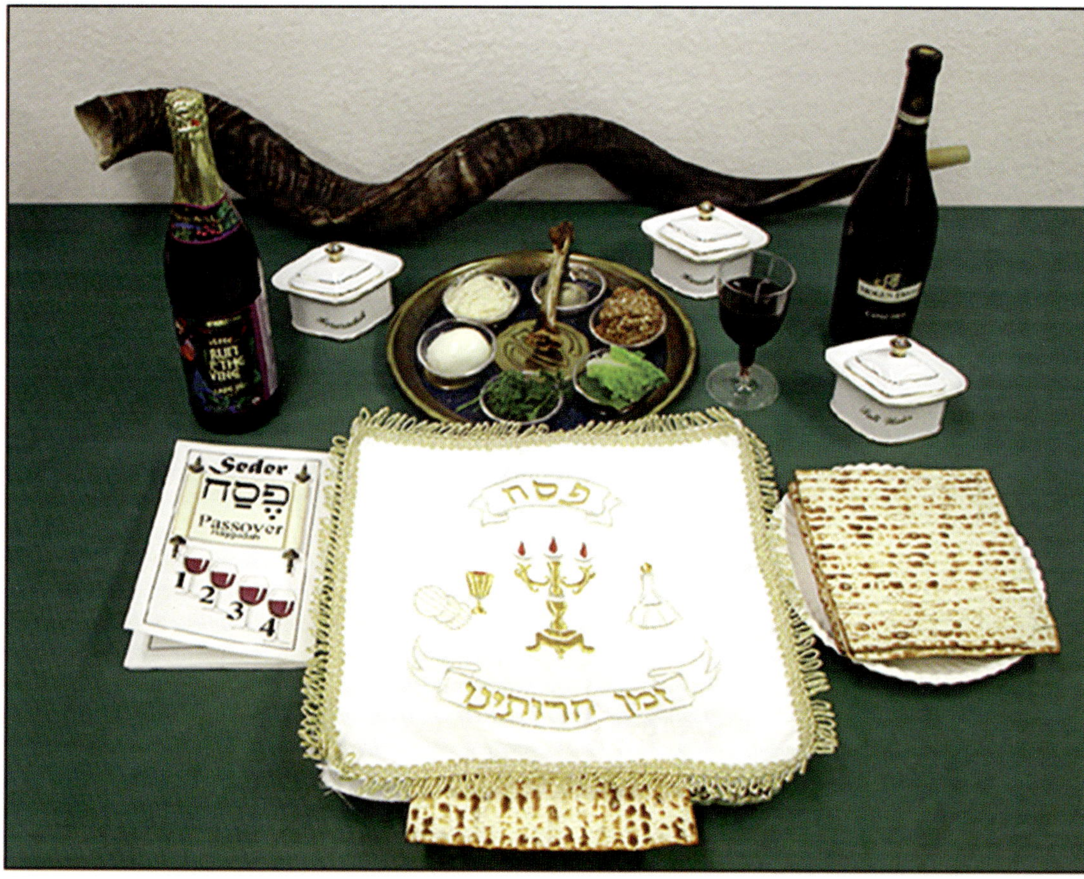

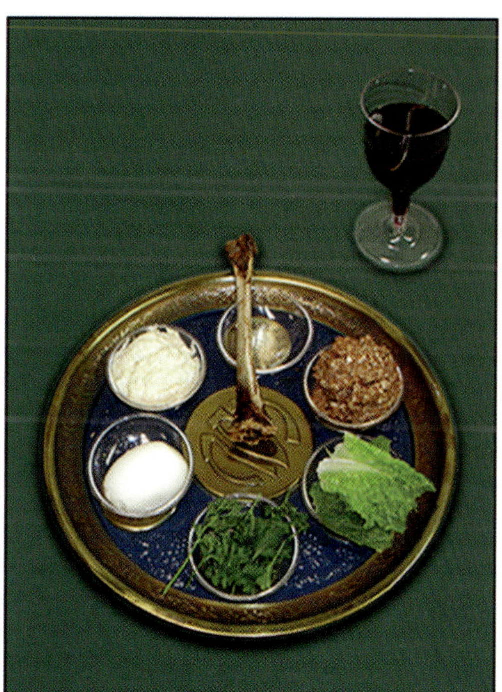

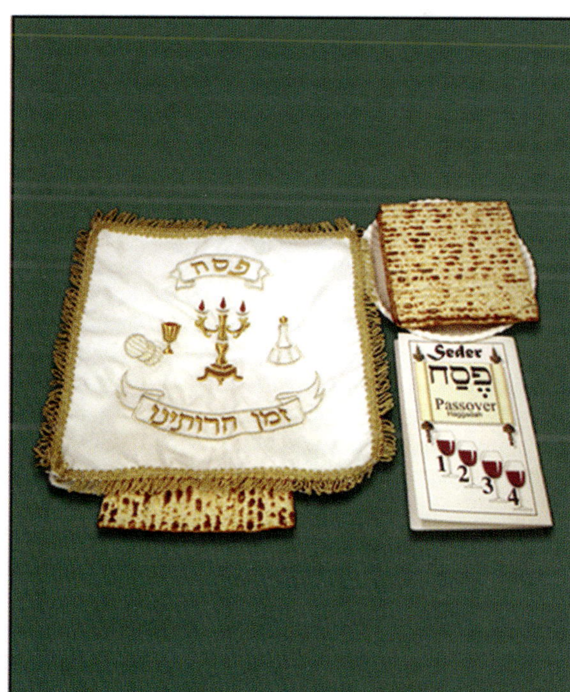

Map 15 – Cities of Palestine

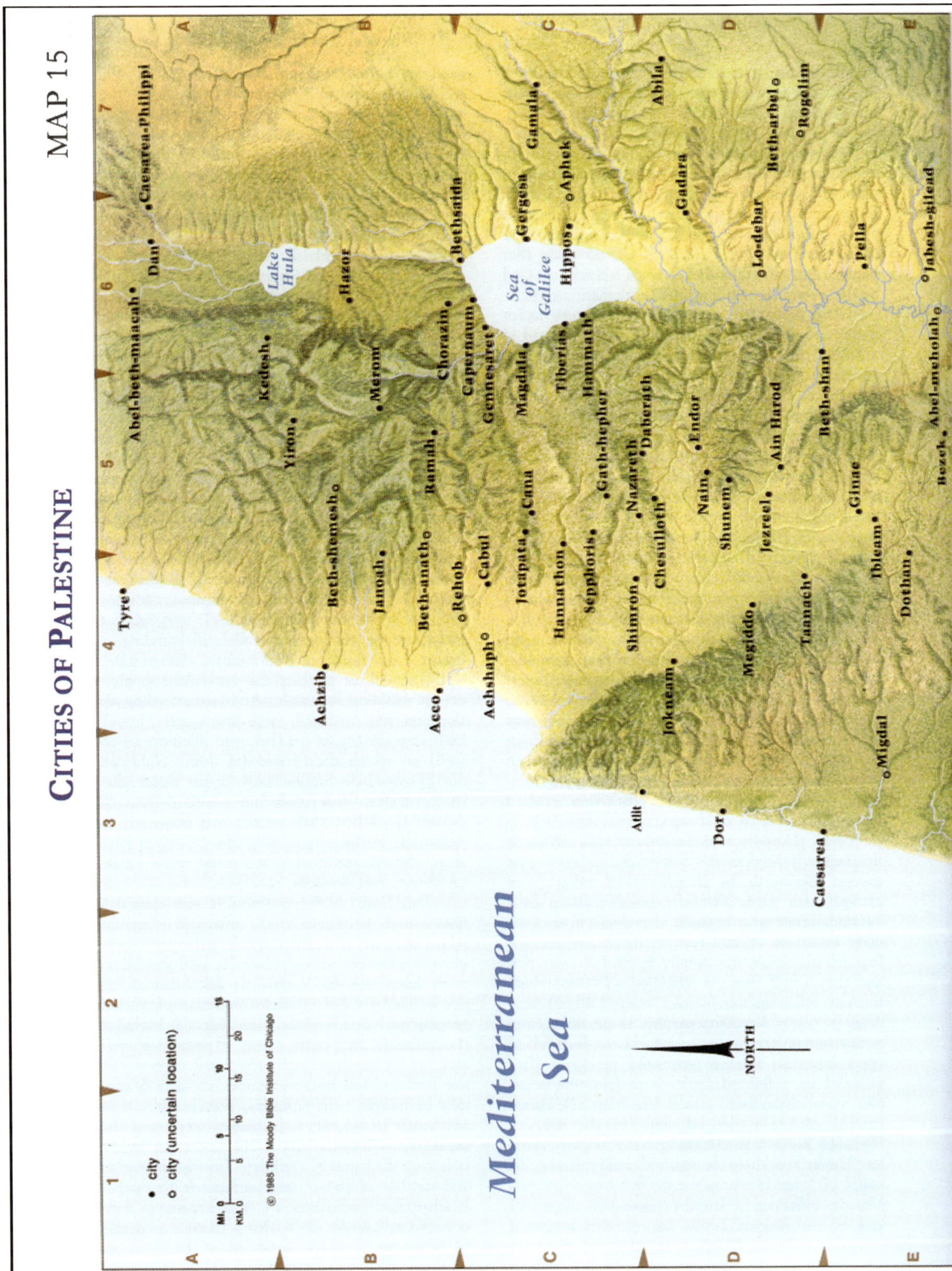

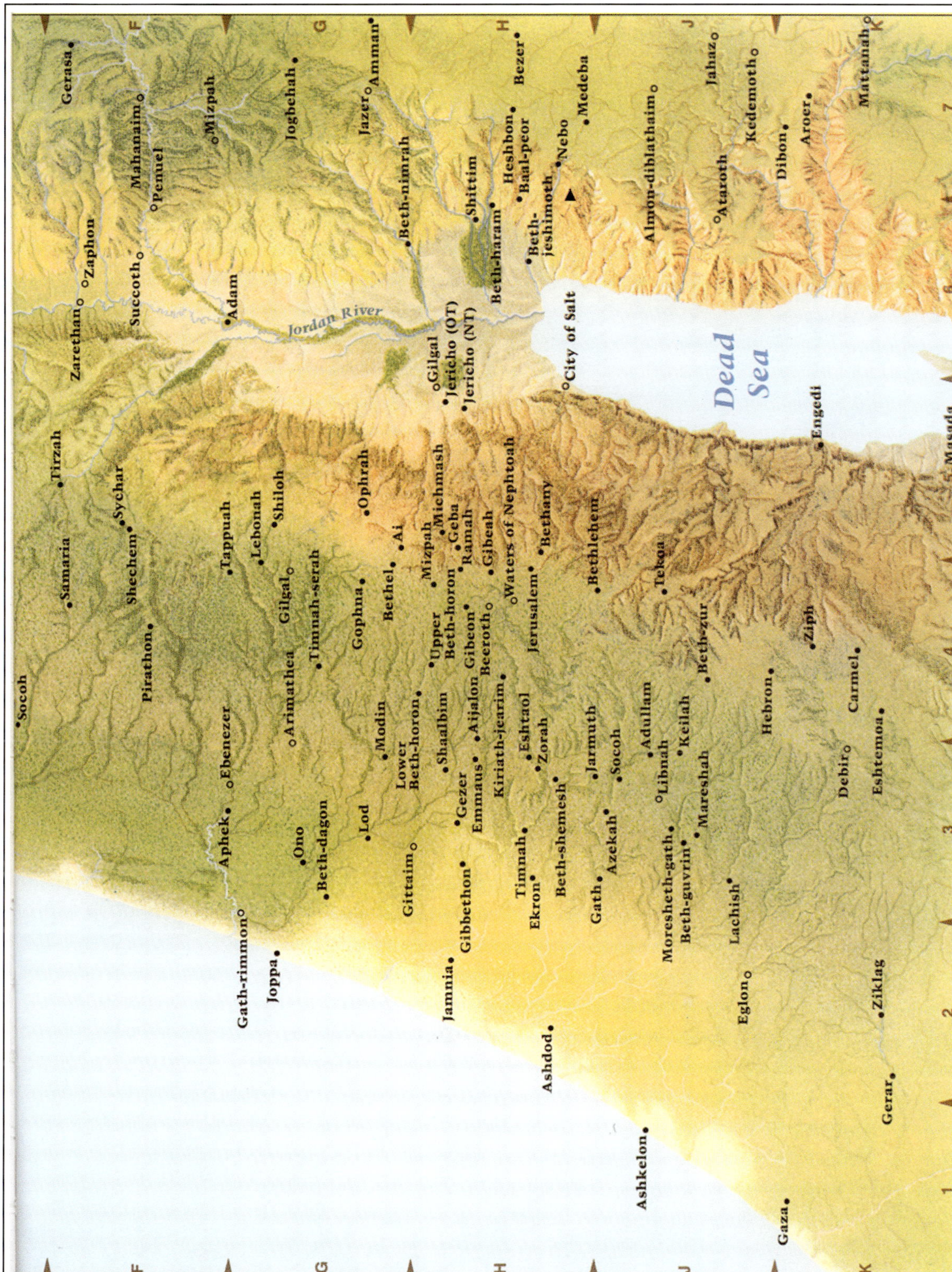
Gerasa
Zaphon
Zarethan
Succoth
Mahanaim
Penuel
Mizpah
Adam
Jogbehah
Jazer
Amman
Beth-nimrah
Jordan River
Shittim
Beth-haram
Heshbon
Baal-peor
Bezer
Medeba
Nebo
Beth-jeshimoth
Almon-diblathaim
Jahaz
Kedemoth
Ataroth
Dibon
Aroer
Mattanah
Dead Sea
City of Salt
Gilgal
Jericho (OT)
Jericho (NT)
Engedi
Masada
Tirzah
Sychar
Samaria
Shechem
Tappuah
Lebonah
Shiloh
Gilgal
Timnah-serah
Ophrah
Gophna
Bethel
Ai
Michmash
Mizpah
Geba
Ramah
Gibeah
Upper Beth-horon
Gibeon
Beeroth
Waters of Nephtoah
Bethany
Jerusalem
Bethlehem
Tekoa
Beth-zur
Ziph
Carmel
Hebron
Eshtemoa
Debir
Socoh
Pirathon
Ebenezer
Arimathea
Modin
Lower Beth-horon
Shaalbim
Aijalon
Kiriath-jearim
Eshtaol
Zorah
Emmaus
Gezer
Beth-shemesh
Jarmuth
Socoh
Adullam
Keilah
Libnah
Mareshah
Azekah
Aphek
Ono
Beth-dagon
Lod
Gittaim
Gibbethon
Timnah
Ekron
Gath
Moresheth-gath
Beth-guvrin
Lachish
Gath-rimmon
Joppa
Jamnia
Ashdod
Eglon
Ziklag
Gerar
Ashkelon
Gaza

The Author's Activities

Photos of the 1983 VOSH trip to Colombia, S.A., and working at the computer in 2000⁺.

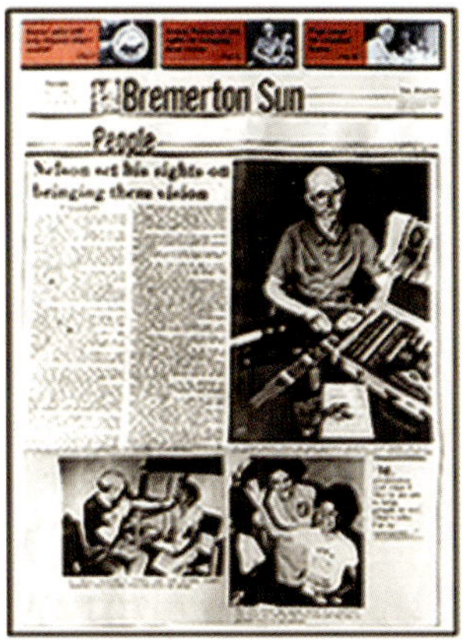

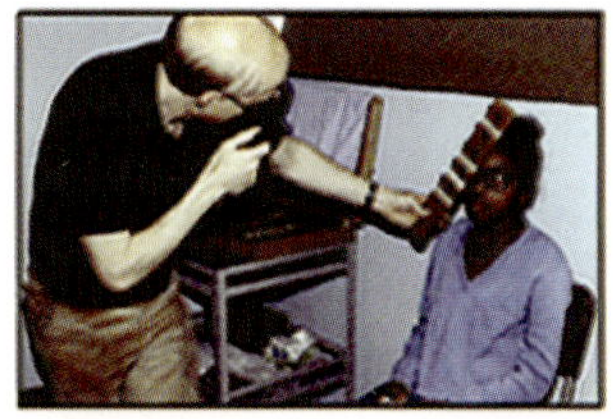

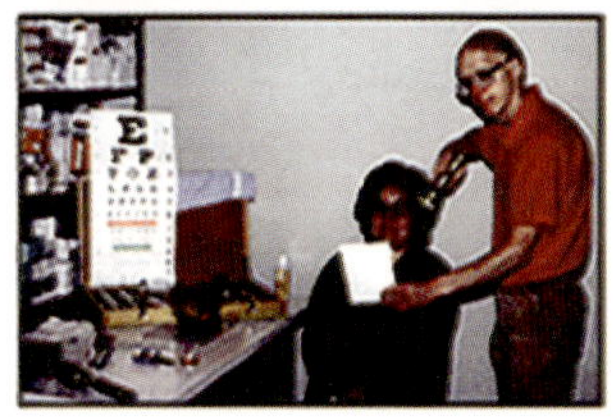

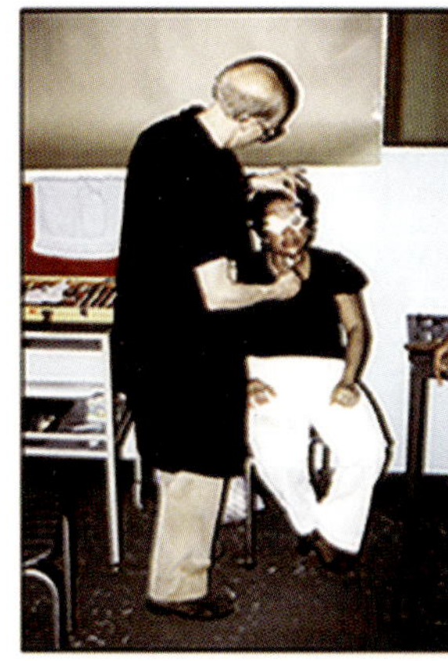

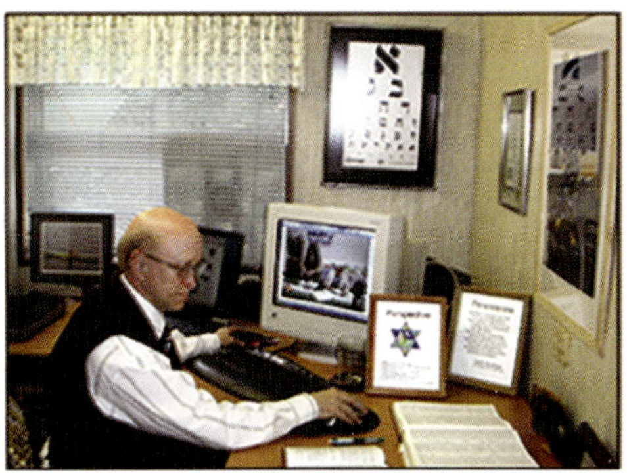

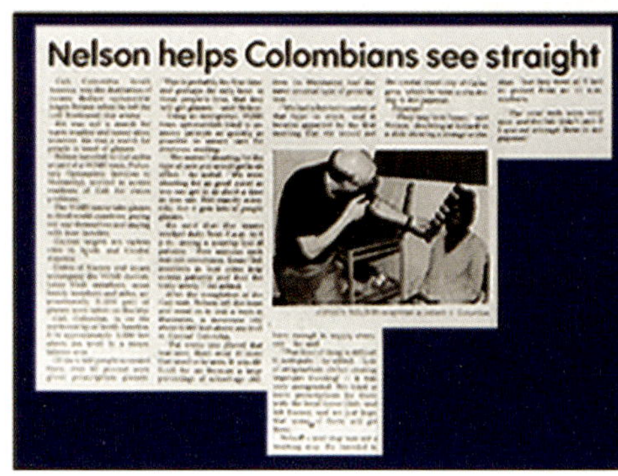

The author's out-of-round left hip.

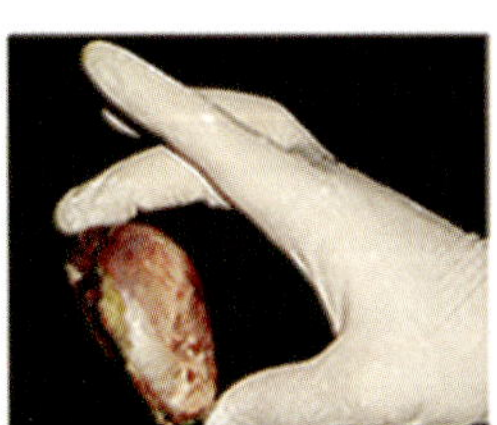

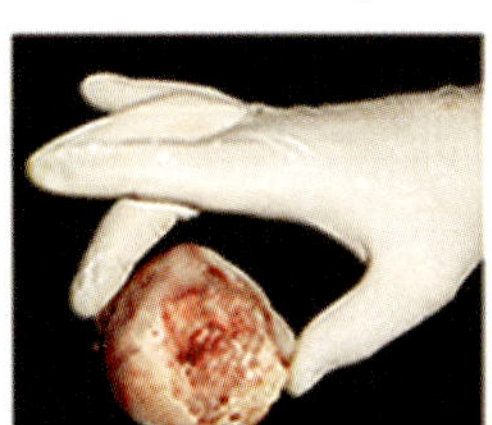

Photos of the author's out-of-round left hip and a normal hip carved in wood by Jeff Iller.

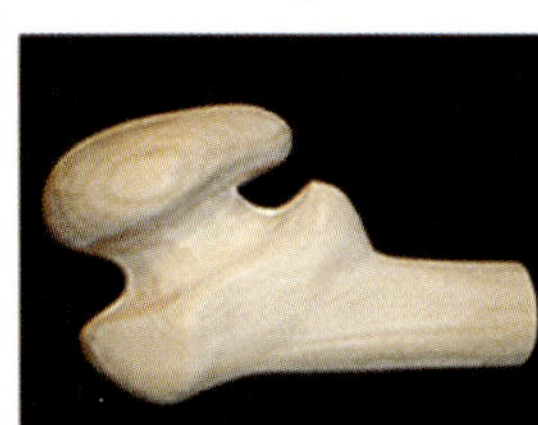

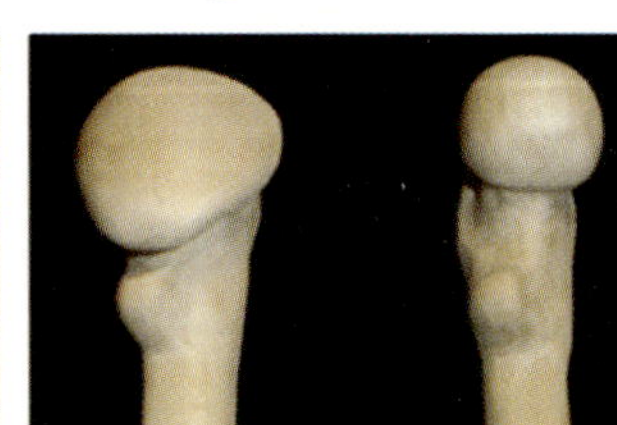

The author kayaking on the Puget Sound

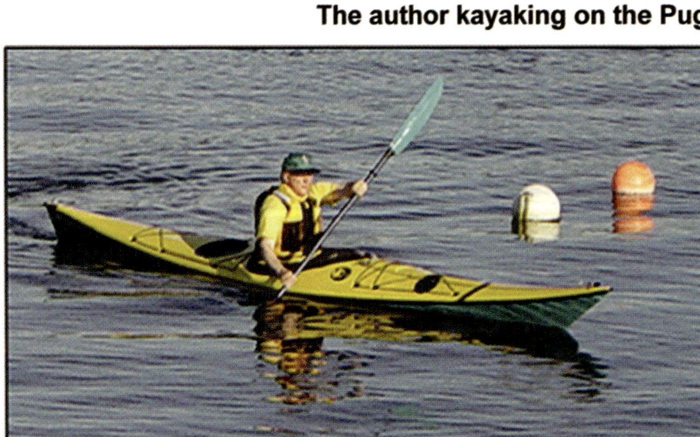

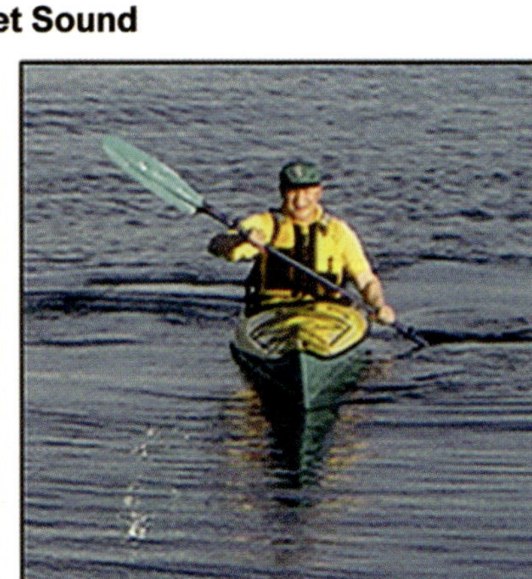

– Israeli Folk Dance CD – and – Folk Dancing Photos –

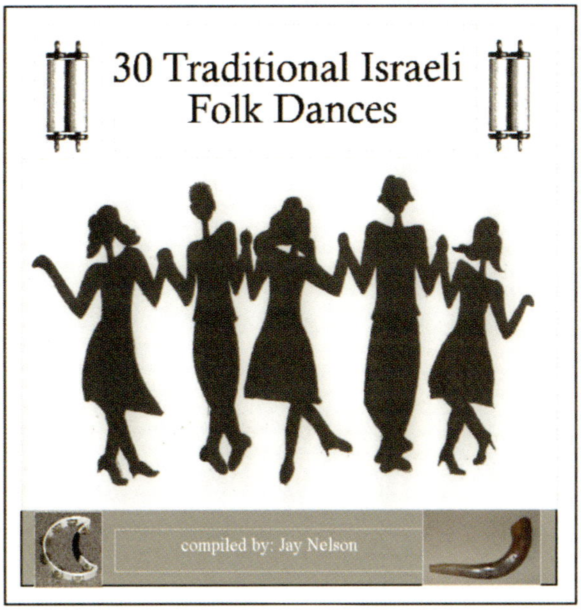

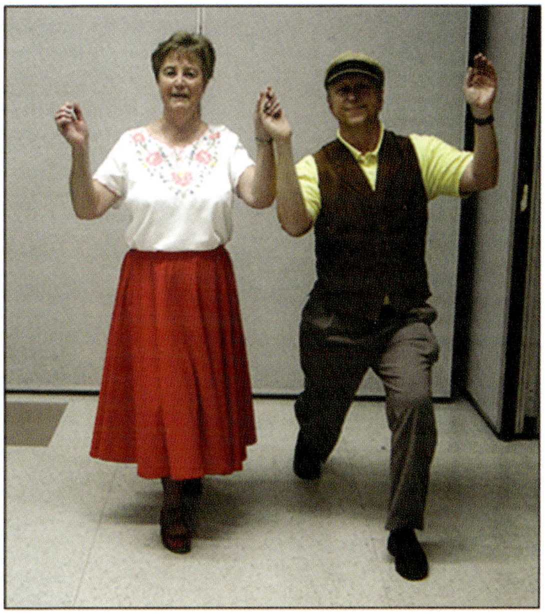

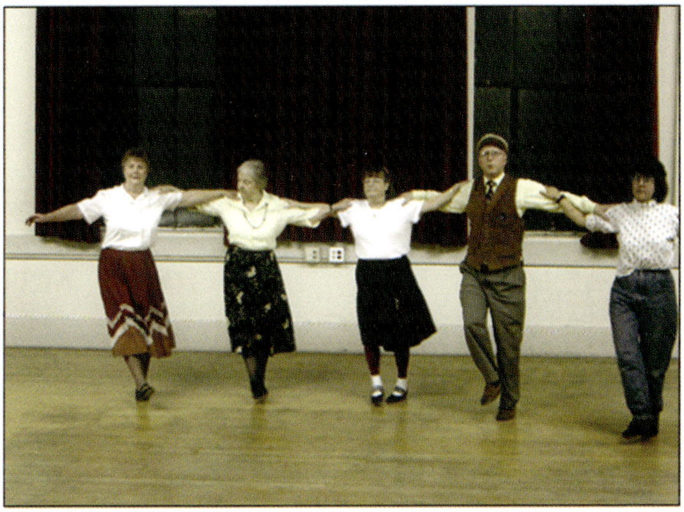

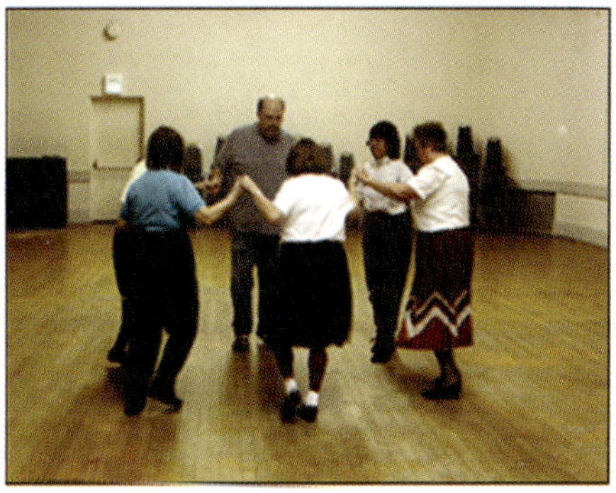

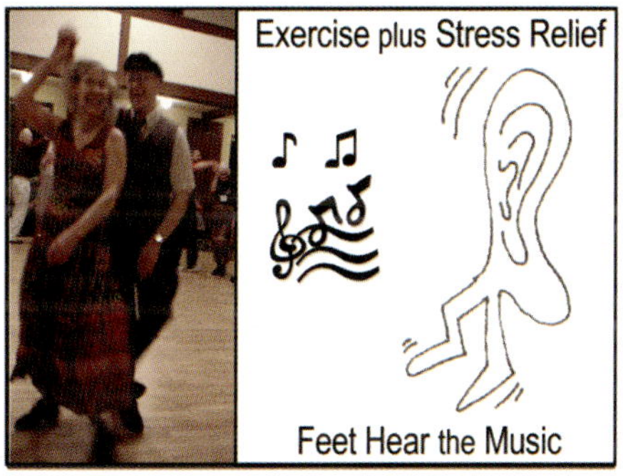

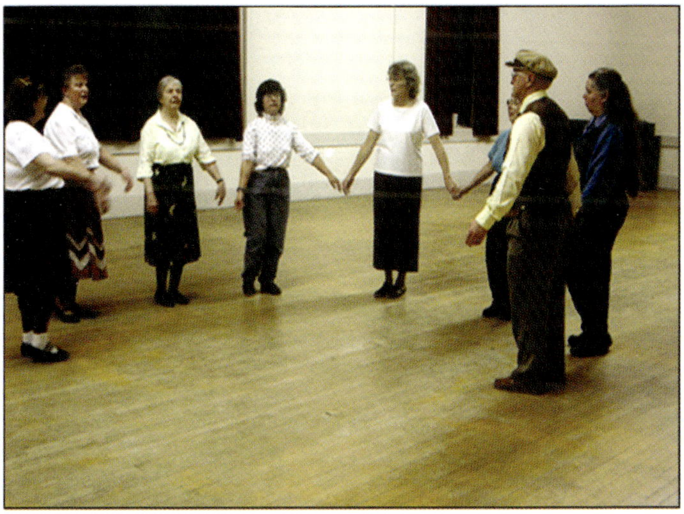

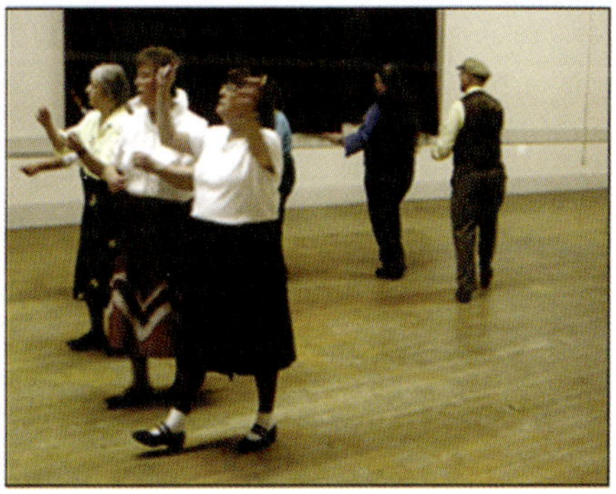

The author has enjoyed folk dancing, especially Israeli folk dancing, for nearly 25 years.

Anatomy of the Human Eye

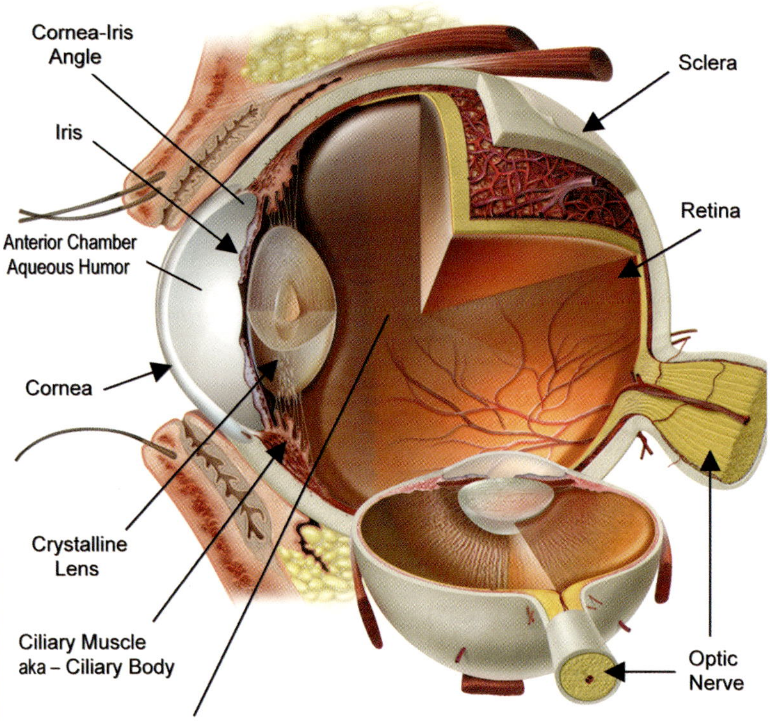

Eye Cross Section 3

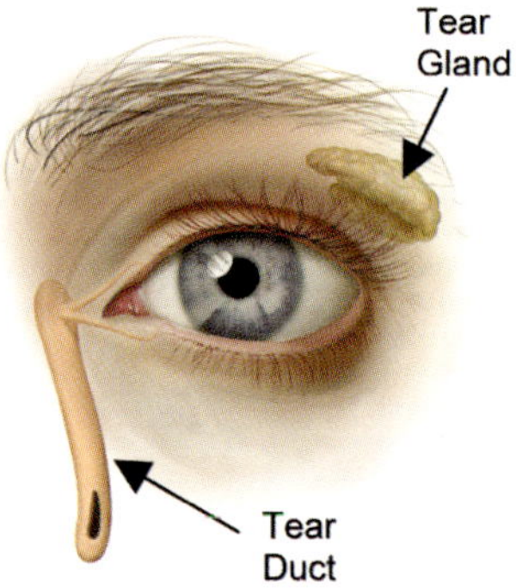

Outer Eye 1

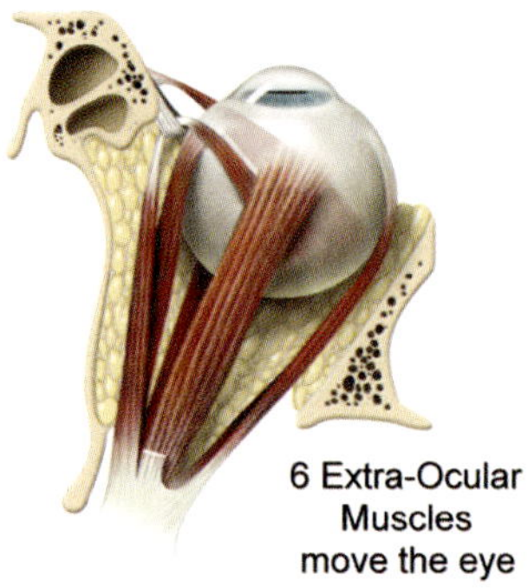

Eye Muscles 2

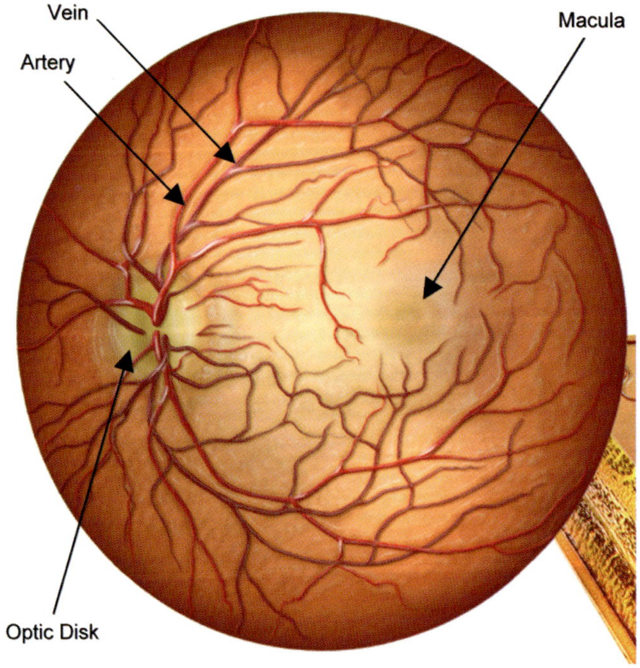

Retina 4

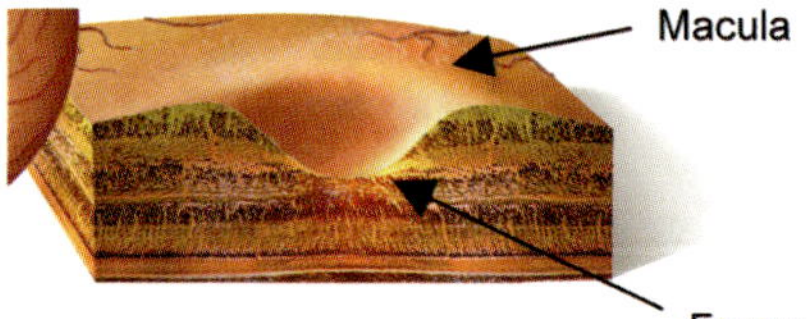

Macula and Fovea 5

The Macula is the center of vision, and it has a pit in the center called the Fovea. Rods and Cones are the cells in the Retina that gather light. Rods are superior for night vision. Cones are superb for daylight sight. The pigmented Macula-Fovea has only tightly grouped Cones, which allow high-resolution 20/20 vision. The Macula requires many nutrients for ideal function, including vitamin A (i.e. – from beta-carotene in carrots). The Macula is damaged by oxidation. Age Related Macular Degeneration (ARMD) that reduces sight is caused by poor nutrition + oxidative stress.

Eye Anatomy pictures #1, #2, #3, #4, #5 & #6 produced by and used with permission from Anatomical Charts Company – Skokie, Illinois – Lippincott Williams & Wilkins

Optical Status of the Human Eye & Cataract (*sketches*) – plus – Visual Pathway

Normal Sight

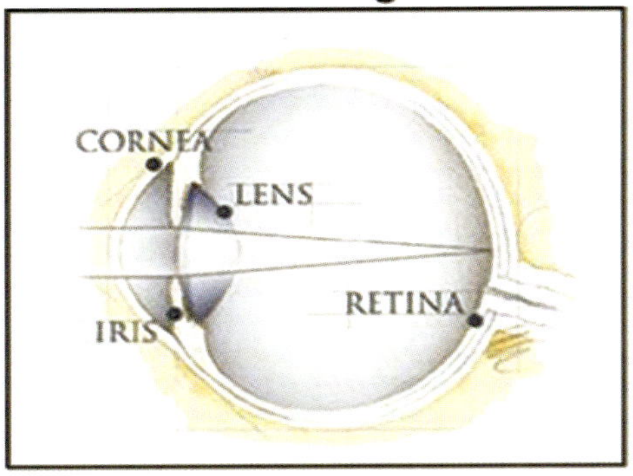

Far-Sighted

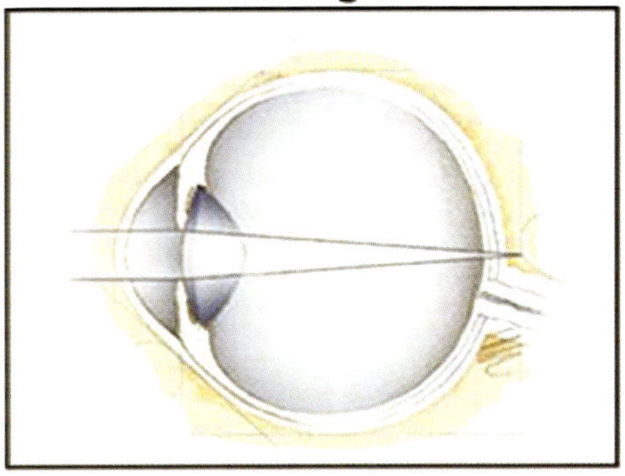

Near-Sighted

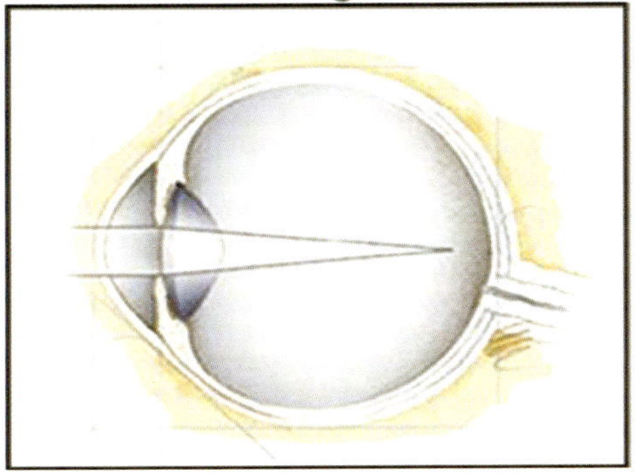

Astigmatism

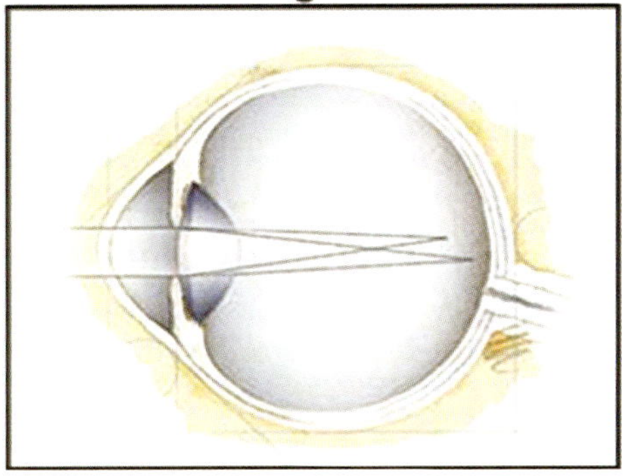

Presbyopia

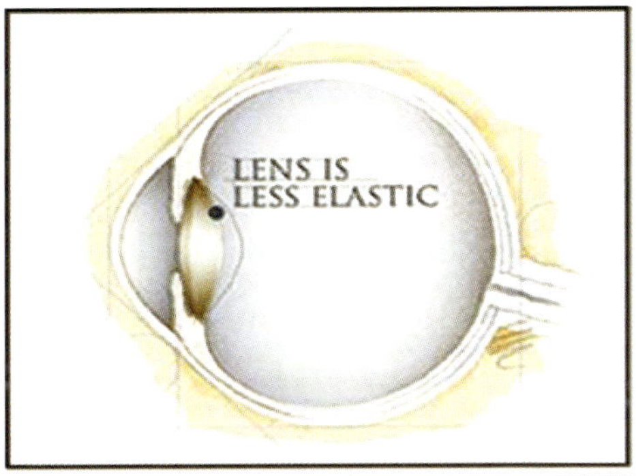

Cataract

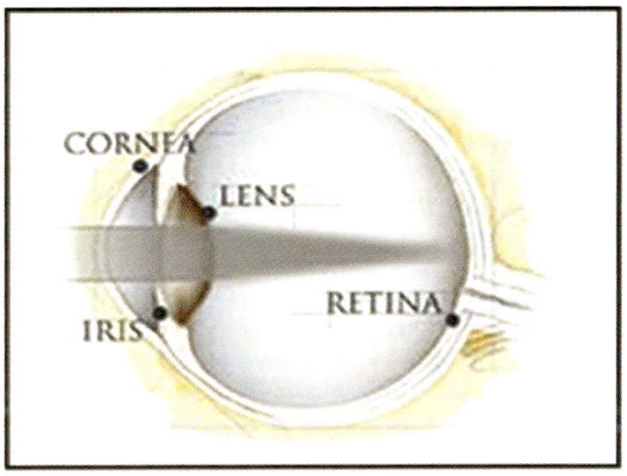

Visual Pathway 6

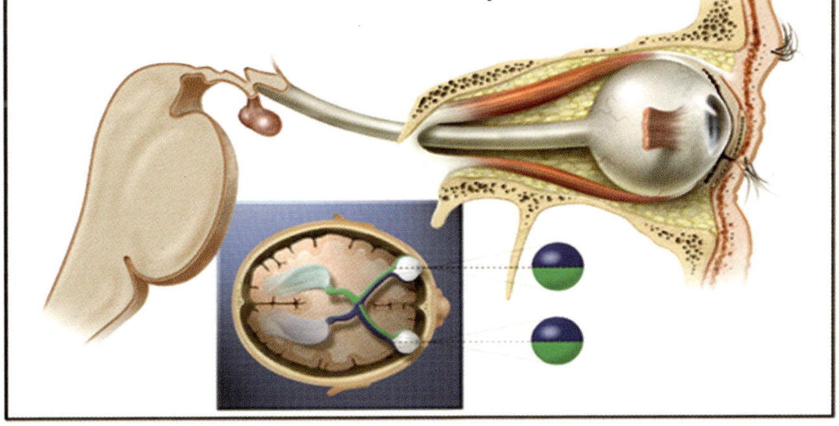

Eye Sketches reproduced with the permission of Pacific Cataract and Laser Institute (1-800-888-9903) w[3].pcli.com

COAG – Chronic Open Angle Glaucoma

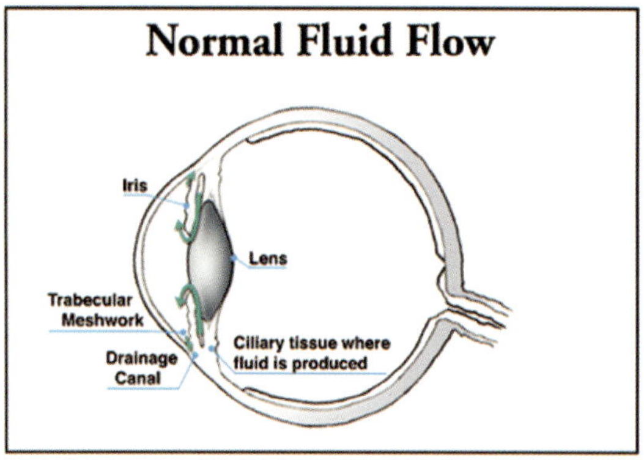

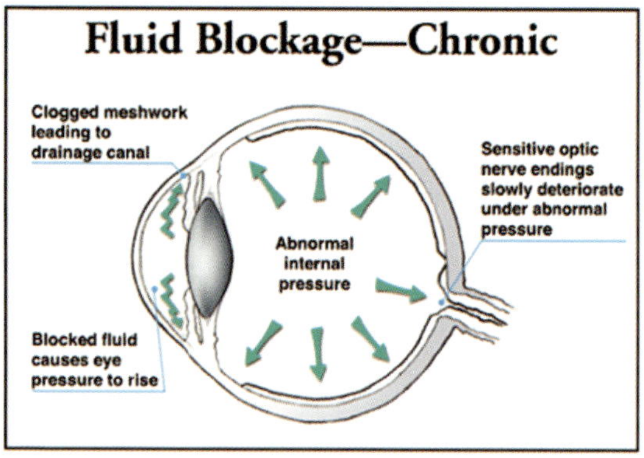

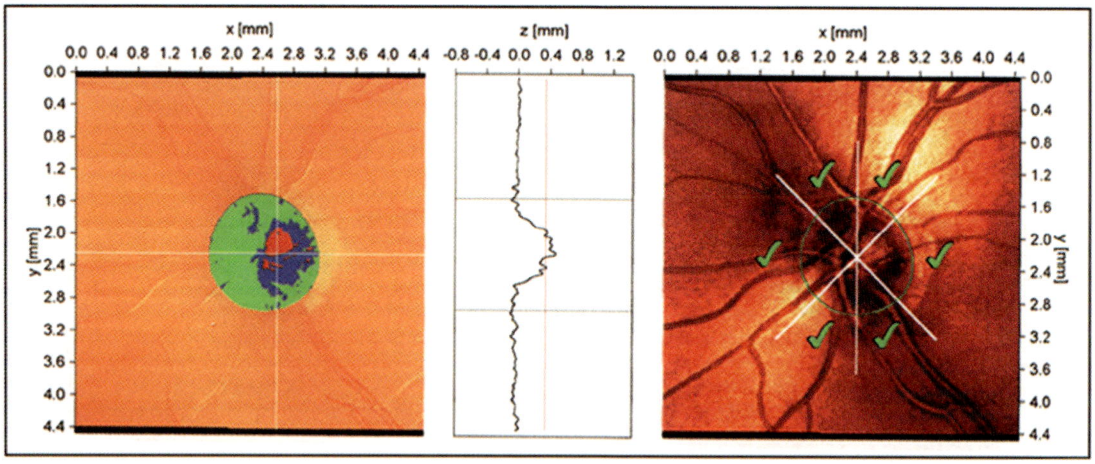

Recent computer imaging of the optic disk help the physician evaluate the optic disk and assess the disk's state of health. The author's optic disk and cup (shown above) are normal and healthy. COAG damages the optic disk and diminishes eyesight, especially reducing the peripheral vision. The small pit in the center of the optic disk is the optic cup. COAG often results in enlargement of the optic cup. The advanced COAG image (shown below) likely results in greatly reduced vision.

The optic disk images (above & below) were taken at PCLI using a Heidelberg II Retinal Tomograph.

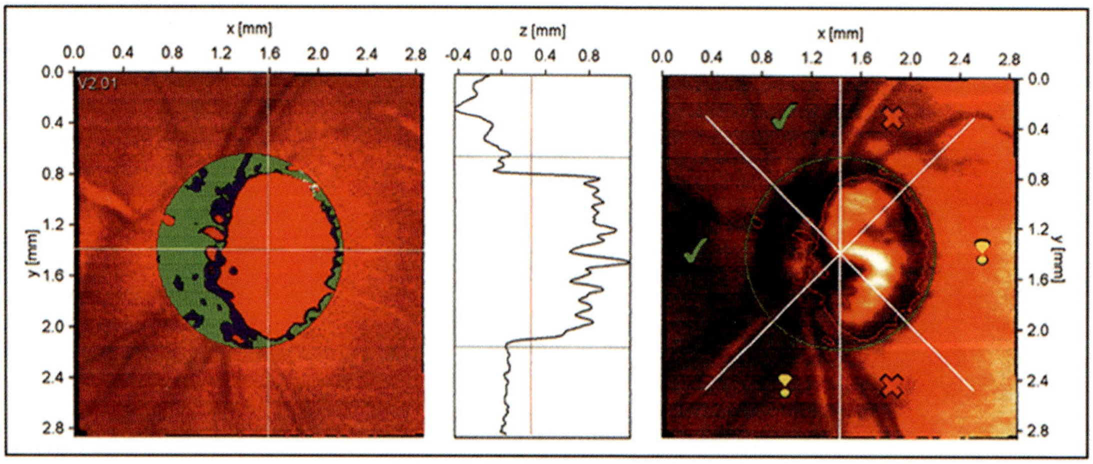

The Heidelberg (HRT) images of the optic disk are on the left and the disk is photographed on the right. In the HRT images– green is flat healthy disk tissue – red shows evacuation ofdisk tissue and blue is intermediate between green and red. The author's disk shows a common small central (red) evacuation. As COAG progresses, the red portion of the HRT image enlarges and the loss of visual field increases.

Glaucoma sketches, photos and Heidelberg images courtesy of Pacific Cataract and Laser Institute.

Chapter 51 The Eyes and Vision

When Moses was 120 years old and in good health, his vision (***ayin***) was not dim. (Deut 34:7)

People come into my office with vision problems including farsightedness, nearsightedness, astigmatism, presbyopia and visually related learning disabilities; as well as eye diseases, such as cataracts, glaucoma, macular degeneration, retinitis pigmentosa, keratoconus, and weeping or dry eye; as well as systemic illnesses that affect the eye, such as diabetes and high blood pressure. This chapter discusses concepts and theory concerning the onset and treatment of eye conditions.

-------------------- **Farsightedness or Hyperopia** ----------------------------------

The normal condition for eyes at birth is to be farsighted. A farsighted eye is often a short eye. Ideally, as a person matures, the eyes lengthen, so that in adulthood the eyes have lengthened the exact amount necessary for the resting focusing system to focus light from a distant object precisely on the retina; this is ideal, but rare. This person is usually blessed with great vision. Farsighted eyes need to use some focusing effort all the time to focus light from distant objects on the retina. Moderate farsightedness in youth usually is not a problem. Eyes that are extremely short at birth may require the focusing system to work very hard to focus, which may cause the eyes to become crossed by 1 or 2 years old. Crossed eyes should be treated <u>soon</u> with glasses so the eyes may develop normally. In a cross-eyed scenario, one eye is often routinely crossed, while the other eye usually remains straight. In this scenario the straight eye may develop normally, while a crossed eye does not develop normally and becomes a 'lazy eye' or amblyopic. The retina has a special area of central vision called the macula, and the center of the macula is an even more specialized area called the fovea. The fovea is the only area of the retina in which detailed 20/20 vision can take place. The neural pathway between the fovea and the brain is not complete at birth and requires a clearly focused image at the critical stage of life (before age 7) to develop normally. The amblyopic or lazy eye never gets the clearly focused picture at the early age it needs to see properly, and may <u>never</u> see normally unless treated at an early age. An eye does not need to be crossed to become amblyopic. Part of vision involves learning to point the eyes at an object so the image falls on both foveae. If this pointing skill is not developed the eye may become 'lazy'. If one eye is significantly more out of focus than the fellow eye, the more out of focus eye may become amblyopic. Thus, even an eye that is anatomically well formed may become amblyopic, if it is significantly out of focus as compared with its fellow eye. Well baby checkups could easily include a simple screening test to see if both eyes are developing normally. <u>A simple screening test anyone can do is: cover one eye and then, later, cover the other eye.</u> The best occluder is often the index and middle finger held closely together. (Any object used as an occluder may attract attention to the object itself and interfere with the test.) If each eye is developing normally, then the baby will not mind when one eye or the other eye is covered and the vision in the covered eye is blocked. Iff, however, there is one well-functioning eye and one poorly-functioning eye, then covering the poorly seeing eye will not produce any response, while covering the well-functioning eye will consistently produce aversion. If the youngster has only one well-functioning eye, he will not like having the only well-seeing eye covered and will quickly turn the head to look past the fingers occluding vision. <u>A consistent aversion response is a sign of a poor-seeing eye that needs a professional evaluation.</u> An eye care professional can look inside each eye and evaluate eye health and appropriate farsightedness. <u>If neither eye shows aversion to being covered and the eyes show normal attention to visually stimulating objects, then both eyes are most likely developing normally.</u> Fortunately, if a functional lazy eye, in which one eye is significantly more out of focus as compared with the fellow eye, is detected early; then treatment is often successful. 1st Both eyes may need glasses so the light is properly focused on the foveae. 2nd A program of alternately patching the well-seeing eye along with vision therapy exercises, followed by patching the poor-seeing eye will encourage each eye to independently point at an object so the image falls on the fovea. Later, when both eyes are seeing well on their own, the eyes can be taught to see well together. An Optometrist who specializes in vision therapy is ideally suited to coordinate a program for lazy eye or crossed eye. For crossed eyes, some health care providers may recommend surgery as the first option; however, the author recommends that surgery for crossed eyes should be the last option. For most people, every attempt to get crossed eyes straightened with proper lenses, prisms and vision therapy should be exhausted and found not successful before surgery is performed. Surgically altered eye muscles may result in eyes that appear cosmetically straight and seeing together, but surgically straightened eyes only rarely develop the two-eyed, stereo (binocular) vision of which most normal healthy eyes are capable.

* **Ideally, most eyes are farsighted at birth, less farsighted in youth, and slightly farsighted for adults.**

------------------- **Nearsightedness or Myopia** -----------------------------------

Nearsighted eyes are generally longer than normal. Very few eyes begin life being myopic. In countries in which reading is not emphasized, myopia is quite rare. The lens of the eye is a variable focus lens, whose power is adjusted by the activity of the ciliary muscle. In the world of three dimensions, the ciliary muscle and lens are constantly adjusting to adapt to various focusing demands from objects at different distances from the eyes. The ciliary muscle changes focus involuntarily and is at rest when looking at optically far distant objects. The ciliary muscle works or uses effort to see objects closer than optical infinity. When reading for long periods of time or staring at a computer VDT, this adaptive focusing process is short circuited and replaced by a fixed, unchanging focusing demand. This can result in fatigue and ciliary muscle eyestrain. Ciliary muscles that are deficient in vitamins/trace minerals may have difficulty focusing for a long time on near objects. This can result in the ciliary muscle working harder than normal for reading and computer work, and then not relaxing properly for distance vision. <u>When the ciliary muscle and lens do not relax properly for viewing distant objects, this results in blurred distance vision and functional myopia</u>. Most myopia (90^{+}%) begins this way. Initially, most myopia is functional because relaxing the focusing ciliary muscle may restore clear distance vision without lenses. Dilating drugs used during vision testing force inactivity of the ciliary muscle in functional myopia.

∗ Vision therapy eye exercises, if begun soon after diagnosis may often reverse functional myopia.

∗ Functional myopia is often progressive when conditions that caused myopia are not changed. Stopping functional myopic progression often requires changing reading habits. Focusing causes the circular ciliary muscle to pull against the globe of the eye to exert force on the crystalline lens. The globe of the eye including the clear cornea is made of collagen protein. For all near vision, the circular ciliary focusing muscle pulls to exert its force against the collagen structure of the globe.

∗ Normal healthy collagen tissue is likely slightly <u>elastic</u> in nature, which means it may be slightly deformed by pressure, but when the pressure is released it will spring back into its original shape.

∗ Progressive myopia often results in lengthening of the posterior portion of the globe of the eye.

∗ The author theorizes: the collagen tissue of the globe in eyes that are progressively nearsighted is protein and/or mineral deficient and likely more <u>plastic</u> in nature. Plastic tissue if distorted by pressure, won't quite rebound all the way back to its original shape when all pressure is removed.

∗ The protein and/or mineral-deficient eye that is subjected to inordinate stress from prolonged focusing activity of the circular ciliary muscle, may become progressively longer and structurally myopic (nearsighted). This structurally nearsighted eye is not likely to regain its ideal shape after vision therapy. The length of the normal eye is ≈24 mm. Lengthening the eye ≈1 mm results in ≈3 lens diopters of myopia. The balance of forces resulting in a normal shaped eye are very delicate. The same reading habits that may have been appropriate to prevent the development of myopia may also be used to arrest further progression of or sometimes even reverse functional myopia. (<u>Relax</u> is my magic word for kids when reading.) 1st All reading, writing, drawing, and computer work should be done with the material at least elbow distance (about 1 cubit) away from the eyes. 2nd Good lighting or contrast on the VDT is essential for relaxed vision. 3rd Everyone should take frequent breaks from close work. (Adults should learn to rest in the LORD about 5 minutes/hour.) (Children should have about 5 minutes of break time for every ½ hour to 45 minutes of reading.) 4th Caffeine may interfere with the proper activity of the focusing muscle and should be avoided. 5th Since vitamin/mineral deficiencies in the ciliary muscle may be part of progressive myopia, vitamin/mineral-deficient foods such as white sugar and white flour should be avoided. 6th Since protein/mineral-deficient collagen may contribute to progressive myopia as the globe lengthens, nutrient-deficient food should be avoided. The author suggests including mineral-rich foods and supplements in the diet. Many healthy human body fluids have an almost identical mineral balance to salt water. The author suggests that people treat their body as a mineral bank and deposit more minerals than are used up. SeaSalt or other well-balanced salts are good mineral supplements. Since salt water has an ideal mineral balance, seaweed and kelp powder are fine supplements. Other mineral supplements must be evaluated on individual merits. The author theorizes: healthy, slightly elastic collagen is required for a globe that resists being pulled out-of-shape. The author theorizes: collagen protein of the globe should be rich in silicon to have a healthy slightly elastic property. Silicon elements are found in abundance in the bran of whole grains such as wheat. Including whole grains in the diet may encourage the formation of mineral (silicon)-rich collagen.

∗ Myopia and myopic progression may be encouraged by excessive reading and by poor nutrition.

-------------------- **Astigmatism or Astigmia** --

Astigmatism results when the cornea or crystalline lens of the eye is out-of-round. A basketball is round, and if sliced is round or symmetrical. A football, if sliced lengthwise, is oval or astigmatic or asymmetrical. Astigmatism produces distortion in vision like a mirror in the house-of-mirrors. Astigmatism in the eye, like farsightedness or nearsightedness, may be present in only a slight amount or a very large amount. A household mirror that is mounted improperly may be slightly distorted, while the mirrors in the house-of-mirrors are purposely distorted to a large amount. The orientation of the mirror determines the shape of the distortion. In the house-of-mirrors, you may look tall and slender like the center of a basketball team in one mirror, or short and wide like a sumo wrestler in another mirror. A slight distortion of a mirror is often only a minor annoyance, while a major house-of-mirrors type distortion causes a significant detriment to good vision. Astigmatism is usually not progressive like nearsightedness, but often changes slightly with time. The front and back surfaces of the cornea and of the crystalline lens determine total astigmatism. Most often, if the eye has a large amount of astigmatism, it is found on the front of the cornea. The cornea is made of identical collagen as the opaque, white globe. The cornea is clear only because the collagen fibers are very regular in the way they are distributed and the collagen is in a proper state of hydration. (Water is continually pumped out of the cornea to keep it clear.) Collagen in a clear cornea is regular in distribution, like length-wise and width-wise fibers in fabric. The white globe is made of the same collagen, but it is random ordered, like spaghetti on a plate. Six external eye muscles that move the eyes in the socket exert strong forces on the cornea and may distort the cornea into an out-of-round astigmatic shape. A protein/mineral-deficient and slightly plastic collagen is likely more subject to astigmatism than a protein/mineral-rich collagen. Once a cornea is significantly distorted, it isn't likely to resume a round normal symmetrical shape. Astigmatism may be significantly altered after surgery for crossed-eyes or walled-eyes, as surgery significantly changes the forces exerted on the cornea by the six extraocular eye muscles. Bran from whole grains may help keep the cornea collagen and globe collagen mineral (silicon)-rich. (Cross-eyed is when one eye is turned in; and wall-eyed is when one eye is turned out.)

-------------------- **Presbyopia and the need for bifocals** ------------------------

The focusing system of the eye consists of the ciliary muscle and the crystalline lens. The lens is very flexible in youth; and in youth, the eye also has a tremendous range of focusing power. There is a steady decline in focusing ability of the lens with time, so by the time a person is nearly 60 years old, the focusing capability of an eye is nearly zero. The loss of the eyes' focusing power in age is directly related to the crystalline lens becoming less flexible through oxidative damage. After the lens loses its flexibility, the activity of the ciliary muscle also decreases. Presbyopia is treated for most people with bifocals or reading lens. In countries with poor nutrition, the onset of presbyopia may begin at an earlier age than for people in better health. People in superior health may become presbyopic much later in life. Moses may not have been presbyopic at 120 years old. Vitamin C is very concentrated in the crystalline lens. Vitamin C-rich foods such as raw milk, fresh fruit, along with plenty of antioxidant minerals may slow the onset or development of presbyopia.

-------------------- **Visually Related Learning Disabilities** ------------------------

Learning Disabilities in children may also be labeled as 'dyslexia' and are often characterized by an inability of the visual system (eyes to brain) to process visual information, even though the eyes are seeing clearly. These children continue to have difficulty separating b's and d's or p's and q's or left from right. Copying a simple figure may be nearly impossible. These children often benefit from a visual rehabilitation therapy program. Good vision is more than just seeing 20/20. Some learning-disabled kids are labeled Attention Deficit (Hyperactivity) Disorder or AD(H)D. These children are frequently very mineral deficient. Some children develop mineral deficiencies from conception or in neonatal life or in youth from a high sugar, vitamin/mineral deficient diet. Joel Wallach, ND, DVM has successfully treated dozens of AD(H)D children with a change in diet that includes eliminating white sugar and a supplement of minerals and other essential nutrients. In time, AD(H)D children with multidisciplinary help often develop normal reading/learning skills.

-------------------- **LASIK Surgery or Laser Refractive Eye Surgery** -----------

LASIK uses a laser to reduce myopia, hyperopia or astigmatism by reshaping the cornea. Calcium and vitamin C promote healing and corneal collagen re-growth after LASIK eye surgery. The author advises that eating calcium and vitamin C-rich food, and taking calcium and vitamin C rich supplements before and after LASIK surgery, or any surgery, may encourage proper healing.

∗ Stress placed on eyes by books, papers and computers may encourage vision problems.

Macular Degeneration or ARMD

Macular Degeneration destroys the integrity of the macula and fovea of the retina, in which all 20/20 vision takes place. Macular Degeneration can be devastating to normal vision, and was first diagnosed in US servicemen who were released from Japanese prisoner of war camps in the South Pacific at the end of WWII. The servicemen were served a minimum sustenance diet consisting mostly of polished, white rice and were forced to perform hard labor in the bright sun. The large amount of UltraViolet-b (UV-b) light the servicemen were exposed to, along with an absolute absence of many vitamins and minerals, undoubtedly led to Macular Degeneration. Vitamin and mineral deficiencies (vitamin C, vitamin E + trace minerals) that are known to contribute to Age Related Macular Degeneration – ARMD – are all part of the antioxidant biochemistry. **Smoking decreases oxygen and increases free radicals, encouraging antioxidant disease.** Macular Degeneration is an antioxidant-type disease. Plants and supplements rich in absorbable vitamin C, vitamin E, antioxidant minerals – copper, selenium, zinc, etc. – and carotinoid pigments – lutein + zeaxanthin – are useful to prevent or treat Macular Degeneration. Lutein and zeaxanthin are pigments normally found in the macula/fovea that are often missing in Macular Degeneration. Lutein and zeaxanthin are found in plant foods, such as, kale, corn and spinach. People at risk for ARMD should avoid prolonged exposure to UV light and include a UV filter in their glasses.

Cataracts

A cataract gradually blurs eyesight, when the crystalline lens becomes translucent with age. Proper nutrition, including vitamin C-rich foods, may delay the onset of cataracts. The crystalline lens is rarely as clear at age 60, as at age 20. Long-lived people often develop old age cataracts. Cataract surgery replaces a cloudy crystalline lens with a clear plastic intraocular lens (IOL). Cataracts usually progress slowly, and cataract surgery may be delayed until the reduced vision restricts normal/required day-to-day activities. Hopefully cataracts are found only in very old age.

Dry Eye and Weeping Eye

Tears have three components: a mucus layer adherent to the cornea; a voluminous middle watery layer; and an external oil layer to prevent the watery layer from evaporating. Too little of any tear layer may cause a dry eye and corneal irritation. Paradoxically, tear glands may produce too much many watery tears to the point of weeping, yet the cornea may still suffer from dry eye. A dry–yet weeping eye may be caused by poor quality tears, causing the tear glands to produce more tears than usual! An excess of poor quality tears is an attempt to maintain a moist cornea. Dry eye may be helped with nutritional supplements providing oil-soluble vitamins and essential fatty acids such as olive oil. Artificial tears don't cure dry eye, but may help to reduce symptoms.

Keratoconus

In keratoconus, a cornea becomes progressively steeper and progressively thinner, which is debilitating to vision and may cause the cornea to perforate on its own. Rigid contacts may help stabilize the cornea. The author theorizes: protein/mineral–deficient corneal collagen is part of progressive keratoconus. Advanced keratoconus may eventually require a corneal transplant.

Floaters

Floaters appear as a coiled piece of string, but are debris in the vitreous – a protein gelatin. A floater is seen only when it casts a shadow near the center of vision and it is usually benign. The author theorizes: floaters may be caused by a protein deficiency of the vitreous humor.

Detached Retina

In a retinal detachment or tear, the retina has separated from the posterior globe, causing a complete loss of vision to part of the vision field – as if someone pulled a window shade down. Floaters from a detached retina or retinal tear are often numerous like a July 4th fireworks show, and are often accompanied by flashes of light that may not stop even when the eyes are closed. This may be sight threatening and may require emergency surgery. Call an Ophthalmologist now!

Retinitis Pigmentosa or RP

Retinitis Pigmentosa (RP) is a progressive destruction of the peripheral retina characterized by poor night vision and poor peripheral vision. RP is often discussed as a vitamin A deficiency.

Discussion

Eye diseases, like many other diseases, do not always lend themselves to a simple cure by just taking a vitamin or mineral pill. Good nutrition always begins with the best food and continues with high quality food-based supplements. Many poor quality supplements are not well absorbed and not well used by the body. Poor quality supplements may do more harm to health than good.

∗ Everyone on Earth to some degree is vitamin, mineral, essential fatty acid and/or protein deficient.
∗ All nutritional therapy must ensure the body is getting adequate amounts of all essential nutrients.

-------------------- **Glaucoma** (COAG) ---

Chronic open angle glaucoma (COAG) is a disease characterized by high pressure inside the eye, a loss of healthy optic nerve tissue, and a loss of visual field. COAG is insidious in onset, progressive in nature, and may be difficult to treat. Aqueous fluid is produced by the ciliary body, flows around the lens, through the pupil, and drains at the angle between the iris and cornea. Normal intraocular pressure (IOP) is maintained at ≤ 20 mm Hg, as compared with 120/80 mm Hg for blood pressure. There is not one exact threshold for IOP below which nobody has glaucoma and above which everyone has glaucoma. When the IOP rises to >20 mm Hg and is destructive to nerve cells of the retina, which shows up on a vision fields test and optic nerve examination, this is COAG. Most COAG is diagnosed with IOP from 25 to 30 mm Hg, although paradoxically some people with IOP < 20 mm Hg are diagnosed with COAG. The aqueous fluid that creates IOP is produced in the anterior half of the eye, yet the destruction of the retinal nerve fibers occurs in the posterior retina of the eye. The aqueous pressure that exerts force on the cornea, and is measured as IOP, also exerts the same force on the vitreous and finally on the retina. COAG is gradual, insidious, usually painless and very difficult for a patient to self diagnose. For a patient, the gradual vision field loss from COAG may seem analogous to a person living in a room lighted by a single lamp with a dimmer switch, and the lamp's rheostat is very slowly being turned down. By the time a person notices the light is dimmer than remembered, the loss of brightness would be significant – and so it is with COAG: by the time someone usually notices vision has become dim, the vision loss is often great. The smallest arterioles nourishing the retina pass through the optic nerve of the eye. The optic nerve has no rods and no cones, and is not responsive to light. The optic nerve causes the normal small blind spot in each eye. The first areas of vision loss in COAG are reduced peripheral vision and an enlargement of the blind spot. In COAG, the IOP becomes pathological, the optic nerve loses healthy neural tissue, the size of the blind spot is increased and retinal nerve fibers stop functioning normally. The loss of peripheral visual field and enlargement of the blind spot may be due to constriction of delicate capillaries nourishing these tissues, causing death of nerve cells. As COAG progresses, more of the retina is affected and more retinal nerve fibers die. Like other nerve cells, once retinal nerve fibers are dead, they are usually lost forever. Eventually, untreated glaucoma will progress to include the entire retina, with the exception of the macula, which has a slightly different blood supply. In the end, COAG results in 'tunnel vision' and a very restricted area of central vision still capable of 20/20 sight, even while losing all peripheral vision. This is very debilitating. Unlike cataracts, early detection of COAG is critical to the final result. Medical treatment of COAG uses drugs that reduce IOP by – reducing aqueous production of the ciliary body or stimulating aqueous outflow through the cornea/iris angle and/or surgery to create a permanent new aqueous drainage. Medical COAG therapy is effective to reduce IOP, but it may not stop all nerve cell death nor stop all visual field loss. COAG is often attributed to reduced aqueous drainage through the iris/cornea angle as the primary cause of elevated IOP. Reduced aqueous drainage will elevate IOP; but reduced drainage alone can't explain all COAG.

The author's theory is: Chronic Open Angle Glaucoma (COAG) is often a nutritional disease as the ciliary body is deficient in key essential nutrients and produces excess, poor–quality, aqueous. The glaucomatous (COAG) response of the ciliary body is to produce more poor–quality aqueous fluid than would ordinarily be required! More aqueous production than is necessary elevates IOP! This glaucomatous (COAG) ciliary body activity may be similar to the response of the tear glands. (Tear glands that are lacking key nutrients may produce an excess quantity of poor–quality tears.) (If the ciliary focusing muscle is deficient in trace minerals it may over-work, encouraging myopia.) The author doesn't know which nutrient deficiencies may cause poor–quality aqueous and COAG. This COAG theory may also explain why medical/surgical COAG therapy is not always successful. When medicine/surgery is used to reduce aqueous production or eliminate existing aqueous, the unhealthy response of the ciliary body in COAG remains to produce more, poor–quality, aqueous. If a ciliary body in COAG produces excess, poor–quality, aqueous, the benefit of medical/surgical therapy to reduce existing aqueous volume is limited, as the ciliary body produces more aqueous. Proof that excess, poor–quality, aqueous may cause COAG is non-existent; but anecdotally, a few people with COAG have documented a reduction in IOP after following an improved quality diet. Proper nutrition may help the ciliary body produce high-quality aqueous that lowers IOP, and may improve aqueous drainage to lower IOP, and may help retinal nerve fibers better survive high IOP.

Marijuana smoke decreases IOP for ≈4 hours, but the mechanism for its action is unknown.

∗ Glaucoma, a leading cause of blindness in the world, may often be a nutritional deficiency disease.

-------------------- **Diabetes** --

In the history of the world, glaucoma and cataracts are the two leading causes of blindness. In the US, diabetes is the leading cause of blindness from age 20 to 75. When I tell my patients how to minimize their risk of developing diabetes they are attentive, as I say: historically, diabetes is very rare prior to the sugar plantations of the 1500s AD that introduced nutrient-deficient, white table sugar into the common diet. ∗ **To help prevent diabetes – don't eat white table sugar!**

∗ **Today, people in the US may ingest their body weight (≈150 lbs) of white table sugar each year!**
The human pancreas and liver were not designed to process huge volumes of processed sugar apart from the vitamins, minerals, enzymes and fiber that are found in sugar beet or sugar cane. Sugar from one yard of sugar cane is often found in a single serving of ice cream with a syrupy sauce and a soft drink; but where are the vitamins, minerals, fiber or enzymes? After 30 or 40 years of eating high sugar foods the pancreas is simply worn out ahead of its time, and is unable to produce the insulin necessary to process table sugar. Hypoglycemics often have a pancreas on the brink of exhaustion, in which the nearly worn-out pancreas isn't able to produce enough insulin to balance sugar intake. When blood sugar rises to dangerously high, diabetic-like levels, an alarm goes off and the pancreas overproduces insulin, causing a drastic hypoglycemic drop in blood sugar. An overworked pancreas may soon stop producing enough insulin, and then people often develop type 2, adult-onset diabetes. In type 2 diabetes, the pancreas still makes some insulin, and oral medicine simply prolongs the action of the little insulin that the pancreas does produce. Insulin normally acts at the cell wall, to take sugar out of the blood, and move sugar into the cell. Formula-fed, rather than breast-milk-fed infants, may be at greater risk for adult-onset diabetes.

Type 1 diabetes is often autoimmune: as a person's immune system destroys its own pancreas. Type 1, juvenile-onset, diabetes may be triggered between age 5 to 15 by a difficult-to-diagnose unspecified toxin, resulting in a non-functional pancreas that requires insulin injections to control blood sugar. A type 1 diabetic may spend up to $250,000.00 over his lifetime, just to treat diabetes! Type 1 diabetics often develop hemorrhagic retinal complications later in life that lead to blindness.

∗ **Diabetes is almost an epidemic in the US today, as nearly 15% of the people are affected.**
Even honey, the LORD's perfect sweetener, should not be consumed in huge volumes. (Pr 25:27) The consequence of insulin not removing sugar from blood and transporting sugar into the cells is elevated blood sugar (100 mg/ml is normal, but 200^{+} is often found in diabetes), which causes the blood to become thick like syrup. In diabetes, cells are starved for the glucose they require, while blood vessels and capillaries struggle to transport the syrup-like blood overloaded with glucose. Diabetes for tissues, results in 'Starvation in the Midst of Plenty'. Diabetes becomes a vascular disease: in the extremities tissues are starved for oxygen and are at risk for gangrene and/or amputation; the kidneys are stressed and may require dialysis; and capillaries in the retina often hemorrhage blood, which may lead to blindness. The increased viscosity and subsequent difficulty in blood moving through blood vessels plays a huge part in the devastation to health from diabetes. New fragile blood vessels form in the retina to aid circulation, but these new vessels are fragile and often bleed. New fragile vessels may hemorrhage into the vitreous, this blood coagulates and puts traction on the retina, leading to retinal detachment, which leads to blindness. To prevent the diabetic retinal disease, large areas of the retina are destroyed with laser photocoagulation, which reduces the retina's demand for oxygen and minimizes the risk of blinding retinal hemorrhages.

∗ **White table sugar and alcohol place a nutritional tax on the body that no one should be forced to pay.**

-------------------- **High Blood Pressure or HBP** -----------------------------------

High blood pressure that is not controlled may cause retinal hemorrhages and reduced vision. A balanced mineral diet helps the kidneys balance blood minerals and control of blood pressure.

--- Nicotine from smoking cigarettes/cigars constricts blood vessels, which reduces blood flow, which reduces oxygen to the eye and retina, which may make HBP or any eye condition worse. ---

-------------------- **Sty and Irritated Eyelid Glands** --------------------------------

Eyelid glands produce oil for tears. A Sty is usually a red irritated clogged infected eyelid gland. Alternating hot and cold, is often a helpful therapy for eyelid/skin disorders. Repeated applications to eyelids of a washcloth soaked in hot water followed by an ice-cube wrapped in a washcloth, will often help expand and contract eyelid glands, encouraging better drainage to help relieve a sty. Eyelid scrubs with a mild shampoo or herbal soap may be helpful to keep eyelids clean and healthy.

∗ **If poor nutrition contributes to an illness, then better nutrition may help to restore health.**

Digestion and Supplements

Motility is everything for a healthy digestive system, and exercise/activity promotes motility. The authors' diet includes lean clean meat, fish and fowl; raw milk from a trusted source and raw milk cheese; free-range fertile eggs; fresh fruit and fresh vegetables, or fruit and vegetable juices; raw nuts and seeds; beans; purified water; whole grain bread and pastries; SeaSalt; and honey. The author avoids coffee, cigarettes, white table sugar, ***shekar*** alcohol and all microwaved food. The author eats frequently, eats well and regularly takes a variety of food-based supplements such as are listed below and occasionally takes other vitamin-mineral supplements as needed.

Powdered and Concentrated Foods as Supplements

Alfalfa
Barley
BlueGreen Algae – Chlorella
Bone Meal
Gelatin – Beef (never pork)
Kelp or Dulce – (i.e. - Sea Weed)
Liver (Beef and/or Chicken)
Milk, Egg, Soy – and other protein-rich foods
Psyllium Seed – and various other fiber-rich foods
Wheat Germ and Sprouted Wheat
Whey and other cultured dairy products

Fruit juices — Apple, any fresh Citrus, Grape, etc
Vegetables juices — Carrot, Beet, Celery, etc
Honey — Royal Jelly – Honeycomb – Bee Pollen
Olive Oil (Extra Virgin) and Evening Primrose Oil
Sunflower Seed Oil and Sesame Seed Oil
Pumpkin Seeds and Pumpkin Seed Oil
Flax Seed and Flax Seed Oil
Soy Oil and Liquid Soy Lecithin
Fish oil – such as Cod Liver Oil
Wheat Germ Oil
Brans — Oat, Rice, Wheat

Good digestion is critical to continued good health: chew food thoroughly – drink fluids slowly. Enjoy eating and drinking, it's healthy. Start each day with a hearty breakfast. The author has an under-acid stomach. SeaSalt eaten with meals is often helpful for proper stomach acidity–activity. Fresh ripe acid fruit (citrus - such as Orange) or fruit juice before eating proteins may help digestion. Pineapple chunks or canned pineapple juice that is not made from concentrate are both excellent. Pineapple juice, rings, chunks and bits all supply both acids and enzymes that aid ideal digestion. A poor diet may encourage excess acidity, while alkaline vegetables tend to restore pH to normal. The gall bladder releases bile salts into the small intestine. Extra Virgin Olive oil along with citrus (especially ripe fresh Lemon) and Apple juices may keep the gall bladder from developing stones. The healthy digestive system must maintain at least seven different pH levels, from the highest acidity of the stomach, decreasing through the small intestines, to the lowest acidity in the colon. Fresh vegetable or fruit juice, especially not-from-concentrate Concord Grape juice, is great to help keep the pH balanced throughout the intestines. (Sadly, most grape juice is 'from-concentrate'.) Coffee, many teas, soft drinks and beer may disrupt the ideal pH balance of the digestive system. Friendly bacteria are also very important to digestion, and the proper pH allows them to flourish. The colon (large intestine) is the largest reservoir of friendly aerobic bacteria. Yogurt, buttermilk or cheese (ideally raw milk) adds friendly bacteria (acidophilus, biffidus, etc.) to the digestive system. Disbiosis, which is common, is a reduced ratio of aerobic (acidophilus) to anaerobic (E. coli) bacteria.

The health of the colon is often a great indication of the health of the entire body. A colon is like a city sewer system; you must dispose of wastes efficiently to promote a clean digestive system.
∗ Soluble Fiber acts to absorb toxins and Insoluble Fiber acts like a brush, to keep the colon clean. An ideal balance of minerals promotes proper contraction of the strong muscular intestinal walls.
∗ Strong intestinal wall contractions + friendly bacteria + fiber = large, frequent, soft, healthy stools. One or two large soft well-formed stools ≈ the volume of food eaten per day is generally proper. Many people who have not had a healthy diet for some time have parasites living in their colon, and a disproportionately large number of unfriendly *e-coli* bacteria and *candida* yeast, and often between 5 and 15 pounds of impacted fecal matter, and diverticuli (ballooned intestinal wall) or constrictions of the colon. All the above can create an environment suitable for colon disease. Mercury that leaches out of 'silver–amalgam' dental fillings may interfere with proper digestion. The author used colonics to flush the mercury out of his colon, after replacing his 'amalgams'. Colonics (water irrigation of the colon) are often crucial for restoring proper colon health/function. Herbal preparations and regular hand and/or foot reflexology may be helpful for proper digestion.

∗ Disease often begins in the colon! — The road to health is paved with good intestines!

The author suspects that microwaved food isn't well digested and may encourage poor colon health. The author occasionally checks his food transit time by eating a meal containing several large beets. A beet red color in a stool allows calculation of the transit time from the meal to the bowel movement. A 24 to 30 hour transit time is generally normal. Salads with dinner encourage a proper transit time.

∗ Proper digestive function and a clean, active colon are crucial to health and longevity.

Tobacco – and other Oxidants

Tobacco was only native to the Western Hemisphere, and Moses wrote no warning against it. Coffee was first brewed in ≈1,000 AD, and Moses also wrote no prohibition against drinking coffee. In 1492, Columbus found the New World natives smoking, chewing and snuffing tobacco leaves. Tobacco comes from *tobago*, the name of the pipe the Caribbean natives used for smoking. Native Americans cultivated tobacco before Columbus arrived and they traded it with Europeans. In 1612, tobacco was first cultivated in the 'colonies' in Jamestown, Virginia. Tobacco plantations, like sugar plantations, were very labor intensive and encouraged using Black Africans as slaves. In ≈1840, Ellen G. White, author of *Councils on Diet and Food* wisely warned against tobacco use. When a study medically delivered an equal dose of several popular recreational drugs, nicotine was voted 'most popular and most addictive' – nicotine both elevated depression and calmed anxiety. A small amount of nicotine is a stimulant – but in large quantities nicotine may act as a depressant. Nicotine from tobacco is addictive – cessation from smoking produces an unpleasant withdrawal. The majority of adults who smoke tobacco began smoking as teenagers, and many adults who attempt to quit smoking soon resume due to the physical/psychological addiction to the nicotine. Nicotine from smoking tobacco may not be as harmful to health as tars and carbon monoxide (CO). The tip of the burning cone of the center of the cigarette is a miniature blast furnace of ≈2000°F. Chronic smoking results in a loss of elasticity of lung tissue, reduced efficiency of small alveoli lung sacs to deliver oxygen to the blood and eliminate carbon dioxide, and cellular changes that leaves lung tissue resembling tanned leather; which may cause emphysema or pulmonary disease (COPD). Carbon monoxide (CO) in tobacco smoke limits the ability of hemoglobin in red blood cells to carry oxygen (O_2) to cells and carry carbon dioxide (CO_2) away from cells – this reduces oxygen to the heart and other body tissues may increase risk of heart attack, stroke and other heart-lung diseases. Toxic heavy metals, tar, carbon monoxide and nicotine in tobacco reduces lung capacity, constricts blood vessels and reduces oxygenation of tissues, which can make any health condition worse.

Tobacco, marijuana, wood and coffee beans contain naturally occurring oils that are chemically changed during burning/roasting. When wood, tobacco or marijuana is burned and coffee beans are roasted, the oils become a variety of sticky polycyclic aromatic hydrocarbons (P{C}AH). Creosote is a complex family of these gums, tars and resins (P{C}AH)s that result from burning most organic oil. Wood burned in a stove produces creosote that may collect inside a stovepipe/chimney. Creosote is not easily biodegraded, which makes it ideal to preserve wood such as railroad ties or docks. Industrial creosote often has other chemicals added to enhance its wood preservation properties. Today, industrial creosote is labeled bio-hazardous and it has only very restricted applications. Creosote is found in every cup of coffee and is recognized as the black film on the inside of a cup. Tobacco leaves contain ≈300 compounds before burning that become ≈5,000 (tar-like) compounds in cigarette smoke. [R23] 'Tar' on a label measures everything in tobacco smoke except nicotine/water.

> "Cigarette smoke contains such chemicals as arsenic (poison), ammonia (toilet cleaner), carbon monoxide (car exhaust fumes), methane (swamp gas), acetone (nail polish remover), and formaldehyde (used to preserve dead bodies) among thousands of others, and would be a serious health risk in the absence of nicotine." [R24] pg 33

∗ One deadly chemical change in the burning of tobacco is when relatively harmless nitrates (NO_3^-) become reactive nitrites (NO_2^-), which combine with nicotine to become carcinogenic nitrosamines. Nitrosamines can enter a cell and alter its DNA, causing genetic defects, and nitrosamine damaged DNA can encourage rapid, uncontrolled cellular multiplication that is often characteristic of 'cancer'.

∗ Tar gives tobacco smoke its characteristic taste, while nicotine gives smokers the desired high.

In 1964, the Surgeon General issued the first warning linking smoking tobacco to 'lung cancer'. In 1964, 52% of men - 34% of women over 18 smoked, but in 1991, 28% of men - 24% of women smoked. Since tars and other toxins in smoke are more harmful to health than the desired nicotine, filtered cigarettes were designed to be a healthier cigarette. In the 1950's, one cigarette filter used asbestos (briefly) in its filter. "Light cigarettes' reduce nicotine from 2 to 1 mg and toxic tar from 37 to 14 mg, but 'light cigarettes' often encourage more cigarettes to be smoked to get the same 'nicotine-high'.

Maternal smoking during pregnancy increases the risk of birth defects and undersized babies. Nicotine is a physically and psychologically addictive drug. Nicotine withdrawal includes cravings for nicotine, irritability, nausea, anxiety, difficulty concentrating, restlessness and increased appetite. 'Secondhand' tobacco smoke may increase the risk to non-smokers of smoker's health problems. Smokeless tobacco may lead to very similar health problems as those from smoking tobacco. Tobacco use causes 'nicotine drug tolerance', where more nicotine is required for the same effect.

∗ Tobacco smoke is a powerful oxidant — creating free radicals that may damage all body tissues.

Marijuana – Hype or Hope for treating GOAG

Marijuana contains the hallucinogenic drug THC. Marijuana smoke lowers IOP for ≈4 hours – but the psychoactive drug TCH, if isolated and administered by needle or pill does not lower IOP. Most research concerning the IOP lowering effect of marijuana still concentrates on the drug, THC. The author theorizes: Marijuana toxins in smoke may be ciliary body poisons that inhibit the ability of the ciliary body to produce aqueous fluid and the toxins are deactivated by the liver in ≈4 hours. Marijuana leaves contain more oil than tobacco leaves. Smoking marijuana likely creates as many, if not more, toxic compounds as smoking tobacco; some of which are likely toxic to the ciliary body. The most likely ciliary body toxins from marijuana smoke are a mixture of (P{C}AH)s, that are similar to the mixture of gums, tars and resins that are found in tobacco tar, coffee creosote or the byproducts of burning wood or processing crude oil. Smoke happens! Avoid smoke for good health.
* Marijuana smoke likely contains chemicals that are toxic, not therapeutic, to briefly reduce IOP.

Minerals and Vitamins are essential for good vision and are essential for good ocular health.

> "Vitamins and minerals are organic food substances. They have no caloric value but are required as co-factors of enzymes. They regulate metabolic rate, convert fat and carbohydrate into energy, and are vital for healthy body tissues. The function of vitamins and minerals is to stimulate biochemical reactions catalyzed by enzymes. In a diseased person, these reactions may not occur or may occur too slowly without high amounts of the vitamin or mineral. In some diseases or hereditary conditions, biochemical reactions can be overcome with high dosages of a particular vitamin or mineral. In over 3,000 nutritional examinations I have yet to find anyone without vitamin or mineral deficiencies, even in those following excellent diets. In order to get the same amounts of vitamins and minerals your grandparents did, you would need to consume six large meals per day. Since that would overload the calories, it is necessary to take supplements of vitamins and minerals. (This overloading of calories in people who do not supplement their diets often accounts for irrational food cravings, binging on junk foods, and the resulting obesity.) Supplements should only be taken on the basis of biochemical individuality testing." [R25]

* If it could be measured, a valuable index to access a person's risk of developing many modern Chronic Degenerative Diseases (CDD) would be the ratio of the accumulated 'toxic' Oxidants as compared to the stored 'protective' Anti-Oxidants. The list of toxic Oxidants is long and includes – heavy metals, trans-fats, pesticides, tars, alcohol, dental toxins and homotoxins in unclean meats; while the list of protective Anti-Oxidants includes – vitamin C, vitamin E and numerous trace minerals. Dentistry often introduces several toxic Oxidants including: fluoride, silver-mercury amalgams, and thio-ethers from root canals/cavitations, as discussed by Hal Huggins, DDS and Paul Genung, DDS.

Human Health in the Balance

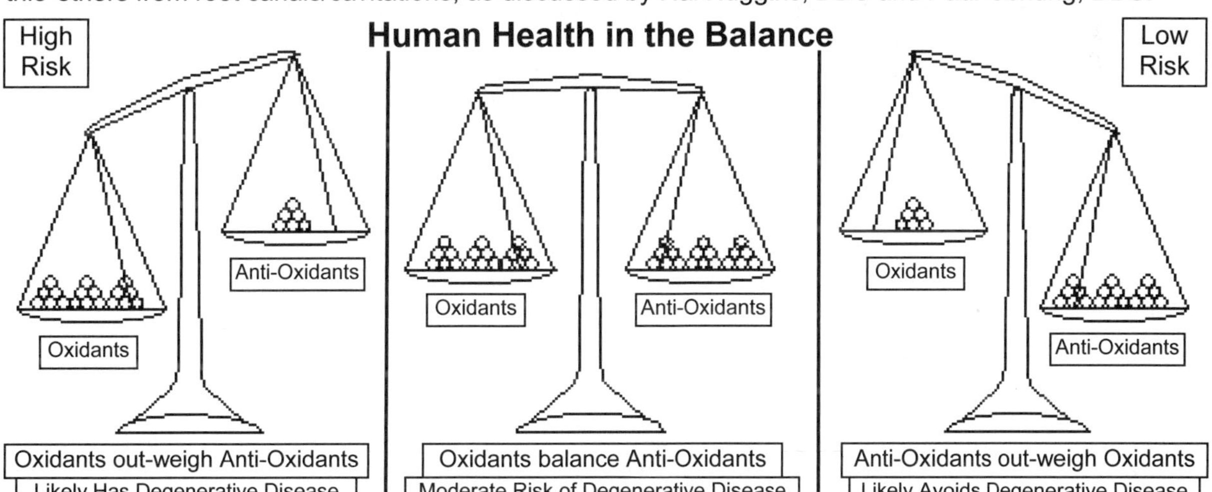

People may feel that they are in 'good health' and they won't get a 'Chronic Degenerative Disease' – such as: Heart Attack, Stroke, Diabetes, Cancer, Auto-Immune Disease, Chrone's, ARMD, COAG, etc. In truth, many people are rapidly accumulating Oxidants and not storing protective Anti-oxidants, such that they are really walking 'time bombs' just waiting to develop a CDD. Once a CDD diagnosis is made, then relating a single 'cause to the effect' of the disease is often very difficult, as Dr. Jensen said:

"It often takes 20 years of abuse to cause the body environment that allows a cancer to develop."

* Eating the 'Kosher Diet', as written by Moses and as discussed in this book, may be the best formula to minimize toxic Oxidants, to maximize beneficial Anti-Oxidants, and to promote health and longevity.

The Dental Connection

In the 1950's, Ralph Steinman, DDS researched the cause of dental caries and tooth decay. Dr. Steinman found that healthy teeth have a (osmotic) flow that goes from the pulp outward toward the surface (enamel) of the tooth. In teeth that were undergoing decay and developing cavities this flow was found reversed, and the flow moved from the surface of the tooth inward toward the pulp. Dr. Steinman found several key blood chemistry indicators for when this critical reversal in flow in the tooth would take place, including a drop in the blood serum phosphorous level below 3.4 mg%. When Dr. Steinman experimentally fed rats a high white sugar diet through a tube that bypassed the teeth and went directly into the stomach, he found that all rats soon developed dental caries. Dr. Steinman concluded that tooth decay was a symptom of systemic disease, resulting from eating white table sugar and other nutrient deficient foods that upset the normal biochemistry of the blood. The common explanation for dental caries is that the bacteria that live in the mouth and on the surfaces of teeth feed on sugar from food, creating acids that initiate the erosion of tooth enamel. Dr. Steinman's research indicates that prior to decay of tooth enamel, the tooth's normal physiology must be <u>first</u> be compromised by a nutrient deficient diet including high amounts of white sugar and other nutrient deficient food; while bacterial involvement with already decayed teeth is <u>secondary</u>.

Dr. Steinman's model of tooth decay may be similar to viewing osteoporosis as primarily a blood chemistry disorder; where nutrient deficient blood results in calcium and other minerals being taken from bones to satisfy the needs blood chemistry, leaving the bone structure weak and brittle.

In 1943, Dr. Heard in Hereford, Texas found that his patients had remarkably few dental caries. The dentist tested the water and found 1.5 to 2.5 ppm fluoride in the water along with unusually high amounts of calcium and other minerals. Local soils and foods grown on these soils were also found to have high amounts of calcium, phosphorous, magnesium, iron and other essential trace minerals. In 1951, Dr. Heard wrote a follow up article for the Lee Foundation for Nutritional Research.

> "It is not true that Hereford, Texas, is a 'town without a toothache'. This phrase has been used effectively by people interested in marketing sodium fluoride all over the country. I practiced dentistry here for years and the incidence of tooth decay originally was very low. Considerable research by some dental authorities brought the suggestion that the relatively high content of natural fluoride in the water might be the reason. I accepted this conclusion for a time. However, as the town grew and people began to live on processed foods … tooth decay increased by leaps and bounds. The increase persisted in spite of the fact that the people were drinking the same water they drank when they were eating natural and unadulterated foods. The dental investigators made a serious mistake when they gave fluoride the credit for our good teeth. They overlooked the food grown in our rich, well-mineralized soil. It is those minerals, of which processed food robs the body, that build health and good teeth. That goes for trace minerals as well as for nitrogen, calcium, potash, and phosphorous. It takes all these elements to build sound bodies …" [R8]

Excess fluoride often causes 'mottled teeth' that are called 'Texas teeth' in the SW United States. [R9]

Weston Price, DDS in his book *Nutrition and Physical Degeneration* also documented that poor nutrition, not a lack of fluoride, caused many musculo-skeletal defects and a poor tooth structure.

When dental caries occur the material used to fill the cavity is often a silver-mercury 'amalgam'. Amalgam dental fillings are a mixture of ≈50% mercury, combined with silver, copper, tin and zinc. A mercury based preservative, thimerosal, was used in the ophthalmic solutions 25 years ago, until it caused many people allergic reactions. Thimerosal is now discontinued in ophthalmic solutions. People who are sensitive to mercury in dental amalgams often have the amalgam fillings replaced. The mercury in one amalgam filling is about the same amount as in one hand-held oral thermometer. Mercury has been used in dental fillings for ≈150 years. Mercury is liquid nature at room temperature. Mercury combined with other metal powders makes an amalgam that begins soft, yet cures to be very hard, which is necessary/ideal for dentistry. Question #1 – Is mercury bound with the other metals in a manner that the mercury can't slowly leach out; or does mercury gradually escape from an amalgam? Today, conclusive evidence demonstrates that mercury does leach out of amalgam fillings over time. Question #2 – Is mercury that is leached from dental amalgams toxic to health? For people who develop toxic or allergic reactions to mercury leached from amalgam dental fillings, the list of possible symptoms, contribution to disease and body tissues affected is virtually unlimited. Hal Huggins, DDS and Thomas Levy, MD, JsD in their book *Uninformed Consent* and Hal Huggins, DDS in his book *Its All in Your Head* and my friend Paul Genung, DDS on his website – <u>w^3.toothwisdom.net</u> discusses these dental issues, plus how thio-ethers from a root canal or cavitation may damage overall health.

∗ White Sugar, Fluoride and Mercury in '<u>amalgam</u>' dental fillings may all cascade people to poor health.

Science and the Miracle of Vision

In the 1700's, belief in 'Divine Creation' for the origin of life and the 'Noachian Flood' to account for most geological features on Earth was almost universally accepted by the educated western world. ('Naturalistic explanations' for the origin of life are as old as the Greek civilization of ≈1,200 to 50 BC.) In 1687, Isaac Newton wrote his book *Principia Mathematica* in which he discussed motion of planets, stars and earthly objects according to the natural law of 'gravity', yet Newton affirmed 'Divine Creation'. (In the 1800's, some scientists sought other natural laws to explain of all phenomenon apart from Divine Creation.) In 1750, Carolus Linnaeus, MD wanted to understand how the biblical term 'kind' (***myin***) of Genesis 1 related to known plants and animals, so he formulated the now universally used system of taxonomy {Kingdom, Phylum, Class, Order, Family, Genus, Species, Variety} to classify all plants and animals. In ≈1830, Charles Lyell, a lawyer, discussed in his book *Principles of Geology* how geological features of Earth whose origins were already explained by Divine Creation and catastrophe (such as the Flood) may otherwise be explained by ordinary, low energy events, acting through immense periods of time. (∗ Catastrophe is defined as a geological event of rare occurrence, intense energy and short duration.) In 1831, Charles Darwin sailed from England on *H.M.S. Beagle* for a 5 year voyage as a naturalist with a copy of Lyell's book *Principles of Geology*, thoughts of biological evolution from his grandfather Erasmus Darwin, and a dislike for the biblical theology that he had just recently studied at Cambridge. In 1835, Darwin visited the Galapagos Islands, where he 'observed' tremendous variety in animals. Darwin used the Linnaean system of plant/animal taxonomy to help organize his factual 'observations'. Darwin observed that a physical trait, such as beaks, varied from one finch to another and one beak size may be advantageous for a finch in a specific environment. Darwin reasoned, in the struggle of life, finches with beaks well adapted for a particular ecosystem were better suited to survive and pass a beneficial trait on to offspring. ∗Thus, Darwin developed the biological principle of 'natural selection'. 'Natural Selection' discusses variation within a population (***myin***); and, how, in the struggle for survival advantageous traits will be passed on to offspring, causing them to be well adapted to the ecosystem. Darwin observed natural selection within a ***myin*** many times in many places during his 5 year voyage. But, natural selection has never been demonstrated to cause evolution from one ***myin*** to a new ***myin***. In 1866, Gregor Mendel formulated genetic laws that added mathematical predictability to inheritance. Mendel was a catholic monk and naturalist, which gave him similar training and experience to Darwin; yet Mendel and Linnaeus believed in a 'fixed ***myin***' and genetic variability only within a biblical 'kind'. To the author: variety, only within a 'fixed ***myin***', is necessary to explain the 'survival of the species'. To Darwin the struggle to survive was sufficient to stimulate evolutionary change and suggest how one ***myin*** may become a new ***myin***. Darwin's advocate friend, Thomas Huxley, tried to include mutation to better suggest how new organs and new ***myin*** may have evolved; but Darwin firmly rejected mutation. Modern neo-Darwinian's add mutation to natural selection to attempt to explain evolution of new ***myin***.

To Darwin an organ, such as the eye, must change slightly from one generation to the next, each time becoming more complex to develop functional vision. Darwin wrote about the origin of the eye.

> "To suppose that the eye with all its inimitable contrivances for adjusting the focus to different distances, for admitting different amounts of light, and for the correction of spherical and chromatic aberration, could have been formed by natural selection, seems, I freely confess, absurd in the highest possible degree."

[Darwin should have stopped here, but then he speculated and theorized on how an eye may have been formed by natural selection.]

> "Yet, reason tells me, that if the numerous gradations from a perfect and complex eye to one very imperfect and simple, each grade being useful to its possessor, can be shown to exist. If further the eye does vary ever so slightly and the variations be inherited, which is certainly the case and if any variation or modification in the organ be ever useful to an animal under changing conditions of life. Then, the difficulty of believing that a perfect and complex eye could be formed by natural selection, though insuperable by our imagination, can hardly be considered real." [R24-64-69] [This is pure theory without proof!]

Darwin might be forgiven for theorizing beyond his initial thoughts of 'absurdity' that an eye that is non-functional in one generation, may via natural selection become functional in future generations. Darwin didn't have the advantage of studying the mathematical probability of inheritance with Mendel. Darwin didn't have the advantage of studying DNA with F. Crick, PhD and J. Watson, PhD in 1962. Darwin didn't have the advantage of studying eyesight with D. Hubel, MD and T. Wiesel, MD in 1981; as the sophisticated neurology of vision is more complex than the latest Microsoft computer program. Darwin didn't have the advantage of studying 'irreducible complexity' with Michael Behe, PhD in 1998. Dr. Behe, in his book *Darwin's Black Box* discusses the principle of 'irreducible complexity', which states: if any part of a functional system is missing, then the whole system is useless and wouldn't be inherited. Eyesight, like a mousetrap, requires all parts to be working in the beginning, if it is useful in any way.
∗ Theorization that vision evolved by natural selection, as opposed to Divine Creation, is unsubstantiated!

Vision must begin with all parts fully functioning, not progress to slowly develop complexity.

Chapter 52 The Author Recently

My Brother, Jeff – pt 1

When my brother, Jim, Jeff's fraternal twin, was in 3rd grade, and I was in 7th grade, Jim began to limp. Later the same year, I was also seen to limp. Our orthopedic physician sent the whole family to the University of Washington for a genetics study. Jim and I were diagnosed with a rare, autosomal recessive genetic bone disease resulting in a poor blood supply to the developing head of the bone. Jim's disease was caught early and was limited to his right hip. Jim was on crutches for 2^+ years to relieve pressure, while swimming developed a good blood supply and allowed normal bone growth. My bone disease involved avascular necrosis of both hips and both ankles. The damage–distortion to my left hip and my left ankle was already far advanced, at the time of diagnosis. Jeff was normal. Jeff somehow felt left out from all the special attention that the physicians showed to both Jim and I.

When I was in High School and Jeff was in 6th Grade, Jeff helped me solve Math logic problems. When I was in College and Jeff was in High School, I was failing English class until Jeff helped me. Jeff always earned straight A's in school, while I usually struggled to earn B's. Though I was 4 years older than Jeff, I could never help Jeff with anything, while Jeff always helped me with everything. We brothers were very competitive, but it soon became clear that Jeff was more talented than Jim or I. Our whole family all enjoyed summer vacations at Cheerio Lodge on Hood Canal, where we rented a cabin and went swimming, boating, water-skiing, sang songs, and where Jeff and Jim played tennis. I learned to play chess 5 years before Jeff. After I taught Jeff to play chess, we played once and I won. Jeff never played another game of chess with me, Jeff settled for beating me at every other game. One summer break from Optometry College, I had nasal surgery for a congenitally deviated septum. Jeff was attending Stanford, and taking a night Calculus class at the U. of Washington that summer. Jeff stopped by the hospital in Seattle to visit me before his class and just after I got out of surgery. Jeff went on to his class and I fell asleep. When I awoke, Jeff was back after his class to wish me well. To me it was as if Jeff had never left; Jeff was always there for me – a funny family story ever since. Jeff was superb in many sports, including winning the '76' Kitsap county Men's Tennis Championship. Jeff played on the Claremont Men's College tennis team that finished 4th in Division II in the nation. Jeff took up golf after college, and Jeff soon became good golfer despite having little time for practice.

In 1980, Jeff married his Stanford sweetheart, Margot. Their minister advised Jeff and Margot to: Take time out from the demands of life to: 1) spend time alone with the LORD each day in prayer 2) spend time together, just the two of you alone 3) do the personal activities that you most enjoy. This advice is similar to the message of Moses to love the LORD, love your neighbor and love yourself. These three commandments were also repeated by Jesus. (Deut 6:4 /Lev 19:18 /Matt 22:37-40) In 1990, I showed Jeff parts of my book and I told Jeff, "I wrote as I learned and learned as I wrote." Jeff encouraged me to write in the book about how Jim and I overcame our bone disease in our hips. Jeff was always the strong healthy brother. Although Jeff read many chapters of my book recently, he didn't embrace or practice all its nutritional concepts. I understood Jeff not practicing all the health principles that I did, especially while Jeff seemed to be perfectly healthy. Jeff never smoked tobacco or marijuana, or used drugs. Jeff drank some beer and wine, but never to an excess. Jeff was a very good athlete. Jeff was always physical fit. Jeff always appeared to be an ideal role model for health.

Jeff enjoyed playing tennis and Jeff enjoyed riding in endurance cycling events and Jeff also enjoyed playing golf.

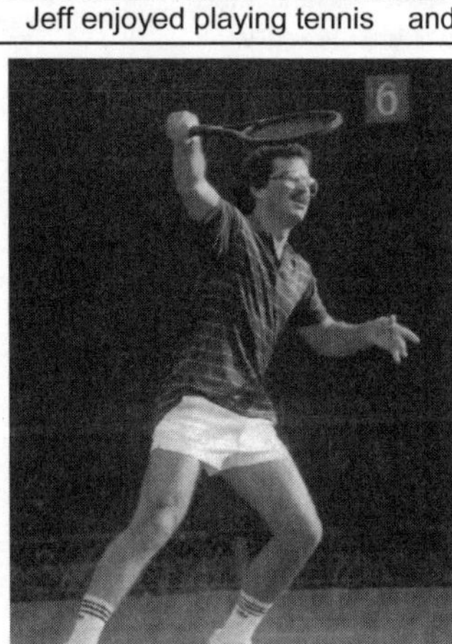

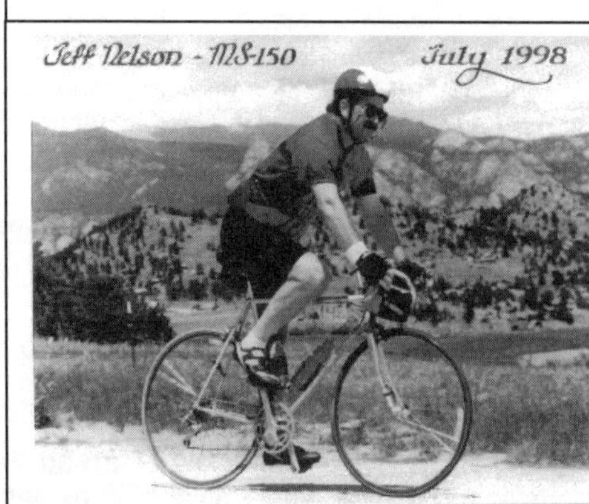

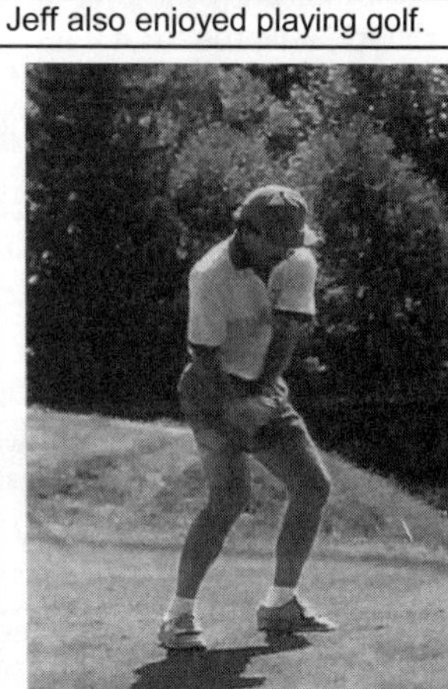

1985 Tennis + 1998 Bicycling + 1992 Golf

While finishing this book after Jeff died of cancer, my emotions may have been similar to Richard Carpenter as he finished the last Carpenter's album after his sister, Karen, died from anorexia.

My Brother, Jeff – and Cancer

Jeff developed a small brain tumor in the spring of 1997 and later that year the low-grade tumor was surgically removed. The surgery was successful and Jeff was convinced that he was strong and healthy, that medicine had the answer for cancer, and that once the brain tumor was removed it would not return. I visited Jeff in Colorado each of the following three winters and we discussed my rehabilitation from hip replacement surgery. We went skiing each of those years. Jeff skied the Blue Squares and some Black Diamonds, while I skied the Green Circles and some Blue Squares. Our time talking as brothers will always be remembered by me as many our fondest times together. I knew health principles that I wanted, as a big brother, to share with Jeff and him help beat cancer. But each winter I discussed health concepts with Jeff that Jeff felt were unnecessary to implement. Andrew Weil, MD discusses that surgery is effective for cancer, but radiation and chemotherapy are often not effective for cancer. In 1998, Jeff played golf with Paul Azinger in the ProAm of Arnold Palmer's Bayhill Classic. Paul Azinger had just recovered from bone cancer and was a hero to Jeff. Jeff scored a natural birdie 4 on a par 5; the hole where John Daily later hit 5 balls in the water. Jeff's brain tumor caused him seizures before the surgery that returned after surgery, and each year Jeff required more medicine to prevent the return of seizures. I knew instinctively that Jeff's tumor was returning, even while Jeff did not want to discuss the possibility. Medicine has helped people survive cancer for 5 years after diagnosis, but the cancer survival rate beyond 5 years is no better today than it was 25^+ years ago, when the Surgeon General declared 'War Against Cancer'. I suggested to Jeff that he visit Francisco Contreras, MD at the Oasis Clinic in Tijuana, Mexico, who routinely treats cancer with long term success, but Jeff felt this unnecessary. Some doctors, such as our childhood friend Steven Masley, MD, discuss antioxidants that are disappearing from food, as important to prevent and/or treat cancer. I attempted to discuss Steve's book with Jeff, but Jeff often preferred to discuss the lasted software development that our friend Bill Gates was promoting. In the spring of 2000, Jeff's brain tumor returned, but the surgeon could not remove all the tumor. Our last dinner in Bremerton, Wash. was at Jeff's favorite waterfront restaurant, where Jeff ordered shellfish that I didn't approve of. After Jeff's second partially successful surgery, and chemotherapy, and radiation, it was apparent that Jeff would never recover. My brother, Jeff, died on Aug 14, 2001.

From the winter of 1997 after Jeff's first successful brain cancer surgery until the summer of 2001, chronicling Jeff's health and conversations about Jeff's health included statements such as the following.

Thanks for your concern Jay the surgeons got it (the brain tumor) all. When Jeff had another seizure after his surgery, Jeff took medication to prevent more seizures. Whenever Jeff was not experiencing a seizure, Jeff felt fine, as a primary brain tumor doesn't spread outside the brain. (Steve Masley, MD, wisely informed me that scar tissue after brain surgery could cause seizures.) As I look back on things, feeling fine when not have a seizure gave Jeff a false sense of security. Jeff was now playing golf as well, if not better than ever, as his score in the ProAm demonstrated. Jeff said, Jay the medications are working fine, all is well, don't worry. It's not your problem Jay! After Jeff was free from seizures for several months Jeff had his driver's license was re-instated. Then, Jeff had another seizure and now required multiple medications to prevent further seizures. Jay, my doctors say everything is fine. Eventually, when Jeff was on multiple seizure prevention medications, Jeff experienced partial complex seizures as the brain tumor re-appeared. Jay they need to do another surgery. Jay they couldn't get it all. Jay I need chemo. Jay I need radiation. After months of more chemo and more radiation, Jeff called to say, "Jay, I'm dieing." Now I had to abandon hope that Jeff would pursue 'alternative cancer therapy', and just help Jeff prepare to die. The only time that I was happy to lose at anything to Jeff was our last game of backgammon, while Jeff was on his deathbed. The scene was similar to Wyatt Earp and Doc Holiday playing poker in the movie *Tombstone*, while Doc Holiday was dieing in a Tuberculosis Sanitarium in Colorado.

How could Jeff help me format my book on computers, and encourage me to publish it, yet not embrace its principles? That question haunted me for months as I watched *Gulliver's Travels* on TV. On the show Gulliver's wife was asked if she believed her husband's story – she quietly answered; "I believe in my husband." Then, I quickly realized that that was how Jeff had always felt about me. Recognizing that Jeff always believed in me, even when there wasn't much reason to believe in me, was always comforting. Having people who believe in you is essential to developing a 'full vessel'. As an adult I now knew why, after vacations/visits with Jeff, I always left feeling like I would succeed. Jeff was a natural born leader, who excelled at most everything thing that he undertook. Jeff always encouraged and led by example, helping others to succeed in business, sports, life and loving God. Many of Jeff's friends and co-workers showed up to the small Church in Littleton, Colorado from both the Atlantic and Pacific coasts for the 2 hour memorial service to honor the life of my brother, Jeff. Jeff was a devout family man to his wife, Margot, and to his two teenage daughters, Laura and Lisa.

Health, Nutrition and Surgery

Good nutrition, from food and supplements, may help make any eye condition less traumatic, and may prevent many conditions from developing, but good nutrition by itself will not cure every condition. This author began studying and implementing principles of good nutrition 25^+ years ago. Good nutrition has helped stabilize my hypoglycemia, when my blood sugar was going up and down like a yo-yo; and my nutrition program has likely prevented me from developing diabetes. Improving my diet and practicing my rules for reading helped stabilize my prescription for glasses. Diet didn't cause my nearsightedness or astigmatism to go away, but my prescription was stable for 20^+ years, until I had laser eye surgery. LASIK eye surgery reduced my myopia and astigmatia so I can participate in many activities (kayaking and folk dancing) without spectacles. Diet helped me recover from eye surgery quickly and, as expected, I healed quickly. Audrey Talley, MD preformed my left eye LASIK at NW Eye Surgeons in March of 1999 and Paul Shenk, MD preformed my right eye LASIK at PCL-Tacoma in April of 2000. After both surgeries, I was back to work the next day. A good diet is great for health, but good nutrition may not cause all medical conditions to vanish.

My brother, Jim, and I each had a bone disease in youth, causing the ball of the femur to became soft and distorted from weight-bearing stress/activity. A genetics study at the University of Washington helped explain the rare genetic disease in two siblings as being autosomal recessive. We were both diagnosed as the disease was just beginning for Jim; and a treatment of no weight bearing plus swimming allowed Jim's hip to develop normally. I was 4 years older than Jim, and I was not nearly as fortunate, since my left hip was already grossly distorted at the time of diagnosis. My physician said, "Plan on a less than active life." I followed this advice for a while. Later, I wore out my left hip mountain climbing. Diet helped me function reasonably well for the last 25^+ years with a grossly distorted left hip, but diet did not cause my distorted hip to become more round like a normal hip. In November of 1998, I had hip joint-replacement surgery. I continued to dance until two days before surgery despite moderate joint pain. My physician, Paul McCullough, MD, said my hip was "the most distorted piece of bone he had ever seen". Dr. McCullough prescribed coumadin prophalactically as a blood thinner during my hospital recovery time and every day my blood was evaluated for the coumadin's effectiveness. Dr. McCullough remarked upon my release, "I have never seen anyone so resistant to coumadin." My liver and kidneys must have eliminated the coumadin very quickly. My distorted hip caused my left leg to be 1 inch shorter than my right leg, and surgery lengthened my left leg ¾ of an inch as well as replaced my diseased hip with a new steel hip. I initially traded bone pain for muscle, tendon and ligament pain, but I was undaunted. I put a small lift in my right shoe to regain part of the pelvic tilt I was used to, and began a rehab plan of water-aerobics, stretching, walking and massage therapy; and three weeks after surgery I was back dancing and working part-time. My folkdance group didn't believe I'd begin dancing just three weeks after surgery, when three months would have been a good recovery time. When I saw Dr. McCullough four weeks after surgery he was beside himself, as he had told me there was no dancing until I could walk without a limp without using a cane. Dr. McCullough said, "walk down to the end of the hall, and turn around and walk back." As I walked back toward him, Dr. McCullough stood there shaking his head in disbelief. "I don't believe this" were the only words he had for me when he saw that I was walking without a limp. "Go ahead and go folk dancing if you want to." I felt reassured to have Dr. McCullough's blessing. Dr. McCullough had never seen anyone recover from surgery so quickly because he had never had a patient dedicated to nutrition, such as myself. Of course, keeping my muscles, ligaments and tendons in good shape before surgery helped my recovery. I'm now using my left leg better for dancing than before surgery, despite mild discomfort. Massage therapy from Shawn O'Brien, LMT permitted my speedy recovery for dancing and work. Back/waist exercises and chiropractic from Bruce Davis, DC helped to align my neck and spine. Kayaking is another passion in my life. On October 2, 1999, with my good friend Bill Zurbrugg, I finished paddling my kayak around the entire non-ocean, marine coastline of Washington State. Someone told me there are about 2,500 miles of non-ocean, marine coastline for the Puget Sound, San Juan Islands, and Straits of Juan deFuca. Kayaking is a great exercise for anyone with a joint disease in a leg. I've enjoyed and benefited from paddling a kayak very much. This year I plan to begin paddling the Pacific Ocean coastline of Washington State and the western waterways of the Lewis and Clark Expedition from the Clearwater, Snake and Columbia rivers to Astoria, Oregon and the Pacific Ocean. I have less hip discomfort from folk dancing and paddling my kayak now, than before joint replacement. I can now folk dance, paddle a kayak and read a map without spectacles.

∗ Nutrition, massage, chiropractic and surgery have all helped improve the quality of my life recently.

------------------ References Ch 51 Vision and Eyes and Ch 52 The Author ---------------------

[R1] Eyes and Nutrition (Delicious Sept 98)\ by Ben Lane, OD; pg 24-29; nutritional deficiency & myopia

[R2] What Your Doctor Doesn't Tell You (WYDDT journal – UK)\ 10-31-1998 vol 9; N7; pg 8
Case Study: Curing Glaucoma – used nutritional supplements to treat COAG

[R3] Smart Medicine for Your Eyes\ by Jeffrey Anshel, OD; better nutrition reduces risk of eye diseases

[R4] Prevent and Treat Eye Disease with Nutrition\ by Ben Lane, OD; pg 42-46 ARMD – nutrition + supplements

[R5] Toxic Metal Syndrome\ by Dr. Richard Casdorph and Dr. Morton Walker; pg 131-164 Mercury

[R6] It's All in Your Head\ by Hal Huggins, DDS Mercury in amalgam dental fillings

[R7] Uninformed Consent\ by Hal Huggins, DDS and Thomas Levy, MD, 'what you don't know'

[R8] The American Fluoridation Experiment\ by F. B. Exner, MD and G. L. Waldbott, MD; pg 3-7 Hereford, Tx
– The high mineral content of water and soil, not isolated Fluoride, temporally produced good dental health.

[R9] The Town Without a Toothache (Feb 1943)\ in Reader's Digest – Hereford, Tx + fluoride in the water

[R10] Dental Amalgams (12-16-1990)\ by 60 Minutes CBS TV – controversy concerning health risks

[R11] Toxemia The Basic Cause of Disease\ by John Tildon, MD; All degenerative disease begins with toxemia.

[R12] ARED Study (2001)\ Age Related Macular Degeneration and Antioxidant Supplements

[R13] Nicotine an Old-fashion Addiction (video)\ by Schlessinger Videos ≈2000°F blast furnace

[R14] The Encyclopedia of Psychoactive Drugs (series) — Tobacco — Coffee — Marijuana
[R14A] Tobacco [R14B] Coffee The Worlds Most Popular Stimulant [R14C] Marijuana

[R15] PCLI Education Meeting (Tac 01-99)\ by Rick Burk, OD; Marijuana smoke reduces IOP for ≈4 hrs

[R16] Hooked but not Helpless Kicking the Nicotine Addiction\ by Patricia Allison

[R17] Tissue Cleansing Through Bowel Management\ by Bernard Jensen, DC, PhD; keep the colon clean

[R18] Strong's Concordance\ by James Strong, STD, LLD

pg 326	eye	# 5869	H pg 87	***ayin***	Deut 34:7
pg 562	kind	# 4327	H pg 65	***myin***	Gen 1:21 to 25

[R19] Constipation (audio)\ by Brenda Watson, Colon Therapist; impacted feces↑ ⇒ health↓ w^3.renewlife.com

[R20] Health Consequences of Smoking (CANCER-1986-8) + Nicotine Addiction (1988)\ by Surgeon General

[R21] Cigarette Country\ by Susan Wagner // [R21A] Tobacco\ by Iain Gately

[R22] The Cigarette Papers\ by Glantz, Slade, Bero, Hanauer and Barnes

[R23] The Search for a Safe Cigarette (PBS TV & DVD)\ by NOVA – no cigarette is safe to smoke

[R24] Tobacco and Smoking Opposing Viewpoints\ by Greenhaven Press; pg 33 quote

[R25] The Joy of Health\ by Zoltan Rona, MD; pg 60-61 quote on the need for minerals/vitamins

[R26] Men of Science Men of God\ by Henry M. Morris, PhD; pg 27 Linnaeus (Newton, Mendel, Pasteur)

[R27] Great Scientists and the Bible (audio)\ by D. James Kennedy, ThD (Linnaeus – 'kind' = ***myin*** ≈ ?species?)

[R28] The 28-Day Antioxidant Diet Program\ by Steven Masley, MD; antioxidants = protect and/or restore

[R29] Outrage: The Five Reasons O.J. Got Away with Murder\ by Vincent Bugliosi, JsD
(From Vincent Bugliosi the author learned how to purposely present evidence in a manner calculated to support a premise.)

[R30] Iridology Simplified\ by Bernard Jensen, DC, PhD – 'Iris Analysis' to evaluate human health

[R31] A Guide for the Perplexed\ by Rabbi Moses ben Maimon (aka – Maimonides) (aka – Rambam)

[R32] Philosophy Natural Principia Mathematica\ by Isaac Newton (1687) – aka *Principia Mathematica*
(Newton described Gravity – and developed Calculus – yet he devoted more time/energy to writing about Theology.)

[R33] Finding Order in Nature\ by Paul Lawrence Faber; pg 6-13 pg 11 – Carolus Linnaeus, MD (1753)
(In 1753, in *Species Plantarum* Linnaeus discussed the taxonomy of plant 'kinds' (***myin***), as used 10 times in Genesis 1.)

[R34] Linnaeus Nature and Nation\ by Lisbert Koerner; pg 23-4 ***myin*** = kind – *Philosophia Botanica*
(In 1750, in *Philosophia Botanica* Linnaeus related his 'genus – species' nomenclature to Adam naming animals in Genesis 1.)

[R35] Gregor Mendel and the Roots of Genetics\ by Edward Edelson Augustinian monk & naturalist
(In 1866, Mendel's work was 1st published, but it was obscure until shortly after 1900, when it became widely recognized.)

[R36] Principles of Geology Being an Attempt to Explain the Former Changes of the Earth's Surface by Causes Now in Operation\ by Charles Lyell (≈1830) – aka *Principles of Geology*

[R37] The Origin of Species by Means of Natural Selection or the Preservation of Favored Races in the Struggle for Life\ by Charles Darwin (1859); ch VI pg 133 eye quote – aka *Origin of Species*

[R38] Ever Since Darwin\ by Stephen J. Gould, PhD; pg 103-104 Darwin – evolution of the eye

[R39] Darwin's Black Box\ by Michael Behe, PhD; (1998) biological principle of 'irreducible complexity'

[R40] Vision Research\ David Hubel, MD and Torsten Wiesel, MD – 1981 Nobel Prize
(While in Optometry College, the author had the privilege of hearing Dr. Torsten Wiesel speak in Portland, OR.)

[R41] Life Itself\ by Francis Crick, PhD – 1962 Nobel Prize with James Watson, PhD – miracle of life

[R42] Health and Light\ by John Ott; sunlight is a nutrient – sunlight↓ ⇒ Seasonal Affective Disorder (SAD)↑

[R43] Pacific Health Center – (Update #43 Eye Problems)\ by Monte Kline, PhD; ARMD & Anti-Oxidants

[R44] Basin and Range (bk+ado)\ by John McPhee In 1795, James Hutton, MD wrote of geologic time & natural selection.

[R45] In Suspect Terrain (bk+ado)\ by John McPhee (tp1-sd2) In geology, catastrophes are always preserved in rock.

[R46] Omega 3 Oils\ by Donald Rudin, MD; pg 19 – Omega 3 → Prostaglandins → regulate IOP

[R47] Great Pharoahs (3 videos)\ by The Learnig Channel; (v-#1) Egyptian magicians' trick = snake around a stick

[R48] Diet, Science and the Eye (Review of Optometry Sept 15, 2001)\ by Stuart Richter, OD, PhD; pg 76-84

[R49] Diabetes Epidemic (Review of Optometry Sept 15, 2003)\ by Jeffrey Eisenberg; pg 78-89; retinopathy risk

{ } – may be part of name

30 Traditional Israeli Folkdances (80 minute CD)

	Hebrew Name	English Name	Choreographer	Year	Composer	Skill	Set	Time
01	***At Va'ani***	You and I	Uziel	62	Gilad	Bg	Cr	2:56
02	***Bo Iti El Hagalil***	Come with Me to Galilee	Amishai	69	Rosenblum	Bg$^+$	So	1:50
03	***Dodi Li*** (**)	My Beloved {is Mine} (SoS ch2)	Shturman	48	CHen	Ad	Pt	1:59
04	***Eretz Eretz*** {***Eretz***}	Land, Land {Land} (***Eretz*** Israel)	Levy	74	Paikov	Bg	Cr	2:30
05	***Erev Ba***	Evening Comes	Ashriel	60	Levanon	Int	Cr	3:32
06	***Erev Tov***	Good Evening	Sha'uli	77	Hacohen	Int	Cr	2:50
07	Harmonica	(Hebrew-***Mapukeet***) (Mouth Organ)	Shturman	45	Midlim	Int	Cr	2:47
08	***Haroa Haktana***	The Little Shepherdess	Karmon	59	Wilenski	Int	So	1:41
09	***Hava Nagila***	Come Let Us Rejoice	Ashriel	68	Folk	Bg	Cr/Ln	2:16
10	***Hine Ma Tov*** (***)	Behold How Good (Ps 133:1)	Shturman	50	Yacovson	Bg$^+$	Cr	2:09
11	***Hora Agadati***	Agadati's Dance (Israeli twist)	Agadati	20	Boskovitz	Bg	Cr	3:15
12	***Hora CHassidit***	CHassidit's Dance	Shturman	66	Folk	Bg	Cr	2:27
13	Joshua	(Hebrew-***Yehoshua***) (Military dance)	Dassa	67	Zari	Ad	Ln	2:20
14	***Ki Eshmera*** {***Shabbat***}	For I Guard {the Sabbath}	Levy	73	Traditional	Int	Cr	3:47
15	***Klezmer*** (Yiddish)	Band (Instrumental Melody)	Ashriel	70	CHassidic	Bg	Cr	2:31
16	***Kuma Echa***	Arise Brother	Shturman	45	Postolsky	Bg	Cr	2:01
17	***Lakabalat Shabbat***	Welcoming the Sabbath	Alfassy	79	Shevech	Int	Cr	3:05
18	***Lech Lamidbar***	Go to the Desert	Tsimble	79	Argov	Int	Ln	3:07
19	***Ma Navu***	How Beautiful (Is 52:7)	Shturman	62	Spivak	Bg	Cr	2:34
20	***Mayim Mayim***	Waters, Waters (Rain dance)	Dublin	37	Amiran	Bg	Cr	2:11
21	***Numi Numi***	Fall Asleep, Fall Asleep (Lullaby)	Bachar	76	Engel	Bg	Cr	2:07
22	{***Od***} ***Lo Ahavti Dai***	I Have Not Loved Enough	Levy	77	Shemer	Bg	Cr	2:16
23	***Rav B'rachot***	Many Blessings	Bergstein	58	Shelem	Bg	Cr	2:52
24	***Sisu V'Simchu***	Rejoice and Be Glad (***Torah*** dance)	Ashriel	74	Paikov	Bg	Cr	2:02
25	***Sulam Ya'akov***	Jacob's Ladder (Gen 28:12)	Gabay	72	Hirsh	Bg	Cr	2:42
26	***Ta'am Haman***	Taste of the Manna	Ashriel	50	Naron	Bg	Cr	2:45
27	***Tzadik Katamar***	Righteous as a Palm Tree (Ps 92)	Gabay	69	Ne'eman	Bg	Cr	1:45
28	***Tzena Tzena*** (*)	Come Out, Come Out {alt – Go Forth}	Lapson	60	Meron	Bg	Cr	2:20
29	***Ve David***	As David {has Beautiful Eyes}	Shturman	53	Shelem	Bg	Mx	1:55
30	***Yedid Nefesh*** (**)	Soul Friend	Gabay	71	Twing	Int	Cr	2:52
31	***Zemer Atik***	Ancient Melody (very easy)	Shturman	55	Ne'eman	Bg	Cr	3:14

------- This CD is produced For Educational Purposes Only ------- Total Time 79:53

Beginner	Bg – slow, easy dance steps – people skilled in basic footwork usually learn quickly
Intermediate	Int – quicker pace, more precise sequences of steps – more parts – tougher to learn
Advanced	Ad – faster pace, more complex steps, many direction changes – challenging to learn
Expert	Ex – fastest pace, demanding steps – choreographed disco – fun for the best dancers

(Profits from this CD to benefit 'Bridges for Peace', a non-profit organization that supports Jews who are returning to ***Eretz*** Israel.)

Israeli folkdance is 1st mentioned in Scripture after the Red Sea crossing, when Miriam, the prophetess and sister of Moses, with a timbrel lead the Hebrews in song and dance. (Ex 15:20) Since then song and dance have been an integral part of Hebrew health and worship to the LORD. King David emphasized song and dance as part of worship to the LORD, with the Psalms (songs) he wrote and with his dance when he brought the Ark of the Covenant to Jerusalem. (II Sam 6:16). In 1920, Baruch Agadati choreographed steps to Alexander Boskowitz's 1st modern Israeli folkdance. In 1937, Israel's 2nd folkdance - ***Mayim Mayim*** - was composed for a water festival at ***Kibbutz Na'an***. Since 1945, and the return of Jews as a nation to ***Eretz*** Israel from Europe, Russia, Arabia and the 4-corners of the world, Israeli folkdance to worship the LORD and for recreation has blossomed. Modern Israeli folkdance style is an amalgam that was influenced by traditional Hebrew culture as well as the many cultures in which Jews have co-mingled for the past ≈2000 years of the ***Diaspora***.

Many websites under the heading of 'Israeli folkdance' were used to complete these pages, including:
– Australia Israeli Dance – Kesher LeMachol – Beit Tikvah – Beth Emunah – Israeli Dance & – Ken Avner.
(*) Performed on the *Seattle Romania* cassette in 1986 by the Mazeltones, and used with their encouragement.
The author would like to contact anyone involved with these 31 Israeli Folkdances. Moses5in1Torah@msn.com
-------- Sung by (**) Roberta Paulson (***) Roberta and Amy Paulson recorded by Justin Hebert --------
The author is grateful to many Israeli dance teachers since 1980 including Arne Swensen, Ruth Galloway, Kathy Rios, Robin Cowan, Rick Hebron, Belinda Timpke, Jessie Camerer, Ellie Morhaime and Mike Merryman; and to Rabbi Murray Silberling for efforts to restore dance in worship to the LORD with his book *Dancing for Joy*.
The CD is dedicated to the memory of May Robertson, who enjoyed Israeli folkdance – especially **Ma Navu**.

Set

Dance Vocabulary and Glossary

Circle – Cr – All dancers hold hands forming a Circle and facing toward the center of the Circle.
Line – Ln – All dancers hold hands in one Line (often with a leader) or in several shorter Lines.
Partner – Pt – All dancers are paired into Couples (Partners) of one man and one woman.
Mixer – Mx – Partner dance where men and women move to new Partners during the dance.
Solo – So – All dancers dance alone, dancers may be loosely organized in a Circle or in Lines.

Line-of-Direction = L-o-D – often CounterClockWise (CCW)
Reverse Line-of-Direction = R-L-o-D – usually ClockWise (CW)

------- Lf = LEFT foot ------- Dance Footwork Glossary ------- Rt = RIGHT foot ----

Footwork Name {alt..} Steps can begin with the Rt or Lf foot and all steps can be danced to either the right or left.

Ashrei Rt hop-turn 90° CCW – step back on Lf – Lf returns to place [steps usually mirrored to left]
Balance {Sway} Rt and Lf side by side – lean to right – lean back to left (no movement of feet)
Box Rt step ahead {with a hop} – cross Lf in front and to side of Rt – return Rt beside Lf
Brush Lf in place – swing Rt behind Lf – then swing Rt ahead of Lf lightly brushing the floor
Cha Cha {Bumble Bee} Rt small step – Lf closes behind Rt – Rt steps ahead (often repeats)
Change Rt ahead of Lf – quick jump to exchange Rt and Lf feet positions simultaneously
Chug Rt sharp, quick hop (backward or in place) [Rt knee bent – no weight on Lf]
Coupe Rt in place – Lf step across Rt – Rt step in place – Lf step back in place
Cross Rt step ahead and cross in front of Lf (may often be followed by Lf cross in front of Rt)
Debka {Heel-Toe} Rt to front – Rt tap heel + then weight ball of Rt (feet in same place) (2 beats)
Harmonica Hop Lf step across Rt – Rt stationary – Lf returns to place + Hop on Lf (= Coupe + Hop)
Hop Rt hops off floor – come down on Rt
Hora Rt steps to right – Lf steps quickly next to Rt – Rt steps quickly in place
Hook Lf in place – lift Rt in front of Lf and pull Rt back toward Lf – return Rt to place
Join {Close} Rt moves adjacent to Lf (Rt begins laterally separated from Lf)
Joshua Rt step – Lf joins Rt – Rt hops sideways to left – step on Lf – Rt joins Lf (5 beats)
Jump Rt and Lf – both feet jump off floor up at the same time – Lf and Rt land together
Kick Lf in place – lift and kick Rt straight ahead
Klezmer Rt steps ahead & to right on heal – Lf steps behind Rt [both knees bent] (often repeats)
Leap Rt jumps forward or to the side, landing on Rt
Lift Lf in place – lift Rt – pause – bring Rt down
Mayim {Grapevine} Lf crosses Rt – Rt to side – Lf behind Rt – Rt to side (very common step)
Open Mayim Rt to side – Lf crosses Rt – Rt to side – Lf behind Rt {alt. – Mayim on the ½ Step}
Pativah {Hora} Rt step in place – Lf step in place – Rt step in place (3 steps in quick succession)
Pivot {½ Turn} – swivels on one foot to change orientation 180° ((¼ Turn = 90° re-orientation))
(Pivot is usually CW while dance moves CCW. – Reverse Pivot is CCW while dance moves CCW.)
Point Lf in place – tap (touch) Rt toe to floor ahead of Lf – or ahead and to the side of Lf
Rock Rt begins ahead of Lf – transfer weight forward to Rt – back to Lf – w/o moving feet
Scissor[s] Lf cross/hop to front/right of Rt – hop back on Rt (feet remain crossed) – (often repeats)
Shuffle Rt and Lf purposelessly move to keep pace with the circle/line — bad dance form!!
Spin Rt raises on toes and Lf initiates a full 360° turn while staying on toes of Rt
Step Rt steps in front of Lf – like walking
Step-bend Rt steps in front of Lf with deep knee bend of both legs simultaneously
Tcherkessia Rt in front – Lf in place – Rt returns to place {alt. – short graceful Lung}
Touch Lf in place – tap (touch) Rt toe to floor (often beside Lf) – w/o weight on Rt
Turn rotate around (360°) //often '3 Step Turn' Rt – Lf – Rt //rarer '2 Step Turn' Rt – Lf
Twist Rt and Lf jump and rotate ¼ turn in the air – usually followed by reverse direction twist
Yemenite Rt to side – Lf behind Rt – Rt crosses back in front of Lf (very common change-of-direction step)
Back Yemenite Rt steps back – Lf steps farther back than Rt – Rt steps forward and returns to place
Wrap Lf in place – lift and arc Rt in front of Lf and beyond Lf – { alt. – long slow Cross step}

In 1992, the author visited Israel with a tour lead by Rabbi Murray Silberling, the 'dancing Rabbi'. When we played and danced to Israeli folkdance music on a Tel Aviv street corner, it seemed as if we were the 'Pied Piper'. Tourists and Israeli citizens, especially teenagers, gathered in great numbers to

∗ To Sing, Dance and Rejoice before the LORD as Prophetess Miriam and King David did is healthy!

Moses and the Miraculous Staff

The life of Moses was a series of miracles that were often orchestrated by the LORD for His purpose. Some miracles in the life of Moses were ordinary or infrequent events that occurred with exquisite timing, such as: Moses being found by Pharaoh's daughter in the reed basket in the bulrushes of the Nile River. Other miracles in the life of Moses were unique events for which there is no known natural explanation, such as: when Moses tossed his staff to the ground and the staff became a snake, and, later as pictured below, when Moses picked up the snake by the tail and the snake returned to again become his staff.

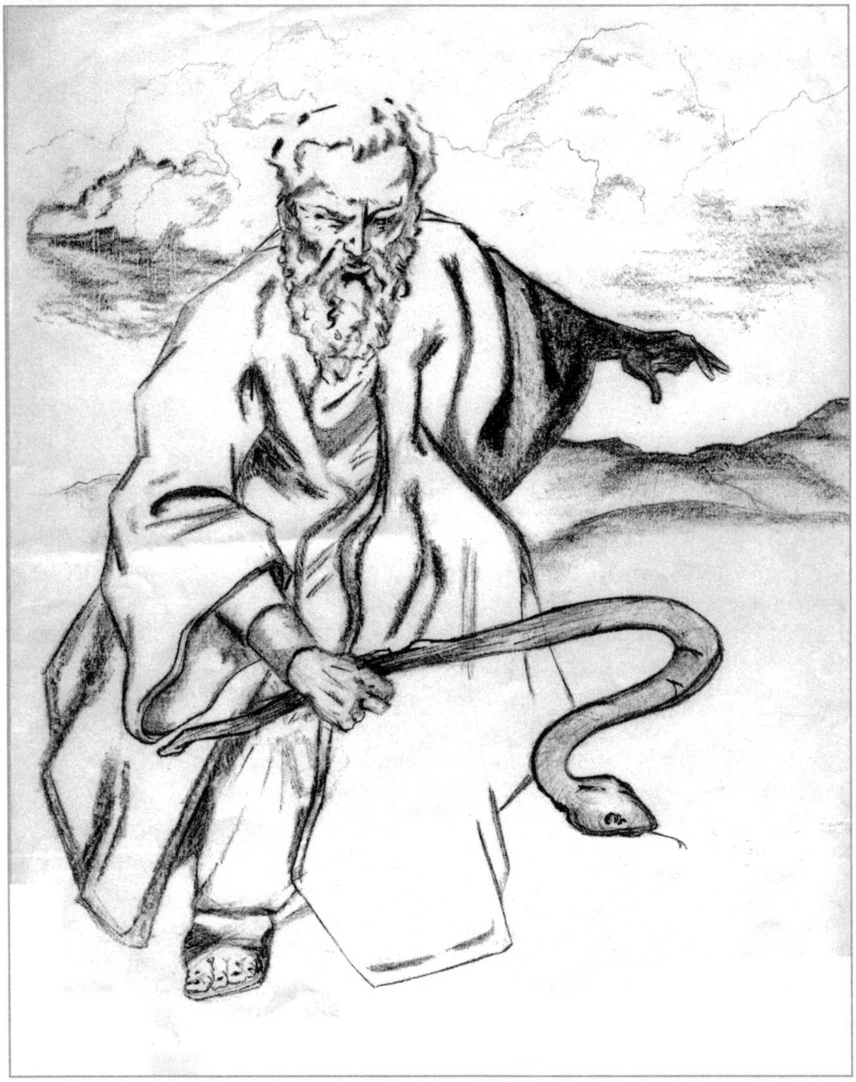

Egyptian magicians may have trained a snake to wrap itself around a stick. When the stick was dropped to the ground, the snake slithered away. Pharaoh may have tried to cheapen the staff–snake–staff miracle of the LORD, when he likened it to the simple 'magician's trick' of training a snake to wrap itself around a stick. [R46]

Chuck Missler jokingly stated before a Bible study on a controversial passage that tonight he promised a presentation that would include 'some material guaranteed to offend everyone'. Although unintentional, perhaps this book has fulfilled Dr. Missler's worst fears. The intent of this book was to enlighten readers. The author apologizes for any presentations in this book that offended, rather than informed, the reader.

The information and perspectives presented in this book are intended for educational purposes only. No discussion in this book should be used to diagnose or treat or prescribe for any medical condition; that is the job of a licensed medical professional. No information or advice in this book should be used to alter dosage of a prescription medication or to alter any medically prescribed therapy. The author assumes no responsibility for anyone who uses this book to diagnose, treat or prescribe for any health condition. Changes to any existing medical prescription or therapy must be made by a licensed medical professional.